Lung Cancer 1

Cancer Treatment and Research

WILLIAM L. McGUIRE, *series editor*

Volume 1

Forthcoming:

2. G. Bennett Humphrey, L.P. Dehner, G.B. Grindley and R.T. Acton, eds., Pediatric Oncology 1 (with a special section on rare primitive neuroectodermal tumors). 1981. ISBN 90-247-2408-2.
3. J. J. DeCosse and P. Sherlock, eds., Gastrointestinal Cancer 1. 1981. ISBN 90-247-2461-9.

series ISBN 90-247-2426-0

Lung Cancer 1

edited by

R. B. LIVINGSTON

Cleveland Clinic, Cleveland, Ohio 44106, U.S.A.

1981

MARTINUS NIJHOFF PUBLISHERS

THE HAGUE/BOSTON/LONDON

Distributors:

for the United States and Canada

Kluwer Boston, Inc.
190 Old Derby Street
Hingham, MA 02043
USA

for all other countries

Kluwer Academic Publishers Group
Distribution Center
P.O. Box 322
3300 AH Dordrecht
The Netherlands

This volume is listed in the Library of Congress Cataloging in Publication Data

ISBN 90-247-2394-9 (this volume)
ISBN 90-247-2426-0 (series)

Contents

Foreword   vii

Preface   ix

List of contributors   xiii

1. Pulmonary carcinogenesis: aryl hydrocarbon hydroxylase   1
   THEODORE L. MCLEMORE, R. RUSSELL MARTIN

2. Adjuvant therapy with surgery: immunotherapy – overview   35
   WILLIAM P. MCGUIRE

3. The immunotherapy of lung cancer   51
   E. CARMACK HOLMES

4. The use of pre-operative radiation therapy in the treatment of lung   63
   carcinoma
   DAVID M. SHERMAN, RALPH R. WEICHSELBAUM

5. Lung cancer – post resection irradiation   75
   NATHAN GREEN

6. The role of radiation therapy in the treatment of regional non-small   113
   (oat)-cell carcinoma of the lung
   JOEL ELLIOT WHITE, MURRAY BOLES

7. Small cell anaplastic carcinoma of the lung: staging   157
   HEINE H. HANSEN, PER DOMBERNOWSKY

8. Small cell bronchogenic carcinoma: a review of therapeutic results   169
   PAUL A. BUNN JR., DANIEL C. IHDE

9. Radiation therapy – new approaches   209
   OMAR M. SALAZAR, GUNAR ZAGARS

10. Pathology of small cell carcinoma of the lung and its subtypes. A   283
    clinico-pathologic correlation
    MARY J. MATTHEWS, ADI F. GAZDAR

Subject index   307

Cancer Treatment and Research

Foreword

Where do you begin to look for a recent, authoritative article on the diagnosis or management of a particular malignancy? The few general oncology textbooks are generally out of date. Single papers in specialized journals are informative but seldom comprehensive; these are more often preliminary reports on a very limited number of patients. Certain general journals frequently publish good in-depth reviews of cancer topics, and published symposium lectures are often the best overviews available. Unfortunately, these reviews and supplements appear sporadically, and the reader can never be sure when a topic of special interest will be covered.

Cancer Treatment and Research is a series of authoritative volumes which aim to meet this need. It is an attempt to establish a critical mass of oncology literature covering virtually all oncology topics, revised frequently to keep the coverage up to date, easily available on a single library shelf or by a single personal subscription.

We have approached the problem in the following fashion. First, by dividing the oncology literature into specific subdivisions such as lung cancer, genitourinary cancer, supportive care, etc. Second, by asking eminent authorities in each of these areas to edit a volume on the specific topic on an annual or biannual basis. Each topic and tumor type is covered in a volume appearing frequently and predictably, discussing current diagnosis, staging, markers, all forms of treatment modalities, basic biology, and more.

In Cancer Treatment and Research, we have an outstanding group of editors, each having made a major commitment to bring to this new series the very best literature in his or her field. Martinus Nijhoff Publishers has made an equally major commitment to the rapid publication of high quality books, and world-wide distribution.

Where can you go to find quickly a recent authoritative article on any major oncology problem? We hope that Cancer Treatment and Research provides an answer.

WILLIAM L. McGUIRE, M.D.
Series Editor

Preface

This volume reviews advances in several areas related to lung cancer: radiation therapy, especially for non-small cell tumors; small cell carcinoma (pathology, staging and treatment); attempts at immunotherapy, often in the 'adjuvant' setting after surgical resection; and carcinogenesis, with special attention to the predictive value of induced aryl hydrocarbon hydroxylase levels. All of these are reviewed by experts, all are controversial, and the reader should not be surprised to discover that there is not unanimity of opinion. What is missing in this volume is material related to chemotherapy for advanced, non-small cell cancers, or to surgery for resectable disease. The reasons are distressingly simple: the former has yet to be shown of proven benefit, and the latter has long since plateaued as a curative modality.

The largest part of this book is devoted to radiation therapy, because it is the editor's opinion (as a medical oncologist) that this is the modality where the application of presently available technology will make the greatest impact on the lung cancer problem in the next few years.

Doctors White and Boles emphasize the value of radiation therapy early rather than late in the treatment of regional non-small cell disease. They cite the data for split and continuous dose-fractionation schemes, and come forth with a recommendation for the continuous approach if radiation is to be used alone. Trials of combined modality approaches with chemotherapy added to radiation are reviewed, and are shown to be of no demonstrated value to date. Of particular interest is their analysis of sites of relapse, and of data suggesting the value of 'prophylactic' cranial irradiation in preventing relapse at this site in *non*-small cell patients.

Doctors Salazar and Zagars have covered new approaches to radiation therapy in a thorough fashion, yet one which is eminently comprehensible to the non-radiation oncologist. That experts do not always agree is implied by their advocacy of split-course over continuous fractionation schemes. Considerable space is devoted to unorthodox, high or varied dose regimens which have been piloted in Europe and Japan, but inadequately studied here. Basic review of such concepts as radiobiologic effectiveness and the oxygen enhancement ratio allows for a clear understanding of the potential advantages to be derived from hypoxic cell radiosensitizers and high-LET radiation, such as fast neutrons. Perhaps the most fascinating section involves Salazar's own extension of the work with hemibody irradiation, originally pioneered in

Toronto. It now appears that this technique is not only usefull for palliation of pain, but may, in conjunction with subsequent local irradiation of the primary tumor and/or chemotherapy, play an important role in reduction of systemic tumor burden.

As Dr. Green points out in his chapter on post-operative irradiation, retrospective data from his own series and that of Kirsch both strongly suggest benefit to patients with clearly resectable disease who have positive hilar or mediastinal lymph nodes. Based on their observations, it has become standard practice in many institutions to perform post-operative irradiation routinely in this setting. Green emphasizes that the appropriate studies to clarify the value of post-operative radiation therapy, namely, prospective, controlled trials with careful staging, have *not* been done. Sherman and Weichselbaum's chapter reviews the data for pre-operative irradiation. They cite previous, large-scale, controlled trials which failed to show any benefit versus surgery alone, and point out that these trials failed to use modern staging, employed lower-dose, protracted radiation therapy, and involved a long period between administration of radiation therapy and the anticipated surgery. Their own pilot trial of short-course, pre-operative radiation therapy, followed in two weeks by surgery, produced encouraging results in a group of patients considered 'marginally resectable' by pre-operative surgical evaluation. Unfortunately, what constitutes 'marginal' resectability varies from one institution to another, and even what makes a tumor 'T3' and therefore 'Stage 3' may vary: the usual criteria cited involve invasion of the mediastinum, diaphragm or chest wall and/or too close a margin to the main carina, but in Sherman's series, involvement of the main pulmonary artery was also considered a criterion for classification as 'T3'. Such patients did particularly well in their combined modality pilot.

A second major topic in this volume is small cell lung cancer, an area in which tremendous changes have taken place. Mary Matthews describes the role of pathologic subclassification among the small cell tumors and makes two extremely important points: 1) among tumors in which small cells are the 'only' tumor cells present, subclassification as to 'lymphocyte-like' versus 'spindle,' 'fusiform,' etc. is of no prognostic value; 2) small cell tumors in which there is a significant admixture of large cells (more generous cytoplasm, clearing of nuclear chromatin, prominent nucleoli) should be *treated* like other small cells, but analyzed separately. The reason for this is that many more will respond to chemotherapy than would be expected for large cell tumors in general, and some will even have long-term complete remissions. but median survival and overall long-term survival are compromised, relative to 'pure' small cell.

Hansen and Dombernowsky review the staging of small cell lung cancer. Especially noteworthy is their observation that blastic new bone formation often accompanies marrow involvement in this disease, unlike the other types of lung cancer, and that it may persist in the absence of demonstrable tumor after therapy. This could lead to a problem with the interpretation of sequential bone scans and/or radiologic bone surveys, especially in patients who present with marrow metastasis. Bunn and Ihde exhaustively review the therapeutic results in treatment of small cell lung cancer, and add some suggestions for future directions if we are to progress beyond the present plateau. It is unquestionably clear that chemotherapy has improved the results of treatment for the average patient with this disease, and it is probable that any of several combinations are superior to single-agent cyclophosphamide. Far from resolved are the questions of how (or if) radiation therapy should be integrated with chemotherapy in management of these patients.

An area of major interest in recent years has been the immunotherapy of cancer, now more fashionably referred to as 'biological response modification,' to include the concept that some of the effects mediated by agents such as BCG, Corynebacterium parvum, thymosin and transfer factor may be by mechanisms other than immunologic. McGuire reviews adjuvant immunotherapy for resected lung cancer patients, as well as the trials of immunotherapy which have been carried out in small cell lung cancer. Hints remain of some advantage for intrapleural BCG after surgery in adequately staged Stage I patients: the rest is negative or inevaluable at present. However, several controlled trials in the United States, Canada and Europe should provide definitive answers in the next two to three years.

From a practical point of view, it may be considered as fact that cigaret smoking is causally related to lung cancer development in the vast majority. Yet only 1 in 20 heavy smokers develops lung cancer. Aside from the other health problems associated with smoking, it would be of great potential value to be able to prospectively identify individuals at special risk *in advance* and try to alter their behaviors and/or exposure to a cancer-causing environment. McLemore and Martin provide in-depth consideration of one very promising avenue: the measurement of aryl hydrocarbon hydroxylase (AHH) levels. As with treatment of this disease, controversy abounds as well in carcinogenesis research. In particular, use of the lymphocyte as a tool with which to measure AHH activity has been criticized, since in patients *with* lung cancer other tissues have more frequently shown elevated levels of AHH. As the authors point out, however, the readily available peripheral blood lymphocyte may still be useful for measuring the inducibility of AHH in those individuals who are free of detectable cancer. Certainly, the time has come to put their hypothesis to the test: prospective studies should be done in high risk individuals (e.g., cigaret smokers), classifying them according to AHH inducibility, then measuring the frequency of lung cancer development and correlating this with AHH activity. It might then be possible to focus intensive preventive efforts on the 5 to 10% of smokers who are really 'high risk.'

Dr. Holmes' chapter on immunotherapy of lung cancer indicates a somewhat more optimistic point of view. While one may debate with some of the conclusions regarding the outcome of adjuvant trials with systemic immunotherapy, his observations of the value of intralesional BCG, injected either via the bronchoscope or directly into the tumor through the chest wall, are extremely provocative. They should stimulate confirmatory efforts in other centers.

We are far from preventing lung cancer, although perhaps the tools are at hand to do so. We are far from curing most cases, and probably lack the tools at present to do more than improve modestly on today's results. Even modest improvement, however, would translate into thousands of lives saved each year. What *has* happened in the last decade is a major ferment of interest, and disappearance of the apathy about the problem which once prevailed in the medical scientific community. These are essential first steps to real progress.

List of Contributors

BOLES, Murray, M.D., Chairman, Department of Therapeutic Radiology, Henry Ford Hospital, Detroit, MI 48202, U.S.A.

BUNN, Paul A., Jr., M.D., National Cancer Institute — Veterans Administration Medical Oncology Branch, Division of Cancer Treatment, National Cancer Institute, VA Medical Center, Washington, DC 20422, U.S.A.

DOMBERNOWSKY, Per, Department of Chemotherapy R II-V, The Finsen Institute and Department of Medicine C, Bispebjerg Hospital, Copenhagen, Denmark.

GAZDAR, Adi F., M.D., George Washington University School of Medicine, Department of Pathology, Washington, DC 20037, U.S.A.

GREEN, Nathan, M.D., Chief Division of Radiation Therapy, Valley Presbyterian Hospital, Associate Clinical Professor/Radiation Therapy, LAC/USC Medical Center, Van Nuys, CA 91405, U.S.A.

HANSEN, Heine H., Department of Chemotherapy R II-V, The Finsen Institute and Department of Medicine C, Bispebjerg Hospital, Copenhagen, Denmark.

HOLMES, E. Carmack, M.D., UCLA School of Medicine, Division of Surgical Oncology, 54–140 CHS, Los Angeles, CA 90024, U.S.A.

IHDE, Daniel C., M.D., National Cancer Institute – Veterans Administration Medical Oncology Branch, Division of Cancer Treatment, National Cancer Institute, VA Medical Center, Washington, DC 20422, U.S.A.

MARTIN, R. Russell, Departments of Medicine and Microbiology and Immunology, Baylor College of Medicine, Houston, TX 77030, U.S.A.

MATTHEWS, Mary J., M.D., National Cancer Institute – Veterans Administration Medical Oncology Branch, VA Medical Center, Washington, DC 20422, U.S.A.

McGUIRE, William P., M.D., Department of Medicine, Section of Medical Oncology, University of Illinois, Chicago, IL 60612, U.S.A.

McLEMORE, Theodore L., Department of Medicine, Baylor College of Medicine, Houston, TX 77030, U.S.A.

SALAZAR, Omar M., M.D., Associate Professor of Radiation Oncology, University of Rochester, Strong Memorial Hospital, Cancer Center, Division of Radiation Oncology, Rochester, NY 14642, U.S.A.

SHERMAN, David M., M.D., Assistant Director, Department of Radiation Oncology, St. Vincent Hospital, Worcester, and Assistant Professor, Department of Radiology, University of Massachusetts Medical School, Worcester, MA 01604, U.S.A.

WEICHSELBAUM, Ralph R., M.D., Assistant Professor of Radiation Therapy, Joint Center for Radiation Therapy, Harvard Medical School, Boston, MA, U.S.A.

WHITE, Joel Elliot, M.D., Head Clinical Division, Department of Therapeutic Radiology, Henry Ford Hospital, Detroit, MI 48202, U.S.A.

ZAGARS, Gunar, M.B., B.S., Assistant Professor of Radiation Oncology, University of Rochester, Strong Memorial Hospital, Cancer Center, Division of Radiation Oncology, Rochester, NY 14642, U.S.A.

1. Pulmonary Carcinogenesis: Aryl Hydrocarbon Hydroxylase

THEODORE L. McLEMORE and R. RUSSELL MARTIN

1. INTRODUCTION

Especially during the past two decades, there has been a growing awareness that exposure of individuals to exogenous environmental agents is responsible for various kinds of cancer. Chemical carcinogenesis in man was first documented in 1775 by the British physician Percival Pott, who attributed the high incidence of scrotal cancer in London chimney sweeps to their chronic exposure to soot and coal tars[1]. In the two hundred years following that initial observation, at least 1000 chemicals have been shown to induce cancer in a wide variety of tissues[2]. As our civilization has become industralized, our food, air, and water have undergone increased contamination with a number of cancer producing chemicals. It is currently estimated that approximately 75 to 85 percent of human cancer may be directly associated with exposure to these environmental carcinogens[3].

Probably the best established and the most extensively studied example of human environmental carcinogenesis is the relationship between cigarette smoking and the development of lung cancer. This area has aroused both medical and public concern and is a major interest for investigators involved in the study of chemical carcinogenesis. Prior to 1920, lung cancer was a rare cancer type seen only infrequently by physicians. However, as the quantity of tobacco products (especially cigarettes) consumed in the United States rose, there was a concomitant increase in the incidence of lung cancer. By 1950, lung cancer had become the number one cause of cancer deaths in adult males in the United States. Since that time with a further increase in cigarette smoking by females, lung cancer is now steadily rising in this subpopulation

Supported by a USPHS research grant CA–15784, ACS grant PDT–149, a grant from the Council for Tobacco Research, USA, and a grant from the Veterans Administration Hospital, Houston, Texas.

R.B. Livingston (ed.), Lung cancer 1, 1–34. All rights reserved.
Copyright © 1981 Martinus Nijhoff Publishers bv, The Hague/Boston/London.

as well. In fact, it is estimated that by 1985, lung cancer will be the number one cause of cancer-related deaths in the total United States adult population [4].

Numerous reports have implicated tobacco (specifically components of cigarette smoke condensate) to be carcinogenic in laboratory animals [5–20], and epidemiological studies in man have directly associated heavy consumption of cigarettes with increased risk of lung cancer [21–27]. However, the precise mechanisms responsible for the initiation of pulmonary neoplasia have remained undefined. There is evidence that genetic factors may play a role in human susceptibility to lung cancer. Tokuhata [28] found that the incidence of lung cancer was greater when a family history of cancer was present, either for nonsmokers or smokers. Furthermore, there was an exponential increase in lung cancer risk among cigarette smokers with a family history of lung cancer. The combination of these two factors, smoking and family history, increased the risk of lung cancer several fold. Tokuhata [29] further suggested that the organ site at which a tumor is likely to develop is largely under genetic control. He further indicated that synergism between genetics and environmental factors is of great importance.

The major carcinogenic agents in cigarette smoke condensate are the polycyclic aromatic hydrocarbons (PAHs). These compounds, which include benzo(a)pyrene (BP) and benzanthracene (BA), are products of incomplete combustion and are among the active components of cigarette smoke condensate [21, 23, 30, 31], air pollution [32, 33], coal tar [34–36], and smoked foods [37]. It is now known that many of these PAHs are converted to active forms after their entry into the body tissues [2, 3, 38–42]. PAHs are only weakly carcinogenic before being converted to electrophilic forms which readily favor covalent binding to protein and nucleic acids within the cell [43–45]. These reactive compounds have been implicated in the process of chemical carcinogenesis in man [46–57]. One enzyme system which is responsible for the conversion of these compounds to their active metabolic forms is aryl hydrocarbon hydroxylase (AHH). This membrane-bound, oxygen-dependent, enzyme system is found in many tissues in the human body and is capable of converting components of cigarette smoke to potent intermediates with enhanced mutagenic [43, 45, 58–60] and carcinogenic potential [61–63]. Specific details of the structure and mechanisms for activation of carcinogens by AHH will be discussed later in this chapter.

In order to understand the intricate interactions between PAHs and human lung tissues (particularly the bronchus, which is the target tissue for lung cancer production), we must understand how formation of these potent intermediate compounds could theoretically fit into the overall scheme of pulmonary carcinogenesis in man. As noted in Figure 1, different stages of the carcinogenic process are interrelated. The initial step in this pathway is the

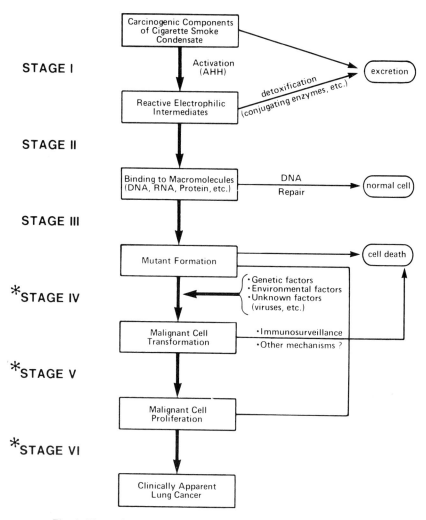

Fig. 1. Theoretical pathways for human pulmonary carcinogenesis.

* Represents those stages requiring long latency periods.

activation of PAH components of cigarette smoke by the AHH enzyme system. The reactive intermediate metabolites which are produced may undergo detoxification (via conjugation and other enzymatic reactions) and be excreted from the body. Metabolites which are not excreted may undergo binding with macromolecules within the cell (stage II), initiating mutagenesis (stage III). These alterations may be rectified by DNA repair mechanisms, in which case normal cellular function would resume. Therefore, in an individual cigarette smoker, many DNA mutations could be formed for a given unit of time, but the efficiency of the individual's DNA repair mechanisms might allow for reversal of these harmful effects. It is only when the DNA repair mechanisms falter that mutations would persist and ultimately lead to malignant transformation (stage IV) in lung tissues. Environmental factors, such as viruses, co-carcinogens (such as asbestos), promoters (such as phorbol esters, which are constituents of cigarette smoke), and various undefined factors may also be involved in promotion of malignant transformation. At some point, the transformed malignant cell may be destroyed by immunosurveillance or other internal protective mechanisms. Alternatively, malignant cell proliferation (stage V) may occur, eventually leading to the appearance of clinically apparent lung cancer (stage VI). Even after proliferation of the malignant cells (before they are clinically apparent) immunosurveillance or other protective body mechanisms may contain the spread or eradicate the malignant tissues. A latency period (as long as 20 years) occurs in progression from stage IV to stage VI, and undoubtedly many abortive progressions through the various stages could occur before the defense mechanisms are overwhelmed and clinically apparent cancer results.

It is apparent that the process of pulmonary carcinogenesis in man is multifactorial and highly complicated in nature. In this chapter, we will discuss in detail only one aspect of this hypothesized scheme for pulmonary carcinogenesis. Biochemical pathways for metabolism of PAHs by human tissues will be reviewed and current concepts defining the relationship between levels of AHH and human lung cancer susceptibility will be discussed, with emphasis on recent reserach developments. This portion of the hypothetical scheme for pulmonary carcinogenesis could be the most relevant since it represents the rate limiting step without which progression to pulmonary neoplasia could not occur (Fig. 1).

2. STRUCTURE AND FUNCTION OF THE AHH ENZYME COMPLEX

AHH represents a labile, multicomponent enzyme system which is tightly bound to membranes and requires NADPH and/or NADH and molecular oxygen for enzymatic activity [64, 65]. Studies by Lu *et al.* [66] and other investigators [67–71] have indicated that the microsomal enzyme is composed of at least three components: 1) a phospholipid portion (intimately associated with the membrane), 2) a reductase (presumably either cytochrome c or cytochrome b5 reductase), and 3) a cytochrome(s) P-450 fraction. It has been proposed that the cytochrome P-450 and the reductase portions of the enzyme are in a halo of phospholipid matrix which is bound to the cell membrane and which allows lateral mobility of these enzymes in the matrix [71]. The substrate specificity of the AHH system is dependent upon the cytochrome P-450 fraction [72–86]. Reducing equivalents for the reactions may be supplied by NADPH and/or NADH, and ultimately reach hydrophobic substrates through cytochrome P-450 or cynanide-sensitive factor[66, 67, 69, 71, 87].

Numerous xenobiotics, including PAH components of cigarette smoke, are highly lipophilic and would remain in the body tissues indefinitely if it were not for enzymes such as the AHH enzyme complex. During metabolism by AHH, one or more polar groups (hydroxyls) are introduced into nonpolar molecules, thereby making them more hydrophilic. These more polar substrates can then be readily conjugated, excreted from cells and eventually cleared from the body[88].

AHH converts PAHs to numerous metabolites by hydroxylation pathways (Fig. 2). BP is the prototype PAH whose metabolism has been extensively studied. The acceptance of one atom of molecular O_2 into an unsaturated BP molecule results in formation of reactive arene oxide (epoxide) intermediates with increased capacity for macromolecular binding. These can undergo nonenzymatic spontaneous rearrangement to form phenols (which may in turn undergo conjugation reactions); be further metabolized by epoxide hydratase to nontoxic dihydrodiols (these may also be conjugated); interact with cellular macromolecules including DNA and RNA; or undergo conjugation reactions (for review see references[89–91]).

Although all epoxide derivatives of BP are electrophilic species capable of binding macromolecules such as DNA, the most reactive of these known to date is the diol epoxide I. As demonstrated (Fig. 2), the proposed pathway for production of the proximate and ultimate carcinogenic BP derivatives involves both primary and secondary metabolism of BP. The 7, 8-dihydrodiol (the proximate carcinogenic metabolite of BP) is produced by initial metabolism of the BP molecule by AHH and subsequent conversion of the 7, 8-epoxide to the 7, 8-dihydrodiol by epoxide hydratase. Further metabolism of this derivative by AHH results in formation of the ultimate carcinogen of BP, the $(+)7\beta, 8\alpha$-dihydrodiol-9 α-10 α-epoxy-7, 8, 9, 10-tetrahydrobenzo(a)-pyrene (diol epoxide I). This molecule subsequently undergoes spontaneous rearrangement to a carbonium ion at the 10 position, which is postulated to then react with cellular macromolecules. Specifically, when this reactive species interacts with DNA guanine base pairs, they form BP-guanine adducts (Fig. 2). Note that at various points along the activation pathways, detoxification pathways can intervene, producing tetrols, triols, and conjugation products which are readily execreted from the cell (Figure 2) (for review see references[89–91]).

AHH is known to metabolize a number of endogenous substrates such as steroids, cholesterol, fatty acids, bilirubin, biogenic amines, indoles, and ethanol. AHH is also essential in the metabolism of a number of xenobiotics. These hydrophobic exogenous substrates include PAHs such as BP, BA, and

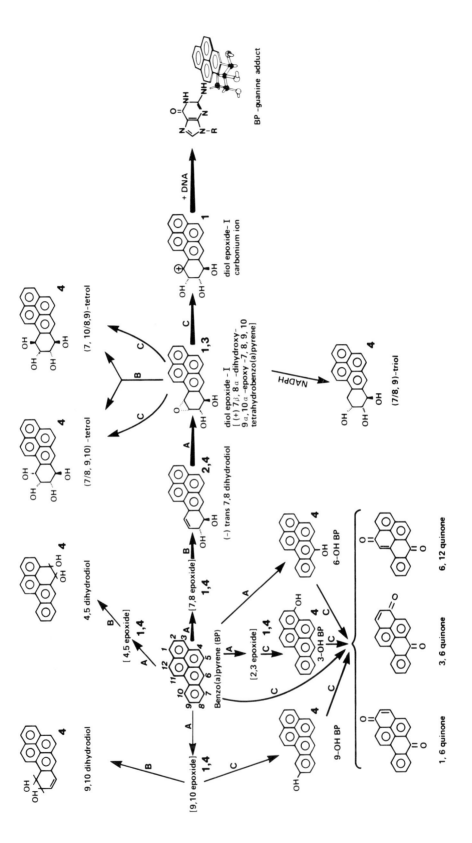

3-methylcholanthrene (MC); halogenated hydrocarbons such as polychlorinated and polybrominated biphenyls, insecticides and ingredients in soaps and
deodorants; strong mutagens such as N-methyl, N-nitro nitrosoguanidine and
nitrosamines; aminoazo dyes and diazo compounds; N-acetylarylamines and
nitrofurans; numerous aromatic amines, such as those found in hair dyes,
nitro aromatics and heterocyclics; wood terpenes; epoxides; carbamates; alkyl
halides; safrole derivatives; certain fungal toxins and antibiotics; many of the
chemotherapeutic agents used to treat human cancers; and most commonly
used drugs [20, 31–37, 41, 87, 88, 92].

An important characteristic of AHH is its inducibility. The levels of the
enzyme fluctuate depending upon exposure to specific inducers which include
the exogenous as well as the endogenous chemicals previously described. The
precise mechanisms whereby AHH inducers increase enzyme action have not
been completely defined, but synthesis of more heme protein is involved [74, 93, 94]. Exposure to inducers produces accelerated *de novo* protein
synthesis and associated increases in the cytochrome P-450 fractions [94].
Poland *et al.* have isolated a cytosol receptor protein molecule which appears
to bind AHH inducers and possibly is associated with initiation of gene
recognition, transcription, and translation of the cytochrome heme proteins [95].

Figure 3 shows a hypothetical scheme associated with the induction of
different P-450s of the AHH system. Inducers, such as the PAHs might bind
the cytosol receptor proteins in the cell. These receptors are themselves under
genetic regulation and can vary with each individual [82, 95, 96]. The binding
of the receptor to inducer molecules activates the genomes thus stimulating
the process of transcription, translation, and ultimately synthesis of the
cytochrome(s) P-450 which are associated with increased monooxygenase
activity [82].

Multiple forms of the cytochrome P-450 heme protein have been identified
in microsomes [94, 97, 103], and various AHH inducers have been associated
with different forms of cytochrome P-450 species. These inducers have been
classified as Type I or Type II depending on the predominant species of the
cytochrome P-450 present [67, 104–107]. Pretreatment of experimental animals with a Type I inducer (e.g. phenobarbital) results in a nonspecific

←

Fig. 2. Pathways for activation and detoxification of benzo (a) pyrene (BP) by the aryl hydrocarbon hydroxylase (AHH) enzyme system. 1 – epoxide intermediates with enhanced macromolecular binding capabilities. 2 – the proximate carcinogen of BP metabolism. 3 – the ultimate carcinogen of BP metabolism. 4 – BP derivatives which may be substrates for conjugation (detoxification)
pathways. A, B, and C represent reactions mediated by AHH, epoxide hydratase, and nonenzymatic rearrangement, respectively. Dark arrows represent the major pathways for activation of
BP.

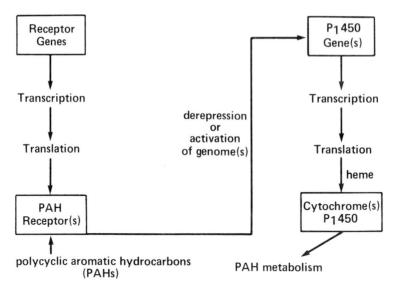

Fig. 3. Hypothetical scheme for polycyclic aromatic hydrocarbon (PAH) induction of different cytochrome P-450s of the AHH enzyme system.

increase in the metabolism of PAH as well as other drugs by the AHH system [72, 73, 75, 77, 78]. Studies utilizing AHH inhibitors [75] or observing metabolite profiles [107] indicate that Type I induced hepatic activity may be only quantitatively different from the constitutive enzyme activity. The liver appears to be the only tissue in which AHH activity is increased by Type I substrates [67, 104–107]. Type II inducers include PAHs and other xenobiotics. Pretreatment of experimental animals with PAHs results in specific increased metabolism of these compounds in hepatic as well as extrahepatic tissues, but AHH activity toward most other substrates remains unchanged [67, 104–107]. Type I induction is associated with an absorbance of the reduced CO-bound cytochrome complex at 450 nm (or cytochrome P-450) [78, 81, 108, 109]. However, Type II enzyme induction has been characterized by an increased absorbance maximum of the reduced, CO-bound complex from 450 to 448 nm (cytochrome P-448) for liver microsomes [109] and from- 450 to 454–446 nm (or cytochrome P_1-450) for nonhepatic tissues [83, 110]. The presence of different heme proteins can also be supported by their electron paramagnetic resonance spectroscopy [78], and by a preferential inhibition of BP hydroxylation *in vitro* [73]. The specific type of cytochrome P-450 induced may influence the distribution of metabolites produced [107–111], as well as the ratios of intermediate products formed [20, 112].

Induction of one or more forms of cytochrome P-450 is associated with induction of numerous monooxygenase activities which are related to PAH responsive portions of the AHH system. These include AHH, p-nitroanisole-O-demethylase,7-ethoxycoumarin O-demethylase,3'-methyl-4-methylaminoazobenzene N-demethylase, zoxazolamine hydroxylase, phenacetin O-deethylase, acetylarylamine (2-aceytlaminofluorine) N-hydroxylase), biphenyl 2-hydroxylase, reduced NAD(P):Menadione oxidoreductase, naphthalene monooxygenase, acetanilide 4-hydroxylase, biphenyl hydroxylase, acetaminophen-N-hydroxylase, p-chloroacetanilide, and ethoxyresorufin O-deethylase activities (for review see ref. [20]). How so many substrates with different chemical structures are oxygenated by a single enzyme-active site is not understood. Kouri *et al.* have suggested that there are probably many forms of cytochrome P-450 heme protein which are responsible for these various activities [20].

3. GENETICS OF AHH

In mice, AHH inducibility can be transmitted either as an autosomal dominant trait [76, 113], or as a co-dominant trait [86]. In most mouse strains studied, data supports the theory that a minimum of six alleles and two loci are responsible for the genetic regulation of AHH [20].

The genetics of AHH inducibility in man is not as easily discernible. Kellermann *et al.* [114] reported that the extent of AHH inducibility in cultured lymphocytes varied among different individuals. After analyzing values obtained from normal Caucasian individuals, these workers concluded that AHH inducibility behaved as an autosomal trait, distributed in a trimodal type of curve, suggesting the presence of a single gene for the control of this enzyme [115]. Other investigators have been unable to confirm the trimodal distribution of AHH inducibility in the normal population. Kouri *et al.* [116] using 2,3,7,8-tetrachlorodibenzo-p-dioxin to induce AHH in lymphocyte cultures, detected a unimodal distribution in the normal population. Atlas *et al.* [117] also failed to demonstrate a trimodal distribution of AHH, but concluded that the capacity for AHH induction in man is in part genetically controlled. Several other investigators have also demonstrated the extent of AHH induction in cultured lymphocytes appears to vary among individuals in the population [46–57, 118–123]. In addition, studies of AHH in other human tissues have demonstrated individual variation in AHH levels [46, 53–56, 124–132].

It appears that genetic control of the AHH system is more complicated than was originally presumed. Presently, it is not clear whether this variation is related to the enzyme control by a single or multiple genes. More elaborate experiments will be required to determine genetic mechanisms responsible for regulation of AHH induction in man.

4. CURRENT THEORIES OF AHH-MEDIATED PULMONARY CARCINOGENESIS

The observation that many environmental carcinogens such as those present in cigarette tar are enzymatically activated to potent carcinogens only after their entry into host tissues [2, 3, 38–42] stimulated interest in the biochemical mechanisms responsible for activation of these compounds. AHH is an enzyme system which has intrigued investigators for the last decade because it is capable of converting hydrophobic PAHs into more hydrophilic products which are more easily excreted and which are usually less carcinogenic. In the process of metabolizing and remetabolizing these hydrocarbons, transient intermediate products are produced with enhanced mutagenic [43, 45, 58–60] and carcinogenic [61–63] potential (see Fig. 2). One of these intermediate compounds, diol epoxide I, is implicated as the ultimate carcinogenic hydrocarbon of the prototype PAH, BP [133–136]. This diol epoxide rearranges to a carbonium ion at the 10 position, a form of the molecule which reacts with cellular macromolecules, including DNA [133] (see Fig. 2). Chronic exposure of the bronchial epithelium to the PAH components of cigarette smoke condensate could initiate malignant transformation in these cells (see Fig. 1). Through production of increased quantities of these intermediate metabolites, high levels of AHH could be detrimental to individuals (i.e. cigarette smokers) chronically exposed to significant quantities of PAHs.

Numerous studies have attempted to define a relationship between carcinogen metabolism (as measured by AHH activity) and lung cancer risk. High AHH inducibility and susceptibility to carcinogenesis by certain PAHs have been investigated in animal models. The incidence of skin tumors in mice exposed to various PAHs is positively associated with tissue AHH levels [85, 137], as is the carcinogenic index and AHH levels in lung tissues from different strains of mice [20, 107]. These relationships in humans are not as well defined, but most reports have implicated AHH as a possible etiological factor in human pulmonary carcinogenesis [46–57].

The remainder of this chapter will concentrate on AHH studies in human tissues. The relationship between AHH levels and lung cancer incidence will be discussed in detail as well as the direction of the thrust for future studies in this area.

5. AHH IN HUMAN TISSUES

Numerous tissues have been utilized for study of AHH in man; however, the peripheral lymphocyte has been the most frequently used and most accessible tissue (Table 1). The remainder of this discussion will concentrate on human tissues which are relevant to the problem of lung cancer.

Table 1. Advantages and disadvantages of utilizing various human tissues for AHH determination.

Tissue	Advantage	Disadvantage
Liver	1. Primary site of drug and xenobiotic metabolism in man (124, 161-176). 2. Highest enzyme activity (124) (in adult) 3. Enzyme activity can be measured on freshly obtained tissue or after further *in vitro* culture	1. Tissue must be obtained by: (a) biopsy (b) surgery (c) autopsy 2. Not a suitable tissue for population studies
Placenta	1. Easy to procure 2. Detectable AHH levels *in situ* (124, 165-168, 170-172, 177-183). 3. AHH is inducible *in situ* in cigarette smoking women (165, 167, 178-181)	1. Obtainable only post-partum or at abortion 2. Select subpopulation (female) 3. Not appropriate for population studies
Blood cells 1. Lymphocytes	1. Readily accessible by venipuncture 2. Suitable tissue for population studies	1. High degree of AHH variability in the lymphocyte culture system (20, 117, 120, 122, 144, 146) 2. Must be cultured and *undergo mitogen activation* before appreciable amounts of AHH activity are present (138, 139)
2. Monocytes	1. Readily accessible 2. This tissue *does not require in vitro mitogen activation* to express appreciable AHH activities (129, 184) 3. Suitable for population studies	1. Requires relatively large quantities of blood 2. Low activity (129, 184-187)
Skin	1. Similar to target tissue in human bronchus 2. May be cultured for *in vitro* enzyme studies (125, 126, 188-190)	1. Tissue must be obtained from (a) foreskins (125, 126) (b) punch biopsies (188) (c) scarification 2. Low activity 3. In the case of foreskins, only a select population of individuals can be tested (male) 4. Not suitable for population studies

Table 1. (Continued)

Tissue	Advantage	Disadvantage
Lung tissue 1. Pulmonary Alveolar Macrophages (PAMs)	1. Directly exposed to environmental carcinogens in the airways of the lung 2. AHH is inducible *in situ* in these cells by cigarette smoke condensate (53, 55, 118, 131, 132) 3. Easily cultured and no mitogen activation is required to obtain appreciable AHH activity (55, 64, 90, 91, 118, 130, 145) 4. Appears to have a low intra-individual day-to-day enzyme variability (47)	1. Can currently be obtained only by bronchopulmonary lavage or at necropsy 2. Limited usefulness for population studies
2. Bronchus	1. Target tissue for carcinogen action 2. Can be cultured for *in vitro* studies (64, 91, 127, 134, 149) 3. Directly exposed to cigarette smoke condensate	1. Obtained by: (a) biopsy (b) surgical resection (c) autopsy 2. Not suitable for population studies
3. Whole Lung Tissue	1. Represents tissue from target organ 2. Directly exposed to cigarette smoke condensate 3. Has measurable AHH activity (128, 191) 4. AHH is inducible in this tissue obtained from cigarette smokers (128)	1. Same as bronchial tissue
Fetal tissue	1. Enables investigator to examine AHH in all organ systems simultaneously 2. Adequate quantities of tissue obtained 3. Can culture tissue for *in vitro* studies (124, 174, 189)	1. Low activity [AHH system is immature in many fetal tissues (124)] 2. Difficulty in sample collection 3. Select subpopulation is involved 4. Not suitable for population studies
Endometrium	1. Accessible 2. Can culture *in vitro* (189)	1. Studies confined to women only 2. Not feasible for population studies

Table 1. (Continued)

Tissue	Advantage	Disadvantage
Kidney	1. Has detectable AHH levels (192, 193) 2. Might be cultured for *in vitro* studies	1. Not easily accessible 2. Not suitable for population studies
Sputum sample	1. Easily obtained 2. Might be suitable for population studies	1. Low number of cells obtained with current sputum collection procedures
Buccal tissue	1. Easily obtained 2. Might be suitable for population studies	1. Collection methods not perfected
Vaginal scrapings or cervical tissue	1. Easily obtained 2. Might be cultured for *in vitro* studies	1. Select population of individuals (females) 2. Not suitable for population studies 3. Collection technique not perfected
Stomach	1. Has detectable AHH activity (192) 2. Might be cultured for *in vitro* studies	See bronchus
Colon	Same as above	See bronchus
Prostate	Same as above	See bronchus 1. Select population of individuals (males)
Aorta	Same as above (192)	See bronchus
Pancreatic duct	Same as above (127)	See bronchus

5.1. Peripheral Blood Lymphocytes

Busbee et al. [138] and Whitlock et al. [139] first reported fluorometric assays for detection of AHH in human lymphocytes. Although fresh lymphocytes have very low AHH activity, culturing in the presence of a mitogen (to stimulate blastogenesis) and PAHs such as BA [54, 55, 118, 128, 140, 141], MC [51, 115, 117, 118, 120–123, 138, 144], or cigarette tars [145] will induce AHH activity. Cigarette smoking has been reported to induce AHH in vivo, whether lymphocytes are cultured with or without the inducer BA in the medium [53, 118, 140]; however, this effect of cigarette smoking has not been consistently found [57].

In an initial study involving human subjects, Kellermann et al. found that approximately half of the individuals in the general population had low AHH inducibility, 40% moderate inducibility, and only 10% high inducibility [51]. In contrast, AHH levels in lung cancer patients were predominantly in the intermediate and high inducibility groups. Subsequently, controversy has arisen regarding the relationship between lymphocyte AHH and lung cancer incidence. Several laboratories have had difficulty establishing a reproducible lymphocyte system for measurement of AHH. Variability appears to be associated with the lymphocyte culture system, rather than with the fluorometric measurement of phenolic derivatives of BP. A number of factors may affect the lymphocyte cultures, including the type and the specific lot of fetal calf serum employed in the medium, the type and lots of mitogens used, the specific PAH inducer employed, the initial cell concentration, and other factors (for review see references [20, 146]). In spite of these problems, the majority of investigators have provided evidence suggesting high lymphocyte AHH inducibility is associated with lung cancer [46–50, 52, 56, 57], while a few reports have been unable to confirm this association [123, 147, 148].

A negative report by Paigen and coworkers [123] examined AHH inducibility among progeny of lung cancer patients and progeny of a matched control group. While there were no differences in AHH inducibility among lung cancer and noncancer progeny, this report did not evaluate sufficient numbers of individuals to determine if an inheritable AHH component was present. Even if the AHH system is controlled by a single gene (which does not seem likely; see AHH genetics section), only 50% of the offspring would receive the gene responsible for AHH induction. If more than one gene were involved, this percentage would be even lower. Therefore, the evaluation of offspring to determine the relationship between AHH inducibility and cancer susceptibility is probably not feasible until the exact genetic variables controlling the human AHH system are delineated.

Further refinements of the lymphocyte AHH culture system may lead to a more reproducible system for measurement of human lymphocyte AHH. Kouri et al. have recently developed a modification of this system which

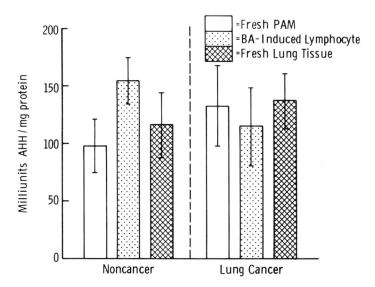

Fig. 4. Aryl hydrocarbon hydroxylase (AHH) activity in freshly lavaged pulmonary alveolar macrophages (PAM), cultured lymphocytes induced by benzanthracene (BA), and fresh, surgically-resected lung tissue from a group of 14 cigarette smokers, 7 with lung cancer and 7 with other pulmonary diseases. Bars represent mean +SE (P>0.05 in all instances).

significantly increases lymphocyte AHH reproducibility[146]. Utilizing this modified system, a double blind study of AHH in lymphocytes from cigarette smokers with and without primary lung cancer has demonstrated a strong association between high AHH levels and lung cancer incidence (unpublished data, R. E. Kouri, T. L. McLemore, D. R. Snodgrass, N. P. Wray, and D. L. Busbee).

5.2. Human Lung Tissues

While lymphocytes are convenient and accessible cells for investigating AHH inducibility, they are not the postulated target tissues for chemical induction of lung cancer. Studies have now appeared utilizing various types of human lung tissues, which may be more directly applicable to the problem of lung cancer. AHH has been induced by BA in explants of cultured human bronchus[64, 91, 127, 134, 149]. A study of the variation among individuals in the capacity to bind BP metabolites indicated that bronchus from patients with lung cancer produced BP metabolites with greater affinity for DNA than bronchus from noncancer patients. The predominant DNA-binding BP metabolite produced by cultured bronchus was the diol epoxide I[91, 134] (for further details see Fig. 2).

McLemore and co-workers have measured AHH activity in homogenates of surgically-resected lung tissue from cigarette smoking noncancer and lung cancer patients [128]. Mean levels of AHH were similar for lung tissue from patients in both groups, and were within the range of enzyme activity reported in cultured human bronchus induced by BA [91, 127, 149]. The lung enzyme levels were comparable to AHH levels measured in either fresh pulmonary alveolar macrophages (PAMs) or cultured BA-induced lymphocytes from the same individuals (Fig. 4). The number of subjects studied was too small to assess adequately the relationship between AHH and lung cancer in humans, but the lung cancer patients generally either had high AHH in PAMs, lymphocytes, or lung tissue [128] (for more details see Fig. 7 in the section on Multivariant Analyses of AHH in Different Human Tissues).

5.3. Pulmonary Alveolar Macrophages

The initial studies of AHH induction in PAMs were performed by Cantrell *et al.* [119, 131–132], who found that AHH activity was elevated 9 to 10-fold in PAMs freshly lavaged from lungs of healthy cigarette smoking volunteers. The increased AHH activity in PAMs from smokers was associated with marked morphological abnormalities, particularly increased ingestion of particulates from cigarette smoke [150–151]. When a normal nonsmoking volunteer initiated smoking 10–15 cigarettes daily for a month, AHH activity in PAMs increased to about 400% above the control (presmoking) levels [131], with decline to normal within two months after smoking ceased. These observations suggested that AHH activity was induced in the lungs of smokers by constituents in cigarette smoke. In subsequent studies employing cultured PAMs, enzyme activity was induced *in vitro* either by BA [64, 90, 118, 130, 140, 152, 153] or by cigarette tars [145].

Utilizing specimens obtained by saline lavage at the time of diagnostic bronchoscopy, McLemore *et al.* found higher AHH activity in cigarette smokers than from nonsmokers, whether or not lung cancer was present [53, 118, 130]. In patients with or without lung cancer, cigarette smoking induced AHH levels in freshly lavaged PAMs which were similar to the levels induced *in vitro* by BA [55, 118]. When only PAM enzyme values were considered, these were not significantly different for noncancer and lung cancer patients [46, 53, 54, 56]. AHH activity in PAMs was normally distributed in a unimodal rather than a trimodal fashion previously reported for lymphocyte AHH activity [51].

Studies of total metabolism of PAHs by cultured PAMs obtained at necropsy from lung cancer or noncancer patients [64, 91] or by saline lavage from normal volunteers [90, 153] indicate that PAMs are capable of metabolizing BP to various derivatives, including potent mutagens. PAMs are also capable of detoxifying these derivatives (via epoxide hydratase, conjugation pathways, etc.; for further details see Fig. 2). Following 24 hour incubation of cells with BP, PAMs have greater metabolizing capabilities than lymphocytes [90] and activity at least as high as that previously reported for cultured human bronchus [64, 127, 149].

Marshall *et al.* have recently demonstrated that metabolism of BP by human PAMs results in significant interindividual variation in production as well as detoxification of various BP metabolites [90, 153]. The same studies have also demonstrated that individuals may have low levels of BP phenolic derivatives and at the same time have high levels of the potent intermediate metabolites such as the 7,8-dihydrodiol (the proximate carcinogen of BP, see Fig. 2). These individuals also vary singificantly in their ability to conjugate (detoxify) various BP derivatives.

These results strongly suggest PAMs play a significant role in PAH metabolism in human lung. By production of increased quantities of the proximate and ultimate carcinogens (see Figure 2), PAMs (which are in close contact with the bronchial epithelium) could render epithelial cells more susceptible to malignant transformation. On the other hand, increased detoxification of these compounds by PAMs could protect epithelial cells from harmfull effects, including carcinogenesis.

5.4. Multivariant Analyses of AHH in Different Human Tissues

The most compelling data implicating AHH as an etiologic factor in pulmonary carcinogenesis has been obtained by utilizing multivariant analyses of AHH in different tissues obtained simultaneously from the same individual. When PAMs and lymphocytes from noncancer patients were simultaneously compared, a positive correlation was noted for AHH values for the same individual (Fig. 5). However, when AHH levels in these two tissue types were compared for individual lung cancer patients, a lack of correlation was noted (Fig. 6). Similar relationships were observed for both nonsmokers and cigarette smokers [46, 53–56]. A similar relationship was noted when three tissues (PAMs, lymphocytes, and lung tissue) from a smaller group of individual noncancer and lung cancer patients were simultaneously compared [128]. AHH levels in one tissue from noncancer patients correlated well with AHH values for another tissue from the same subject. However, enzyme values for the three tissue types obtained from lung cancer patients were poorly correlated (Figure 7). Marshall *et al.* [90], provided further evidence for the consistency of AHH metabolizing capabilities in different tissues by demonstrating that PAMs and lymphocytes from normal volunteers produced similar quantities of both free and conjugated BP metabolites. On the other hand, variation between individuals in both free and conjugated BP metabolite formation was substantial.

The reasons have not been established for the dissociation in AHH values among different tissues from lung cancer patients. Altered enzyme systems have been noted previously in cells of patients with carcinoma [154, 155], and

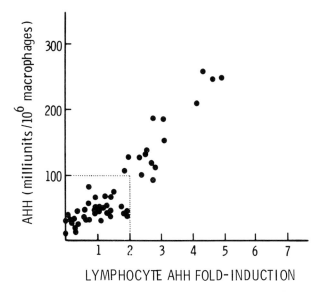

Fig. 5. Comparison of AHH activity in fresh PAMs and fold-induction of AHH in cultured lymphocytes from cigarette smokers without evidence of cancer (r = 0.915), p < .001). Reprinted from [54].

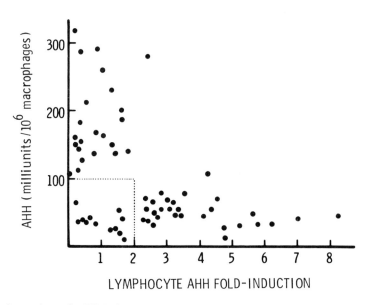

Fig. 6. Comparison of AHH in fresh PAMs and fold-induction of AHH in cultured lymphocytes from cigarette smokers with primary lung cancer. (Linear regression not appropriate for this set of values). Reprinted from [54].

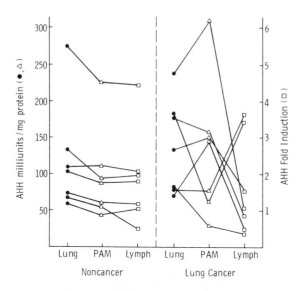

Fig. 7. Simultaneous comparison of AHH in fresh PAMs, fresh lung tissue, and cultured BA-induced lymphocytes from individual cigarette smokers with and without lung cancer. ● = AHH activity in fresh lung tissue; △ = AHH activity in fresh PAMs; □ = cultured lymphocyte AHH fold induction. Connecting lines represent enzyme values for individual patients ($r = 0.987$, $p < 0.001$ for noncancer and $r = 0.701$, $p > 0.25$ for lung cancer patients; multiple regression analysis). Reprinted from [128].

it is not unreasonable to assume that inherent alterations in PAM or lympho-cyte AHH activity could occur as well. In fact, there is additional evidence that PAH metabolism by the AHH system might be altered in cells from lung cancer patients. Studies of binding of BP metabolites to DNA in cultured human bronchus revealed bronchus from individuals with lung cancer gener-ated BP metabolites which more readily bound to DNA than metabolites from bronchus of noncancer patients [149]. Additional studies indicated that the major metabolite bound to DNA was the ultimate carcinogen of BP, the diolepoxide I [134]. The increased binding of BP metabolites to DNA encoun-tered with bronchus from lung cancer patients could be due to an increased rate of diol epoxide I formation in the bronchial epithelium of these individ-uals. In addition, these investigators have demonstrated that the major meta-bolite produced by PAMs obtained at autopsy from lung cancer patients is the proximate carcinogen of BP, the 7,8-dihydrodiol [64], which is further meta-bolized to the diol epoxide I (see Fig. 2). These results are supported by those recently reported by Marshall et al., who studied BP metabolism in PAMs obtained from normal healthy volunteers [90].

The oxidation and elimination of numerous categories of drugs have been documented to be a function of AHH, particularly in the liver[156]. Antipyrine is an example of one drug which has been utilized as a substrate for measuring liver AHH metabolism capabilities. It has been demonstrated that antipyrine plasma clearance is positively correlated with AHH inducibility in cultured lymphocytes obtained from healthy normal subjects (r = 0.947, p < 0.001)[156]. Antipyrine clearance studies on lung cancer patients and on a healthy control group demonstrated a decreased antipyrine half-life (increased antipyrine metabolism) in lung cancer patients. The comparison of both antipyrine half-life and of the metabolic clearance rate in healthy control subjects and in bronchogenic carcinoma patients with histologically different cancer types was reported by Kellermann et al. [52]. The metabolic clearance rate (AHH activity) was higher for any of the lung cancer types than for the control group. The plasma antipyrine half-life was correspondingly lower for the lung cancer patient group than for the healthy control group. These data show that increased rate of plasma antipyrine clearance may be positively correlated with both high AHH inducibility and with the occurrence of bronchogenic carcinoma. The data suggest that high AHH inducibility may thus be correlated with the occurrence of bronchogenic carcinoma. These data provide a direct link between lung cancer occurrence and high AHH inducibility which is not directly dependent on use of the cultured lymphocyte system to measure AHH levels in cancer patients.

The most conclusive studies for establishing a relationship between AHH levels and cancer risk in man have been obtained employing simultaneous analyses of AHH levels in PAMs and lymphocytes from individual noncancer and lung cancer patients. Utilizing multivariant analyses, these studies have demonstrated that the majority of noncancer patients (69%) exhibited low AHH levels in both PAMs and lymphocytes. In contrast, only 19% of the patients with lung cancer demonstrated low PAM or low lymphocyte AHH activity. The difference between these values was quite significant (p < 0.001)[46, 56]. When the noncancer patient population was evaluated for high AHH activity, 31% demonstrated high lymphocyte and high PAM AHH levels. None of the lung cancer patients showed both high PAM and high lymphocyte AHH activity, but 36% demonstrated high PAM and low lymphocyte AHH activity and 45% demonstrated low PAM and high lymphocyte AHH activity. However, when lung cancer patients with either high PAM or high lymphocyte AHH activity were grouped together, 81% exhibited high AHH activity in one of the two tissues. This represents a significant increase in AHH activity in the lung cancer population (81%) above that seen in the noncancer group (31%), (p < 0.001). These results strongly support the theory that high AHH levels are related to lung cancer risk.

5.5. AHH and Lung Cancer Diagnosis

The use of multivariant analysis for investigating AHH levels in multiple tissues could be of diagnostic usefulness in confirming the presence of lung cancer. Because the majority (81%) of lung cancer patients exhibited a dissociation between PAM and lymphocyte AHH values (Fig. 6), (with high levels in one cell type and low levels in the other), and since no noncancer patients in the study group demonstrated this dissociation (Figure 5), determination of enzyme levels in both tissues might be of diagnostic usefulness. Some patients in whom lung cancer is suspected are not correctly diagnosed by initial bronchoscopy with conventional cytology studies. In 21 cigarette smokers previously studied, in whom diagnostic bronchoscopy was inconclusive, 11 out 11 (100%) of the noncancer patients and 9 out of 10 (90%) lung cancer patients could have been correctly diagnosed by examining the patterns of their AHH activity prior to the histologic confirmation of their diagnosis (which required invasive procedures such as thoracotomy, mediastinoscopy, needle biopsy, or necropsy). The one individual who was diagnosed as having lung cancer, but who was not detected by analysing AHH levels in PAMs and lymphocytes, belonged to the group with low enzyme activity in both lymphocytes and PAMs. Such individuals cannot be distinguished on the basis of AHH activity from noncancer patients (Fig. 5). These initial studies suggest a possible role for AHH analysis in combination with other diagnostic procedures for the detection of lung cancer.

McKenzie et al. [157] have recently studied a BP binding protein in human plasma samples. The levels of this protein in human plasma correlated well with the AHH activity in cultured lymphocytes from the same noncancer individual. When levels of BP binding protein in plasma and AHH activity in lymphocytes were compared in individual noncancer patients a positive correlation was observed. However, a lack of positive correlation was noted between the binding protein and lymphocyte AHH activity from lung cancer patients. Although these results are preliminary, it is possible that the measurement of this plasma protein in conjunction with the determination of AHH levels in one or more tissues might be useful as a diagnostic tool for detecting lung cancer.

6. OVERVIEW

One goal of investigation in the field of pulmonary carcinogenesis is the establishment of a set of biochemical criteria for identification of idividuals at high risk for the development of lung cancer. Persons so identified could then be counseled to abstain from exposure to cigarette smoke or other hazardous environmental carcinogens. Based on the current five year survival rates for lung cancer (5–10%)[4, 21] and on the relative resistance of lung cancer types to radiotherapy and cancer chemotherapy[21, 91], the best hope for controlling lung cancer is through prevention rather than treatment of the disease.

Since AHH is responsible for the activation of carcinogenic components of cigarette smoke condensate, this enzyme might represent one of the biochemical markers which could be useful in distinguishing individuals at risk of developing lung cancer. Because AHH appears to be a rate-limiting step in the pathway for pulmonary carcinogenesis (Fig. 1), it has been attractive to hypothesize a relationship between carcinogen metabolism (AHH) and lung cancer risk. While animal studies demonstrate that high AHH levels predispose to PAH-induced carcinogenesis[20, 85, 107, 137], a relationship between carcinogen metabolism and cancer susceptibility in man has not been clearly established. The majority of reports in human tissues do suggest that high AHH levels are related to lung cancer[46–57]. This hypothesis is further supported by the findings that similar potent intermediate compounds are produced by human lung tissues (as well as other human tissues) and animal tissues which have been exposed to various PAH components of cigarette smoke. These initial studies support the hypothesis that similar mechanisms exist for PAH-mediated carcinogenesis in human and animal tissues.

The most widely studied human tissue has been the peripheral blood lymphocyte and although use of the lymphocyte for measurement of AHH has been criticized in the past, it remains the most feasible cell type in terms of accessibility and suitability for large scale human studies. As investigators continue to resolve the problems associated with the variability and reproducibility of the lymphocyte AHH system[146], it appears this cell type will be useful for measuring AHH inducibility in those individuals who are free of detectable cancer. However, in patients with lung cancer, the lymphocyte is probably not the appropriate tissue for measurement of carcinogen metabolism[54–56, 128]. In support of this concept, studies which have employed tissues other than peripheral blood lymphocytes have more consistently demonstrated increased AHH levels in patients with lung cancer compared with the noncancer control groups[46, 54–56, 128].

All investigations of AHH levels in lung cancer patients to date have been retrospective and one cannot conclude whether the increased AHH activity preceded the development of cancer or was a consequence of its development. There is a need for prospective studies utilizing populations of individuals at high risk for development of lung cancer, with classification of these individuals according to AHH inducibility prior to the development of clinically apparent cancer in order to prove or disprove that AHH is related to lung cancer etiology in man.

Another limitation of previous studies is that most have utilized fluorometric assays, which measure only the phenolic BP derivatives for evaluation of AHH activity in human tissues. Although this is generally the major metabolite produced from metabolism of BP, a more comprehensive approach would be to quantitate all metabolites produced by this enzyme system, since formation of BP metabolites such as the diol epoxide I might be a determinant of cancer susceptibility. A major step in secondary BP metaboism is the epoxide hydratase-mediated conversion of BP epoxides to dihydrodiols[158]. The 7,8-dihydrodiol may be further metabolized to the diol epoxide I, presumed to be the ultimate carcinogen of BP ([133,134]; see Fig. 2). Persons with a greater capacity for production of the 7,8-dihydrodiol might, therefore, be at greater risk through further metabolism to ultimate carcinogens.

Concentration of toxic metabolites in the cell depends not only upon synthesis of primary metabolites (epoxides and phenols), but largely upon the further metabolism by conjugation reactions[159,160]. The capacity for production as well as detoxification of intermediate BP derivatives by human lung cells varies among individuals[90,153]. These studies have shown that individuals may have low levels of BP phenolic derivatives while at the same time having high levels of potentially harmful intermediate metabolites such as the 7,8-dihydrodiol. Additionally, the ability to conjugate (detoxify) various BP metabolites may vary among individuals.

The processes of activation and detoxification of PAHs are probably in steady state within the cell and represent a multiplicity of pathways, some of which lead ultimately to activation and others to detoxification and excretion of the compounds from the body. Consequently, future studies of carcinogen metabolism in man should include investigation both of activation and detoxification pathways.

In addition to investigating carcinogen metabolism (AHH), investigators must evaluate other factors which might influence the hypothesized pathways for human pulmonary carcinogenesis (Fig. 1). These variables include the capacity for DNA repair, immunosurveillance mechanisms, synergism among different carcinogens, and other unidentified factors. It appears human lung cancer is a multifaceted process involving numerous biochemical and immunologic regulatory pathways, all of which must be assessed to definitively examine the relationship between carcinogen metabolism and pulmonary carcinogenesis.

REFERENCES

1. Pott P: Chirurgical observations relative to the cataract, the polypus of the nose, the cancer of the scrotum, the different kinds of ruptures, and mortification of the toes and feet. Haues, Clark, and Collins. London, England, 1775.
2. Gelboin HV: Carcinogens, enzyme induction, and gene action. Advances in Cancer Research 1:1-81, 1967.

3. Wagoner JK: Occupational carcinogenesis: Two hundred years since Percivall Pott. Ann NY Acad Sci 271:1-4, 1976.
4. Silverberg E: Cancer statistics, 1979. Ca – A Journal for Clinicians 29:6-21, 1979.
5. Deelman HT and VanErp JP: Beobachtungen an experimentellem tumar wachsrum. Z Krebsforsch 24:86-98, 1927.
6. Berenblum I: Modifying influence of dichloroethylsulphide on induction of tumors in mice by tar. J Pathol Bacteriol 32:425-434, 1929.
7. Auerbach O, Hammond EC, Kirman D, Garfunkel L: Effects of cigarette smoking on dogs. II. Pulmonary neoplasms. Arch Environ Health 21:744-749, 1970.
8. Kinoshita N and Gelboin HV: The role of aryl hydrocarbon hydroxylase in 7,12–dimethyl-benz(a) antracene skin tumorigenesis; on mechanism of 7,8-benzoflavone inhibition of tumorgenesis. Cancer Res 23:1329-1335, 1972.
9. Wynder EL, Graham EA and Croninger AB: Experimental production of carcinoma with cigarette tar. II. Tests with different mouse strains. Cancer Res 15:445-451, 1955.
10. Saffioti U, Montesano R, Sellakumar AR, Cefis F, and Kaufman DG: Respiratory tract carcinogenesis in hamsters induced by different numbers of administrations of benz(a)pyrene and ferric oxide. Cancer Res 32:1073-1081, 1972.
11. Huberman E and Sachs L: Cell-mediated mutagenesis of mammalian cells with chemical carcinogens. Int J Cancer 13(3):326-333, 1974.
12. Kouri RE, Salerno RA and Whitmore CE: Relationships between aryl hydrocarbon hydroxylase inducibility and sensitivity to chemically induced subcutaneous sarcoma in various strains of mice. J Natl Cancer Inst 50:363-368, 1973.
13. Akin EJ, Chamberlain WJ and Chortyk OT: Mouse skin tumorigenesis and induction of aryl hydrocarbon hydroxylase by tobacco smoke fractions. J Natl Cancer Inst 54(4):907-912, 1975.
14. Little JB and O'Toole WF: Respiratory tract tumors in hamsters induced by benzo(a)pyrene and ^{210}Po α-radiation. Cancer Res 34:3026-3029, 1974.
15. Chouroulinkov I and Micheals M: Effects of cigarette smoke condensate (CsC) on rat fetal lung organ culture. In: Karbe E, Park JF (editors). Experimental lung cancer: Carcinogenesis and bioassays. International Symposium, Seattle, Washington, June 23-26, 1974. New York, Springer-Verlag, pp 532-538, 1974.
16. Dontenwill WP: Tumorigenic effect of chronic cigarette inhalation on Syrian Golden hamsters. In: Karbe E, Park JF (editors) Experimental lung cancer: Carcinogenesis and bioassays. International Symposium, Seattle, Washington, June 23–26, 1974. New York, Springer-Verlag, pp 332-359, 1974.
17. Ho W, Wilcox K, Furst A: Pulmonary carcinogenesis by two aryl hydrocarbons on three mouse strains. In: Karbe E, Park JF (editors). Experimental Lung Cancer: Carcinogenesis and Bioassays. International Symposium, Seattle, Washington, June 23–26, 1974. New York, Springer-Verlag, pp 62-71, 1974.
18. Marquandt H, Grover PL and Sims P: *In vitro* malignant transformation of mouse fibroblasts by non K-region dihydrodiols derived from 7-methyl-benz(a)-anthracene, 7,12-dimethylbenz(a)anthracene, and benzo(a)pyrene. Cancer Res 36:2059-1064, 1976.
19. Slaga TJ, Viaje A, Benny DL and Bracken W: Skin tumor initiating ability of benzo(a)pyrene 4,5-7,8- and 7,8-diol-9,10-epoxides and 7,8-diol. Cancer Lett 2:115-122, 1976.
20. Kouri RE and Nebert DW: Genetic regulation of susceptibility to polycyclic hydrocarbon-induced tumors in the mouse. In: H Hiah, JD Watson, JA Winsten (editors), Cold Spring Harbor Symposium on Quantitative Biology: The Origin of Hyman Cancer, pp 811-836. New York: Cold Spring Harbor Laboratory, 1978.
21. Califano JA Jr: Smoking and Health: A report of the Surgeon General. Department of Health Education, and Welfare, Pub No (PHS)79-50066, part I, 1979.

22. Stocks P: Cancer mortality in relation to national consumption of cigarettes, solid fuel, tea, and coffee. Br J Cancer 24:215-221, 1970.
23. Steinfeld JL: The health consequences of smoking. A report of the Surgeon General. The Department of Health, Education and Welfare Publication No (HSM) 71-7513, 239-244, 1971.
24. Korsgaard R: Ar lungcancer artflig? (Is lung cancer hereditary?). Kvartals Skrift 70 (1):13-18, 1975.
25. Caplin M, Festenstein F: Relation between lung cancer, chronic bronchitis, and airways obstruction. Br Med J 3:678-680, 1975.
26. Hammond EC, Selikoff IJ, Seidman H: Multiple interactions of cigarette smoking. Extra-pulmonary cancer. In: Bucalossi P, Veronesi U, Cascinelli H (editors). Cancer epidemiology, environmental factors, Vol. 3, Proceedings of the XI International Cancer Congress. Florence, Oct. 20-26, 1974. Amsterdam, Excerpta Medica 147-150, 1975.
27. Sterling TS: A critical reassessment of the evidence bearing on smoking as the cause of lung cancer. Amer J of Public Health 65:939-953, 1975.
28. Tokuhata GK: Familial factors in human lung cancer and smoking. Amer J of Public Health 54:24-32, 1964.
29. Tokuhata GK: Cancer of the lung: host and environmental interaction. pp 213-232, in: Cancer Genetics, Lunch HT (editor), Charles C. Thomas (Publisher), Springfield, Ill. 1976.
30. Commins BT, Cooper RL and Lindsay AJ: Polycyclic hydrocarbons in cigarette smoke. Brit J Cancer 8:296-302, 1954.
31. Udenfriend S: Fluorescence assay in biology and medicine. Academic Press, New York, p 456, 1972.
32. Falk HL and Kotin P: Chemistry, host entry, and metabolic fate of carcinogens. Clin Pharmacol Ther 4:88-103, 1963.
33. Freeman AE, Price PJ, Bryan RT, Gordon RJ, Gilden RW, Kelloff GJ and Huebner RJ: Transformation of rat and hamster embryo cells by extract of city smog. Proc Soc Nat Acad Sci 68:445-449, 1971.
34. Sawicki E: Airborne carcinogens and allied compounds. Arch Environ Health 14:46-53, 1967.
35. Kennaway EL: The identification of a carcinogenic compounds in coal tar. Brit Med J 2:749-752, 1955.
36. Hammond EC, Selikoff IJ, Lawther PL and Seidman H: Inhalation of benzopyrene and cancer in man. Annals NY Acad Sci 271:116-124, 1976.
37. Kuratsone M: Benzo(a)pyrene content of certain pyrogenic materials. J Nat Cancer Inst 16:1485-1496, 1956.
38. Boyland E: The biological significance of metabolism of polycyclic compounds. Biochem Soc Symp 5:40-54, 1950.
39. Miller OA and Miller EC: Metabolism of drugs in relation to carcinogenesis. Annals NY Acad Sci 271:125-140, 1965.
40. Miller JA: Carcinogenesis by chemical: An overview – GH Clowes Memorial Lecture. Cancer Res 30:559-576, 1970.
41. Heidelberger C: Chemical carcinogenesis. Ann Rev Biochem 44:79-121, 1975.
42. Gelboin H: Studies on the mechanism of microsomal hydroxylase induction and its role in carcinogen action. Rev Can Biol 31:39-60, 1972.
43. Sims P, Grover PL, Swaisland A, Pal K and Hewer A: Metabolic activation of benzo(a)pyrene proceeds by a diol-epoxide. Nature 252:326-335, 1974.
44. Weinstein BL, Jefrey AM, Jennette KW and Blobstein SH: Benzo(a)pyrene diol-epoxides as intermediates in nucleic acid binding *in vitro* and *in vivo*. Science 193:592-595, 1976.

45. Wood AW, Levin W, Lu AYU, Yagi H, Hemandez O, Jerina DM and Conney AH: Metabolism of benzo(a)pyrene and benzo(a)pyrene derivatives to mutagenic products by highly purified hepatic microsomal enzymes. J Biol Chem 251:4882-4890, 1976.
46. Busbee DL, McLemore TL, Martin RR, Wray NP, Marshall MV and Cantrell ET: High AHH inducibility is positively correlated with occurrence of lung cancer. In Cancer: A Comprehensive Survey, Vol 4: Polynuclear aromatic hydrocarbons (eds Jones PW and Freudenthal RI) Batelle, Columbus, Ohio, In press, 1980.
47. Coomes M, Mason W, Muijsson I, Cantrell E, Anderson D, Busbee D: Aryl hydrocarbon hydroxylase and 16αhydroxylase in cultured human lymphocytes. Biochemical Genetics 14:671-685, 1976.
48. Emery AEM, Danford N, Anand R, Duncan W, Paton L: Aryl hydrocarbon hydroxylase inducibility in patients with lung cancer. Lancet 3:470-471, 1978.
49. Gahnberg C, Sekki A, Kouseenem T, Holsti L, Olavi M: Induction of aryl hydrocarbon hydroxylase activity and pulmonary carcinoma. Int J Cancer 23:302-305, 1979.
50. Guirgis HA, Lynch HT, Mate T, Harris RE, Willis I, Caha L: Aryl hydrocarbon hydroxylase activity in lymphocytes from lung cancer and normal controls. Oncology 33:105-109, 1976.
51. Kellermann G, Shaw C and Luyten-Kellermann M: Aryl hydrocarbon hydroxylase inducibility and bronchogenic carcinoma. N Eng J Med 289:934-937, 1973.
52. Kellermann G, Luyten-Kellermann M, Jett J, Moses H and Fontana R: Aryl hydrocarbon hydroxylase in man and lung cancer. Human genetic variation in response to medical and environmental agents: Pharmacogenetics and energetics. Human Genetics (Suppl 1):161-168, 1978.
53. McLemore TL, Martin RR, Busbee DL, Richie RC, Springer RR, Topell KL and Cantrell ET: Aryl hydrocarbon hydroxylase activity in pulmonary macrophages and lymphocytes from lung cancer and noncancer patients. Cancer Res 37:1175-1181, 1977.
54. McLemore Tl, Martin RR, Springer RR, Wray NP, Cantrell ET and Busbee DL: Aryl hydrocarbon hydroxylase activity in pulmonary alveolar macrophages and lymphocytes from lung cancer and noncancer patients: A correlation with family histories of cancer. Biochem Genetics 17:795-806, 1979.
55. McLemore TL, Martin RR, Wray NP, Cantrell ET and Busbee DL: Dissociation between aryl hydrocarbon hydroxylase activity in cultures pulmonary macrophages and blood lymphocytes from lung cancer patients. Cancer Res 38:3805-3811, 1978.
56. McLemore TL, Martin RR, Wray NP, Cantrell ET and Busbee DL: Reassessment of the relationship between aryl hydrocarbon hydroxylase and lung cancer. In press, 1980.
57. Rasco MA, Yamauchi T, Johnson D: AHH in normal and cancer populations. In Griffin AC and Shaw CR (eds). 31st Annual Symposium on Fundamental Cancer Research: Carcinogen identification and mechanism of action. New York, Raven Press, pp 147-156, 1979.
58. Daudel P, Dequesne M, Vigny P, Grover PL and Sims P: Fluorescence spectral evidence that benzo(a)pyrene-DNA products in mouse skin arise from diol-epoxides. Federation European Biochem Soc Letters 57:250-253, 1975.
59. Grover PL and Sims P: K-region epoxides of polycyclic hydrocarbons: Reactions with nucleic acids and polyribonuclecoctides. Biochem Pharmacol 22:661-666, 1973.
60. Pitropaolo C and Weinstein IB: Binding of [^{3}H]benzo(a)pyrene to natural and synthetic nucleic acids in a subcellular microsomal system. Cancer Res 35:2191-2198, 1975
61. Flesher JW, Harvey RG and Sydnor KL: Oncogenicity of K-region epoxides of benzo(a)pyrene and 7,12-dimethyl benz(a)anthracene. Intern J Cancer 18:351-353, 1976.

62. Grover PL, Sims P, Huberman E, Marquardt H, Kuroki T and Heidelberger C: *In vitro* transformation of rodent cells by K-region derivatives of polycyclic hydrocarbons. Proc Natl Acad Sci US 68:1098-1101, 1971.

63. Slaga TJ, Viaje A, Berry DL, Bracken W, Buty SG and Scribner JD: Skin tumor initiation ability of benzo(a)pyrene 4n 5-, 7,8-, and diol-9,10-epoxides and 7,8-diol. Cancer Letters 2:115-122, 1976.

64. Autrup H, Harris CC, Stoner GD, Selkirk JK, Schafer PW and Trump BF: Metabolism of [^{3}H]benzo(a)pyrene by cultured human bronchus and human pulmonary alveolar macrophages. Lab Invest 38:217-224, 1978.

65. Mason HS: Mechanisms of oxygen metabolism. Adv Enzymol 19:79-233, 1957.

66. Lu AYH, Kuntzman R, West S, Jacobson M and Conney AH: Reconstituted liver microsomal enzyme system that hydroxylates drugs, other foreign compounds, and endogenous substrates. The J of Biol Chem 247:1727-1734, 1972.

67. Nebert DW, Robinson HR, Niwa A, Kumaki K and Poland AP: Genetic expression of aryl hydrocarbon hydroxylase activity in the mouse. J Cell Physiol 83:393-414, 1975.

68. Grover PL and Sims P: Interactions of the K-region epoxides of phenanthracene and dibenz(1-h)anthracene with nucleic acids and histone. Biochem Pharmacol 19:2251-2259, 1970.

69. Ulrich V: Enzymatic hydroxylations with molecular oxygen. Angewandke Chemic 11:701-712, 1972.

70. West SB, Levin W, Ryan D, Vore M and Lu AYH: Liver microsomal electron transport systems. The involvement of cytochrome 65 in the NADH-dependent hydroxylation of 3,4-benzpyrene by a reconstituted cytochrome P-448 containing system. Biochem Biophys Res Commun 58:516-522, 1975.

71. Yang CS: Interactions between solubilized cytochrome P-450 and hepatic microsomes. J Biol Chem 252:293-298, 1977.

72. Gielen JE, Goujon FM and Nebert DW. Genetic regulation of aryl hydrocarbon hydroxylase induction. II. Simple mendelian expression in mouse tissue *in vivo*. J Biol Chem 247:1125-1137, 1972.

73. Goujon FM, Nebert DW and Gielen JE: Genetic expression of aryl hydrocarbon hydroxylase induction IV. Interaction of various compounds with different forms of P-450 and the effect on benzo(a)pyrene metabolism *in vitro*. Mol Pharmacol 8:667-680, 1972.

74. Nebert DW and Gielen JE: Aryl hydrocarbon hydroxylase induction in mammalian liver cell culture. II. Effect of actinomycin D and cycloheximide on induction processes by phenobarbital or polycyclic hydrocarbons. J Biol Chem 246:5199-5206, 1971.

75. Nebert DW, Gielen JE and Goujon FM: Genetic expression of aryl hydrocarbon hydroxylase induction. III. Changes in binding of N-octylamine to cytochrome P-450. Mole Pharmacol 8:651-666, 1972.

76. Nebert DW, Goujon FM and Gielen JE: Aryl Hydrocarbon hydroxylase induction by polycyclic hydrocarbons: Simple autosomal dominant trait in the mouse. Nature New Biol 236:107-110, 1972.

77. Nebert DW and Gielen JE: Aryl hydrocarbon hydroxylase induction in the mouse. Fed Proc 31:1315-1325, 1972.

78. Nebert DW and Kon H: Genetic regulation of aryl hydrocarbon hydroxylase induction. V. Specific changes in spin state of cytochrome P-450 from genetically responsive animals. J. Biol Chem 248:169-178, 1973.

79. Nebert DW, Considine N and Owens IS: Genetic expression of aryl hydrocarbon hydroxylase induction. VI. Control of other aromatic hydrocarbon inducible monooxygenase activities at or near the same genetic locus. Arch Biochem Biophys 157:148-159, 1973.

80. Nebert DW, Heidema JK, Strobel HW and Coon MJ: Genetic expression of aryl hydrocarbon hydroxylase induction. Genetic specificity resides in the fraction containing cytochromes P-448 and P-450. J Biol Chem 248:7631-7636, 1973.

81. Nebert DW, Robinson JR and Kon H: Further studies on genetically mediated differences in monooxygenase activities and spin state of cytochrome P-450 iron from rabbit, rat and mouse liver. J Biol Chem 248:7637-7647, 1973.

82. Nebert DW, Benedict WF and Kouri RE: Aromatic hydrocarbon produced tumorigenesis and the genetic differences in aryl hydrocarbon hydroxylase induction. In Chemical Carcinogenesis Ts'O, POP and Dipaolo JA (editors), Marcel-Dekker, Inc., New York. pp 271-288, 1974.

83. Poland AP, Glover E, Robinson JR and Nebert DW: Genetic expression of aryl hydrocarbon hydroxylase activity. Induction of monooxygenase activities and cytochrome P_1-450 formation by 2,3,7,8-tetrachlorodibenzo-p-dioxin in mice genetically 'nonresponsive' to other aromatic hydrocarbons. J Biol Chem 249:5599-5606, 1974.

84. Robinson JR and Nebert DW: Genetic expression of aryl hydrocarbon hydroxylase induction. Presence or absence of association with zoxaxolamine, diphenyl-hydantoin, and hexobarbital metabolism. Mole Pharmacol 10:484-493, 1974.

85. Kouri RE, Ratrie H, Ill, and Whitmire CE: Genetic control of susceptibility to 3-methylcholanthrene-induced subcutaneous sarcomas. Int J Cancer 13:714-720, 1974.

86. Thomas PE and Hutton JJ: Genetics of aryl hydrocarbon hydroxylase induction in mice: Additive inheritance in crosses between C3H/HeJ and DBA/2J. Biochem Genet 8:249-252, 1973.

87. Hayaishi O: Enzymatic hydroxylation. Ann Rev Biochem 38:21-44, 1969.

88. Williams RT: Detoxification mechanisms. The metabolism and detoxification of drugs, toxic substances, and other organic compounds, 796 pages. 2nd edition, Wiley, New York, 1959.

89. Gelboin HV, Selkirk J, Okuda T, Nemoto N, Yang SK, Wiebel FJ, Whitlock JP Jr, Rapp HJ, and Bast RC Jr: Benzo(a)pyrene metabolism: enzymatic and liquid chromatographic analysis and application in human liver, lymphocytes, and monocytes. In: Biological Reactive Intermediates. Ed. Jallow DJ, Kocsis JJ, Snyder R, and Vaino H. (Editors). pp 98-123, Plenum Press, NY, 1977.

90. Marshall MV, McLemore TL, Martin RR, Marshall MV, Wray NP, Busbee DL, Cantrell ET, Arnott MS and Griffin AC: Benzo(a)pyrene activation and detoxification by human pulmonary alveolar macrophages and lymphocytes. In: Cancer: A comprehensive survey, Vol. 4, Polynuclear aromatic hydrocarbons Jones PW and Freudenthal RI. (Editors). Batelle, Columbus, Ohio, In Press, 1980.

91. Harris CC, Autrup H, Trump BF and Stoner GD: Carcinogenesis studies in human respiratory epithelium: An experimental model system. In: Pathogenesis and Therapy of Lung Cancer. Harris CC, (editor), pp 559-607, Marcel Dekker, Inc. NY, 1978.

92. Sims P and Grover PL: Epoxides in polycyclic aromatic hydrocarbon metabolism and carcinogenesis. Adv Cancer Res 20:165-274, 1974.

93. Gielen JE and Nebert DW: Aryl hydrocarbon hydroxylase induction in mammalian liver cell culture. III. Effects of various sera, hormones, biogenic amines, and other endogenous compounds on enzyme activity. J Biol Chem 247:7591-7602, 1972.

94. Haugen DA, Coon MJ and Nebert DW: Induction of multiple forms of mouse liver cytochrome P-450. Evidence for genetically controlled *de novo* protein synthesis in response to treatment with β-naphthoflavone or phenobarbital. J Biol Chem 251:1817-1827, 1976.

95. Poland AP, Glover E and Kende AS: Stereospecific, high affinity binding of 2,3,7,8-tetrachlorodibenzo-p-dioxin by hepatic cytosol: evidence that the binding species is the receptor for the induction of aryl hydrocarbon hydroxylase. J Biol Chem 251:4936–4946, 1976

96. Poland AP and Glover E: Genetic expression of aryl hydrocarbon hydroxylase by 2,3,7,8-tetrachlorodibenzo-p-dioxin: Evidence for a receptor mutation in genetically non-responsive mice. Mol Pharmacol 11:389-398, 1975.

97. Comai K and Gaylor JL: Existence and separation of three forms of cytochrome-450 from rat liver microsomes. J Biol Chem 248:4947-1955, 1973.

98. Alvares A and Siekevitz P: Gel electrophoresis of partially purified cytochromes P-450 from liver microsomes of variously treated rats. Biochem Biophys Res Commun 54:923-929, 1973.

99. Welton AR and Ayst SD: Multiplicity of cytochrome P-450 hemoproteins in rat liver microsomes. Biochem Biophys Res Commun 56:898-906, 1974.

100. Levin W, Lu AYH, Ryan D, West S, Kuntzman R and Conney AH: Partial Purification and separation of multiple forms of cytochrome P-450 and cytochrome P-448 from rat liver microsomes. Adv Exp Med Biol 31:871-879, 1974.

101. Coon MJ, Haugen DA and Van der Hoeven TA: Properties of purified cytochrome P-450 and NADPH-cytochrome P-450 reductase from rabbit liver microsomes. Adv Exp Med Biol 31:972-979, 1975.

102. Haugen DA, Van der Hoeven TA and Coon MJ: Purified liver microsomal cytochrome P-450. Separation and characterization of multiple forms. J Biol Chem 250:3567-3570, 1975.

103. Thomas PE, Lu AYH, Ryan P, West SB, Kawalck J and Levin W: Immunochemical evidence for six forms of rat liver cytochrome P-450 obtained using antibodies against purified rat liver cytochromes P-450 and P-448. Mol Pharmacol 12:746-758, 1976.

104. Jerina DM and Daly JW: Arene oxides: A new aspect of drug metabolism. Science 185:573-582, 1974.

105. Conney AH: Pharmacological implications of microsomal enzyme induction. Pharmacol Rev 19:317-356, 1967.

106. Daly JW, Jerina DM and Witkop B: Arene oxides and the NIH shift: The metabolism, toxicity, and carcinogenicity of aromatic compounds. Experimentia 28:1129-1149, 1972.

107. Nebert DW and Felton JS: Importance of genetic factors influencing the metabolism of foreign compounds. Fed Proc 35:1133-1141, 1976.

108. Peterson JA, Ullrich V and Hildchrandt AG. Metyranone interaction with *Pseudomonas putida* cytochrome P-450. Arch Biochem Biophys 145:531-542, 1971.

109. Ryan D, Lu AYH, West S and Levin W: Multiple forms of cytochrome P-450 in phenobarbital- and 3-methylcholanthrene-treated rats. Separation and spectral properties. J Biol Chem 250:2157-2163, 1975.

110. Owens IS and Nebert DW: Aryl hydrocarbon hydroxylase induction in mammalian liver-derived cell cultures. Stimulation of 'cytochrome P_450-associated' enzyme activity by many inducing compounds. Mol Pharmacol 11:94-104, 1975.

111. Rausmussen RE and Wang YI: Dependence of specific metabolism of benzo(a)pyrene on inducer of hydroxylase activity. Cancer Res (34:2290-2295, 1974.

112. Zampaglione N, Jollow DJ, Mitchell JR, Stripp B, Hamrick M and Gilletze JR. Role of detoxifying enzymes in bromobenzene induced liver necrosis. J Pharmacol Exp Ther 187:218-227, 1973.

113. Thomas PE, Kouri RE and Hutton JJ: The genetics of aryl hydrocarbon hydroxylase induction in mice: A single gene difference between C57Bl/6J and DBA/2J. Biochem Genetics 6:757, 1972.

114. Kellermann G, Cantrell E and Shaw CR: Variation in extent of aryl hydrocarbon hydroxylase induction in cultured human lymphocytes. Cancer Res 33:1654-1656, 1973.

115. Kellermann G, Luyten M-Kellermann and Shaw CR: Genetic variation of aryl hydrocarbon hydroxylase in human lymphocytes. Am J Hum Genet 25:327-331, 1973.

116. Kouri RE, Ratrie H, Atlas SA, Niwa A and Nebert DW: Aryl hydrocarbon hydroxylase induction in human lymphocyte cultures by 2,3,7,8-tetrachlorodibenzo-p-dioxin. Life Sci 15:1585-1595, 1974.

117. Atlas SA, Vesell ES and Nebert DW: Genetic control of interindividual variations in the inducibility of aryl hydrocarbon hydroxylase in cultured human lymphocytes. Cancer Res 36:4619-4630, 1976.

118. McLemore TL, Martin RR, Toppell KL, Busbee DL and Cantrell ET: Comparison of aryl hydrocarbon hydroxylase induction in cultured blood lymphocytes and pulmonary macrophages. J Clin Invest 60:1017-1024, 1977.

119. Cantrell ET, Busbee D, Warr G and Martin RR: Induction of aryl hydrocarbon hydroxylase in human lymphocytes and pulmonary alveolar macrophages — a comparison. Life Sci 13:1649-1654, 1973.

120. Paigen B, Minowada J, Gurtoo HL, Paigen K, Parker NB, Ward E, Hayer NT, Bross IDJ, Bock F and Vincent R: Distribution of aryl hydrocarbon hydroxylase inducibility in cultured human lymphocytes. Cancer Res 37:1829-1837, 1977.

121. Burke MD, Mayer RT and Kouri RE: 3-methylcholanthrene-induced monooxygenase (O-deethylation) activity of human lymphocytes. Cancer Res 37:460-463, 1977.

122. Gurtoo HL, Minowada J, Paigen B, Parker NB and Hayner NT: Factors influencing the measurement and reproducibility of aryl hydrocarbon hydroxylase activity in cultured human lymphocytes. J Natl Cancer Inst 59:787-798, 1977.

123. Paigen B, Gurtoo HL, Minowada J, Houten L, Vincent R, Paigen K, Parker NB, Ward E and Hayner NT: Questionable relation of aryl hydrocarbon hydroxylase to lung cancer risk. N Eng J Med 297:346-350, 1977.

124. Pelkonen O: Metabolism of benzo(a)pyrene in human adult and fetal tissues. In: Carcinogenesis, Vol 1, Polynuclear aromatic hydrocarbons: Chemistry, metabolism, and carcinogenesis (Freudenthal RI and Jones PW eds), Raven Press, New York, pp 9-21, 1976.

125. Levin W, Conney AH, Alvares AP, Merkatz I and Kappas A: Induction of benzo(a)pyrene hydroxylase in human skin. Sci 176:419-420, 1972.

126. Alvares Ap, Kappas A, Levin and Conney AH: Inducibility of benzo(a)pyrene hydroxylase in human skin by polycyclic hydrocarbons. Clin Pharmacol Ther 14:30-39, 1972.

127. Harris CC, H, Stoner G, Yang SK, Leutz JC, Gelboin HV, Selkirk JK, Connor RJ, Barrett, LA, Jones RT, McDowell E and Trump BF: Metabolism of benzo(a)pyrene and 7,12-dimethylbenz(a)anthracene in cultured human bronchus and pancreatic duct. Cancer Res 37:3349-3355, 1977.

128. McLemore TL, Martin RR, Pickard LR, Springer RR, Wray NP, Toppell KL, Mattox KL, Guinn GA, Cantrell ET and Busbee DL: Analysis of aryl hydrocarbon hydroxylase activity in human lung tissue, pulmonary macrophages, and blood lymphocytes. Cancer 41:2292-2300, 1978.

129. Okuda T, Vesell ES, Plotkin E, Tarone R, Bast RC and Gelboin HV: Interindividual and intraindividual variation in aryl hydrocarbon hydroxylase in monocytes from monozygotic and dizygotic twins. Cancer Res 37:3904-3911, 1977.

130. McLemore TL and Martin RR: in vitro induction of aryl hydrocarbon hydroxylase in human pulmonary alveolar macrophages by benzanthracene. Cancer Lett 2:327-334, 1977.

131. Cantrell ET, Warr GA, Busbee DL and Martin RR: Induction of aryl hydrocarbon hydroxylase in human pulmonary alveolar macrophages by cigarette smoking. J Clin Invest 52:1881-1884, 1973.

132. Cantrell ET, Martin RR, Warr GA, Busbee DL, Kellermann G and Shaw CR: Induction of aryl hydrocarbon hydroxylase in human pulmonary alveolar macrophages by cigarette smoking. Trans Assoc Am Phys 86:121-130, 1973.

133. Yang SK, McCourt SW, Leutz JC and Gelboin HV: Benzo(a)pyrene diol epoxides: Mechanisms of enzymatic formation and optically active intermediates. Science 196:1199-1200, 1977.

134. Yang SK, Gelboin HV, Trump BF, Autrup H and Harris CC: Metabolic activation of benzo(a)pyrene and binding to DNA in cultured human bronchus. Cancer Res 37:1210-1215, 1977.

135. Weinstein BI, Jefrey AM, Jennette KW and Blobstein SH: Benzo(a)pyrene diol epoxides as intermediates in nuclecic acid binding *in vitro* and *in vivo*. Sci 193:592-595, 1976.

136. Wood AW, Levin W, Lu AYU, Yasi H, Hernandez O, Jerina DM and Conney AH: Metabolism of benzo(a)pyrene and benzo(a)pyrene derivatives to mutagenic products by highly purified hepatic microsomal enzymes. J Bio Chem 251:4882-4890, 1976.

137. Kouri RE: Relationship between levels of aryl hydrocarbon hydroxylase activity and susceptibility to 3-methylcholanthrene and benzo(a)pyrene-induced cancers in inbred strains of mice. pp 139-151. In: Polynuclear aromatic hydrocarbons: Chemistry metabolism and carcinogenesis, Freudenthal RI and Jones RW, (Editors) Raven Press, New York, 1976.

138. Busbee DL, Shaw CR and Cantrell ET: Aryl hydrocarbon hydroxylase induction in human leukocytes. Sci 178:315-316, 1972.

139. Whitlock JP, Cooper HL and Gelboin HV: Aryl hydrocarbon (benzopyrene) hydroxylase is stimulated in human lymphocytes by mitogens and benz(a)anthracene. Sci 177:618-619, 1972.

140. Kellermann G, Luyten-Kellermann M and Shaw CR: Presence and induction of epoxide hydrase in cultured human lymphocytes. Biochem Biophys Res Comm 52:712-716, 1973.

141. Cantrell E, Abreu M and Busbee D: A simple assay of aryl hydrocarbon hydroxylase in cultured human lymphocytes. Biochem Biophys Res Comm 70:474-479, 1976.

142. Rasco MA, Jacobs MM and Griffin AC: Effects of selenium on aryl hydrocarbon hydroxylase activity in cultured human lymphocytes. Cancer Lett 3:295-301, 1977.

143. Gurtoo HL, Bejba N and Minowada J: Properties, inducibility, and an improved method of analysis of aryl hydrocarbon hydroxylase in cultured human lymphocytes. Cancer res 35:1235-1243, 1975.

144. Kouri RE, Imblum RL and Prough RA: Measurement of aryl hydrocarbon hydroxylase and NADH-dependent cytochrome C reductase activities in mitogen-activated human lymphocytes. In: Proceedings of the Third International Symposium on the Detection and Prevention of Cancer, H. Nieburgs (Editor), pp 1659-1676, Marcel Dekker, New York, 1977.

145. McLemore TL, Warr GA and Martin RR: Induction of aryl hydrocarbon hydroxylase in human pulmonary alveolar macrophages and peripheral lymphocytes by cigarette tars. Cancer Lett 2:161-168, 1977.

146. Kouri RE, Imblum RL, Sosnowski RC, Slomiany BJ and McKinney CE: parameters influencing quantitation of 3-methylcholanthrene induced aryl hydrocarbon hydroxylase activity in cultures human lymphocytes. J Env Path and Toxicol 2:1079-1098, 1979.

147. Ward E, Paigen B, Steenland K, Vincent R, Minowada J, Gurtoo H, Sartori P and Havens M: Aryl Hydrocarbon hydroxylase in persons with lung or laryngeal cancer. Int J Cancer 22:384-389, 1978.

148. Jett J, Moses H, Branum E, Taylor W. and Fontana R: Benzo(a)pyrene metabolism and blast transformation in peripheral blood mononuclear cells from smoking and nonsmoking populations and lung cancer patients. Cancer 41:192-200, 1978.

149. Harris CC, Autrup H, Connor R, Barrett LA, McDowell EM and Trump BF: Interindividual variation in binding of benzo(a)pyrene to DNA in cultured human bronchi. Sci 194:1067-1069, 1976.

150. Martin RR: Altered morphology and increased acid hydrolase content of pulmonary macrophages from cigarette smokers. Amer Rev Resp Dis 107:596-601, 1973.

151. Martin RR and Warr GA: Cigarette smoking and human pulmonary macrophages. Hosp Prac 12:97-104, 1977.

152. Harris CC, Hsu IC, Stoner GD, Trump BF and Selkirk JK Human pulmonary alveolar macrophages metabolize benzo(a)pyrene to proximate and ultimate mutagens. Nature 272:633-634, 1978.

153. Marshall MV, McLemore TL, Martin RR, Jenkins WT, Snodgrass DK, Corson MA, Arnott MS, Wray NP and Griffin AC: Patterns of benzo(a)pyrene metabolism in human pulmonary alveolar macrophages. Cancer Lett 8:103-109, 1979.

154. Weber G: Enzymology of cancer cells. Part I: N Eng J Med 296:486-493, 1977.

155. Weber G: Enzymology of cancer cells. Part II: N Eng J Med 296:541-551, 1977.

156. Kellermann D and Luyten-Kellermann M: Benzo(a)pyrene metabolism and plasma elimination rates of phenacetin, acetanilide, and theophylline in man. Pharmacology 17:191-200, 1978.

157. McKenzie M, McLemore TL, Rankin P, Martin RR, Wray N, Cantrell E and Busbee D. A human plasma component that binds benzo(a)pyrene. Cancer 42:2733-1737, 1978.

158. Yang SK, Roller PP and Gelboin HV: Enzymatic mechanism of benzo(a)pyrene conversion to phenols and diols and an improved high pressure liquid chromatography separation of benzo(a)pyrene derivatives. Biochem 16:3680-3687, 1977.

159. Bock KW: Dual role of glucuronyl and sulfotransferases converting xenobiotics into reactive or biologically inactive and easily excretable compounds. Arch Toxicol 39:77-85, 1977.

160. Depierre JW and Ernster L: The metabolism of polycyclic hydrocarbons and its relationship to cancer. Biochem Biophys Acta 473:149-186, 1978.

161. Kuntzman R, Mark LZ, Brand L, Jacobson M, Levin W and Conney AH: metabolism of drugs and carcinogens by human liver enzymes. J Exp Pharmacol Ther 152:151-156, 1966.

162. Alvares AP, Shilling GP, Levin W, Kuntzman R, Brand L and Mark LC: Cytochromes P-450 and B_5 in human liver microsomes. Clin Pharmacol Ther 10:655-659, 1969.

163. Kapitulnik J, Poppers PJ and Conney AH: Comparative metabolism of benzo(a)pyrene in drugs in human liver. Clin Pharmacol Ther 21:166-176, 1977.

164. Pelkomen O, Kaltiala EH, Karki NT, Jalonen K and Pyorala K: properties of benzpyrene hydroxylase from human liver in comparison with the rat, rabbit and guinea pig enzymes. Xenobiotica 5:501-509, 1975.

165. Conney AH, Pantuck EJ, Hsiao KC, Kuntzman R, Alvares AP and Kappas A: Regulation of drug metabolism in man by environmental chemicals and diet. Fed Proc 36:1647-1652, 1977.

166. Juchau MR, Pedersen MG, Symms KG: Hydroxylation of 3,4-benzpyrene in human fetal tissue homogenates. Biochem Pharmacol 21:2269-2272, 1972.

167. Pelkonen O, Jouppila P and Karki NT: Effect of Maternal cigarette smoking on 3,4-benzpyrene and N-methylaniline metabolism in human fetal liver and placenta. Toxicol Appl Pharmacol 23:399-407, 1972.

168. Schlede E and Scholz H: No differences in benzo(a)pyrene hydroxylase activity in the human immature placenta and in the human fetal liver from cigarette smoking and nonsmoking women. J perinat Med 2:189-193, 1974.

169. Pelkonen O and Karki NT: 3,4-benzpyrene and aniline are hydroxylated by human fetal liver but not by placenta at 6–7 weeks of fetal age. Biochem Pharmacol 22:1538-1540, 1973.

170. Rifkind AP, Bennett S, Forster ES and New MI: Components of the heme biosynthetic pathway and mixed function oxidase activity in human fetal tissues. Biochem Pharmacol 24: 839-846, 1975.

171. Pelkonen O, Arvela P and Karki NT: 3,4-benzpyrene and N-methyaniline metabolizing enzymes in the immature human fetus and placenta. Acta Pharmacol et Toxicol 30:385-395, 1971.

172. Juchau MR, Namkung MJ, Berry DL and Zachariah PK: Oxidative biotransformation of 2-acetylaminofluorence in fetal and placental tissues of humans and monkeys correlations with aryl hydrocarbon hydroxylase activities. Drug Metabol Disp 3:494-500, 1975.

173. Short CR, Kinden DA and Stith R: R: Fetal and neonatal development of the microsomal mono-oxygenase system. Drug Metabol Rev 5:1-42, 1976.

174. Pelkonen O, Korhonen P, Jouppaila B and Karki N: Induction of aryl hydrocarbon hydroxylase in human fetal liver cell and fibroblast cultures by polycyclic hydrocarbons. Life Sci 16:1403-1410, 1975.

175. Pelkonen O, Sotaniemi E and Mokka R: The *in vitro* oxidative metabolism of benzo(a)pyrene in human liver measured by different assays. Chem Biol Interact 16:13-21, 1977.

176. Gelboin HV, Selkirk JK, Yang SK, Wiebel SJ and Nemoto N: Benzo(a)pyrene metabolism by mixed-function oxygenases, hydratases and glutathione-S-transferases: Analysis by high pressure liquid chromatography. In: Glutathione: Metabolism and Function, Arias IM and Jakoby WB, (eds), Raven Press, New York, 1976.

177. Welch RM, Harrison YE, Conney AH, Poppers PJ and Finster M: Cigarette smoking: Stimulatory affect on metabolism of 3,4-benzpyrene by enzymes in human placenta. Sci 160: 541-542, 1968.

178. Conney AH, Welch R, Kuntzman R, Chang R, Jacobson M, Munro-Faure AD, Peck AW, Bye A, Poland A, Poppers PJ, Finster M and Wolff JA: Effects of environmental chemicals on the metabolism of drugs, carcinogens, and normal body constituents in man. Ann NY Acad Sci 179:155-172, 1971.

179. Nebert DW, Winker J and Gelboin HV: Aryl hydrocarbon hydroxylase activity in human placenta from cigarette smoking and nonsmoking women. Cancer Res 29:1763-1769, 1969.

180. Gough ED, Lowe MC and Jauchau MR: Human placental aryl hydrocarbon hydroxylase: Studies with fluorescence histochemistry. J Natl Cancer Inst 54/x819-821, 1975.

181. Kapitulnik J, Levin W, Poppers PJ, Tomaszewski JE, Jerina DM and Conney AH: Comparison of the hydroxylation of zoxazolamine and benzo(a)pyrene in human placenta: Effect of cigarette smoking. Clin Pharmacol Ther 20:557-564, 1976.

182. Jachau MR and Smuckler EA: Subcellular localization of human placental aryl hydrocarbon hydroxylase. Toxicol Appl Pharmacol 26:163-179, 1973.

183. Juchau MR, Lee QH and Blake PH: Inverse correlation between aryl hydrocarbon hydroxylase activity and conversion of cholesterol to pregnenolone in human placentas at term. Life Sci 11:949-956, 1972.

184. Ptashne K, Brothers L, Axline SG and Cogen SN: Aryl hydrocarbon hydroxylase induction in mouse peritoneal macrophages and blood derived human macrophages. Proc Soc Exp Biol Med 146:585-589, 1974.

185. Bast RC, Okuda T, Plotkin E, Tarone R, Rapp HJ and Gelboin HV: Development of an assay for aryl hydrocarbon (benzo(a)pyrene) Hydroxylase in human peripheral blood monocytes. Cancer Res 36:1967-1974, 1976.

186. Okuda T, Bast RC, Miller H, Rapp HJ and Gelboin HV: The half-life of aryl hydrocarbon (benzo(a)pyrene) Hydroxylase in human blood monocytes. Chem-Biol Interac 14:379-382, 1976.

187. Lake RS, Pezzutti MR, Kropko ML, Freeman AE and Igel HJ: Measurement of benzo(a)pyrene metabolism in human monocytes. Cancer Res 37:2530-2537, 1977.

188. Dietz MH and Flaxman DA: Toxicity of aromatic hydrocarbons on normal human epidermal cells *in vitro*. Cancer Res 31:1206-1209, 1971.

189. Huberman E and Sachs L: Metabolism of the carcinogenic hydrocarbon benzo(a)pyrene in human fibroblasts and epithelial cells. Int J Cancer 11:412-418, 1973.
190. Yamasaki H, Huberman E and Sachs L: Metabolism of the carcinogenic hydrocarbon benzo(a)pyrene in human fibroblasts and epithelial cells. II. Difference in metabolism to water soluble products and aryl hydrocarbon hydroxylase activity. Int J Cancer 19:378-382, 1977.
191. Pal K, Grover P and Sims P: Metabolism of carcinogenic polycyclic hydrocarbons by tissues of the respiratory tract. Biochem Soc Trans 3:174-175, 1975.
192. Franklin Cs and Kyegombe DB: The distribution and induction of some drug-metabolizing enzymes in man. Brit J Pharmacol 47:616, 1973.
193. Jakobsson SV and Cinti DL: Studies on the cytochrome P-450-containing mono-oxygenase system in human kidney cortex microsomes. J Pharmacol Exp Ther 185:226-233, 1973.

2. Adjuvant Therapy with Surgery: Immunotherapy – Overview

WILLIAM P. McGUIRE

INTRODUCTION

Bronchogenic carcinoma is today the second most common malignancy and the most frequent cancer killer in man with greater than 100,000 new cases diagnosed yearly [1, 2]. Bronchogenic carcinoma consists of two distinct clinicopathologic entities: small cell or oat cell and non-small cell types. Small cell carcinoma is considered by most physicians as a systemic disease at diagnosis and as such is not amenable to surgical treatment. This type accounts for 20% of all bronchogenic malignancies and primary therapy consists of combination chemotherapy with or without radiation. Thus, immunotherapy is used only as an adjunct to these two non-surgical modalities. The remainder of bronchogenic malignancies are of the non-small cell type where surgery remains the only curative therapy. Unfortunately, less than 30% of the patients have tumors which are able to be totally resected at diagnosis and of these less than one third survive five years after apparent complete surgical removal of all tumor [3]. Use of chemotherapy as an adjuvant to surgery has met with little success [4]. Further, there are no well controlled studies to show a beneficial effect for postoperative radiation in this population.

In the past decade many agents have been developed which alter the immune mechanism of man. These agents may be non-specific stimulators (e.g. BCG) or restorers (e.g. Levamisole) of the intrinsic cellular and/or humoral immune system or specific immunotherapy with 'purified' antigens from tumor tissue which when introduced into man may stimulate production of 1) specific antibodies directed toward the antigen or 2) transformed lymphocytes or macrophages capable of killing tumor cells which contain the same or similar antigens (cellular cytotoxicity).

It is not the purpose of this paper to review the incomplete and poorly understood science of tumor immunology. Rather I shall focus on the rationale for use of these agents, now grouped into a coined category of biologic

R. B. Livingston (ed.), Lung cancer 1, 35–49. All rights reserved.
Copyright © 1981 Martinus Nijhoff Publishers bv, The Hague/Boston/London.

response modifiers, in patients with bronchogenic malignancies and summarize the currently published and ongoing trials in which these agents are used as adjuncts to surgery in the case of non-small cell malignancies or adjuncts to chemotherapy and radiation in the case of small cell carcinoma.

RATIONALE FOR THE USE OF BIOLOGIC RESPONSE MODIFIERS
IN BRONCHOGENIC CARCINOMA

Data Supporting Altered Immunity in Patients with Lung Cancer

In 1968 Krant and associates [5] reported that patients with bronchogenic carcinoma had impairment of delayed cutaneous hypersensitivity to 2,4-dinitrochlorobenzene (DNCB) which stimulated many investigations that unequivocally demonstrate that patients with all stages of lung cancer have defects in their immune system. Holmes [6] and Wells *et al.* [7] have confirmed the defect in DNCB which was directly related to stage of disease and had prognostic implications for both resectability and survival. Wanebo *et al.* [8], on the other hand, showed a less profound defect that was not stage related. In any event, these studies suggested a defect in the afferent and/or efferent limb of the immune system. Simply stated, the host is either unable to process the neo-antigen, DNCB, or unable to 'arm' a lymphocyte to respond to the antigen on restimulation. The defect may be inherent in the host, i.e. it preceded and allowed the development of malignant growth, or it may be secondary to elaboration by the tumor of a substance which interferes with development of cellular immunity as was reported by Hellstrom and co-workers [9]. Recent studies by Inoue *et al.* [10] suggest that the immune defect is in the afferent limb since 15 of 29 patients with resectable disease who were DNCB negative preoperatively became positive postoperatively when resensitized. In contradistinction to this report, however, are reports by Israel [11], Brugarolas [12], and Hughes [13], which show lack of response to recall antigens such as PPD, mumps, dermatophytin and candidin. These studies would tend to implicate the efferent limb of the cellular immune system as defective.

In addition to these *in vivo* correlates of immune dysfunction in the patient with bronchogenic carcinoma, there are a number of *in vitro* tests which demonstrate altered cellular immunity when compared to normal individuals. Investigators have shown that the absolute number of thymic-derived lymphocytes (T cells) are depressed in patients with lung cancer [14]. It is this population of lymphocytes which are probably involved in cell mediated immunity (CMI). Further, the lymphocytes which are present show an altered capability to undergo blastic transformation when cultured with various mitogens such as PPD, phytohemagglutinin, and pokeweed [8, 15, 16] and the degree of impairment seems to relate to prognosis.

Data Supporting Recognition by Patients with Lung Cancer
of Tumor Associated Antigens (TAA)

Even in the face of the impaired cell mediated immunity seen in patients with lung cancer there exists irrefutable evidence that these tumors produce TAA which is recognized by the host as foreign and to which the host can mount a cell mediated response. This subject has been recently reviewed by Herberman[17] and interested readers are referred there for a comprehensive discussion.

Specifically related to lung cancer, however, are studies which show delayed cutaneous hypersensitivity reactions to intradermal injection of autologous tumor extracts[18–20] in lung cancer patients even when there may be impaired or absent DNCB reactivity and response to recall antigens. Further, there is data which shows that lymphocytes from lung cancer patients can proliferate when exposed to TAA in a fashion similar to response to mitogens[21, 22]. This may be especially true when the assay is performed in a medium which is free of host serum that may contain blocking substances.

Effects of Therapy on Host Immunocompetence

Regardless of whether lung cancer is a phenomenon secondary to dysfunction of normal immune surveillance or is primarily responsible for the immune defects due to elaboration of substances which interfere with cell mediated immunity, it seems clear that for any form of immunotherapy to be maximally effective one must begin with a host that has as small a burden of tumor cells as possible[23].

Unfortunately the therapeutic modalities at our disposal have been shown to have immunosuppressive effects themselves. General anesthesia and surgery have a profound and prolonged adverse effect on cell mediated immunity[24, 25] and tumor specific immunity[26]. Radiation therapy has likewise been shown to depress the cellular immune response even when the mediastinum and thymic remnants are not included in the field[27]. Further, many of the cytotoxic agents used today lower the absolute lymphocyte counts and severely depress immunity, with cyclophosphamide being the agent best studied[28]. It is this agent which is most frequently used in the current combination regimens for bronchogenic carcinoma.

Data Supporting a Beneficial Effect on Cell Mediated Immunity
of the Biologic Response Modifiers

If immunotherapy of lung cancer is to have any beneficial effect, the agent which is used must in some way restore or enhance tumor – specific cell mediated immunity without stimulating production of blocking factors. Agent in current use include Bacillus Calmette – Guerin (BCG), methanol extracted residue of BCG (MER-BCG), oil attached BCG cell wall skelton (BCG-CWS), Corynebacterium parvum (C parvum), thymosin, levamisole, and nocardia rubrum which are all non-specific biologic response modifiers, i.e. they generally enhance or restore cell mediated immunity without specifically arming cells toward tumor associated antigen. Other studies have employed specific immunotherapy using antigens extracted from human lung cancer.

It is not within the scope of this review to summarize the data on the immunologic effects of each of these agents. Interested readers are referred to recent comprehensive reviews on two of the best studied modifiers, BCG [29–31] and C parvum [32, 33]. Perhaps the most sobering message that one obtains when reading about these agents is that very little is known about the mechanisms by which they exert the antitumor effects which have been noted in both animal models and humans. In certain animal systems both BCG and C parvum have even been shown to enhance tumor growth. There are studies which demonstrate an improvement in many of the *in vivo* and *in vitro* measurements of immunity such as DNCB sensitization, response to recall antigens, mitogen induced lymphocyte blastogenesis, macrophage infiltration of tumor and T-cell rosette levels with use of BCG or C parvum; however, no one has conclusively shown an improvement in cell-mediated cytotoxicity against tumor cells *in vitro*.

In short, the science supporting the use of biologic response modifiers in lung cancer lags far behind their widespread clinical use. Further, very few of the clinical studies reported to date have evaluated or monitored the changes in host immunity after use of these agents. Nevertheless, many clinical trials have been performed and reported in the literature. The remainder of this paper will briefly review these published studies and comment on their implications for future studies.

REVIEW OF CLINICAL TRIALS IN SMALL CELL CARCINOMA

Only in recent years and with the advent of effective combination chemotherapy has cure or even long-term control of small cell carcinoma been considered. Even with intensive induction chemotherapy and prophylactic CNS irradiation, however, almost all patients with extensive disease and 75–80% of patients with limited disease fail in previous sites of involvement or develop progressive metastatic disease [34]. Since most of these patients have severe derangement of cell mediated immunity when they present and are treated with immunosuppressive cytotoxic chemotherapy, there is a theoretic role for use of biologic response modifiers to restore their immune system. This would be especially true in those patients who attain a complete response clinically and who, therefore, would have a small residual tumor burden.

Three trials have used BCG as an adjuvant. Holoye[35] reported on 31 patients (16 limited, 15 extensive) who received a combination of cytoxan, adriamycin and vincristine (CAV) along with BCG by scarification following each chemotherapy course. There was no difference in survival between limited and extensive disease patients, however, comparison of survival in extensive disease patients who received BCG and historical controls who had received two different chemotherapeutic regimens showed a significant improvement in survival favoring BCG. As is often the case, however, with longer followup this difference disappeared[36].

Einhorn[37] reported on 58 patients (19 limited, 39 extensive) treated with CAV regimen and maintained on cytoxan, methotrexate and CCNU. In addition they received mediastinal and CNS irradiation plus BCG after each chemotherapy course. Of the patients with limited disease the projected median survival was in excess of 80 weeks and of all patients who attained a CR the median survival was in excess of 54 weeks. This shows a tendency for benefit of BCG if survival figures continue, however, the study was not randomized and the number of patients is small.

A single randomized trial has been performed by the Southwest Oncology Group[38]. In this study 94 evaluable patients received one of two drug regimens with mediastinal and brain radiation. Half received BCG by scarification while the others did not. Comparison of patients who did or did not receive immunotherapy showed no differences in survival.

Two studies have used MER-BCG as an adjunct to chemotherapy. Aisner[39] reported on 26 patients who received cytoxan, adriamycin and VP-16. 15 patients also received MER-BCG and there was no benefit in survival for those treated with immunotherapy. The study was not randomized and no comment was made about extent of disease in the two populations so the study is not really evaluable.

Jackson et al. [40] performed a trial which was reported as randomized. 57 patients were treated with CAV plus CCNU and methotrexate and radiation to mediastinum and brain. 24 patients received MER-BCG while 33 did not (suggesting a problem in randomization). There was a tendency for better survival in patients with extensive disease who were treated with MER-BCG. Again the followup time is short and patient numbers small so that benefit from MER-BCG cannot be adequately evaluated.

The other studies evaluated C parvum as an immune adjuvant. Israel[41] conducted a non-randomized trial in 34 patients (18 limited, 16 extensive) using two chemotherapeutic regimens and C parvum in all. The survival results were not superior to other reports with chemotherapy alone. Tenczynski[42] performed a non-randomized trial in 22 patients (12 limited, 10 exten-

sive) using vincristine, VP-16, ifosfamide and adriamycin as the chemotherapy with C parvum used after each cycle. They report a response rate of 90%
but the median followup was less than a year and patient numbers small. The
role of C parvum was not evaluable.

The last study used fraction V of thymosin and reported a beneficial
survival effect for complete responders [43]. In this trial 46 patients (15 limited, 31 extensive) received a complicated chemotherapeutic regimen of six
drugs. Patients were randomized to receive no thymosin or thymosin twice
weekly during the six week induction phase (low dose 20 mg/M^2 or high dose
60 mg/M^2). The investigators reported no difference in induction of complete
response among the three groups, but of those patients attaining a complete
response there was a survival advantage for the group receiving high dose
thymosin. This advantage was due to prolonged relapse free survival. Unfortunately, the survival curves were not actuarial but Kaplan-Meier projections
and the test of significance was one-sided. Further, the patient numbers were
small such that a single relapse in the high dose group would cancel the
survival advantage. Thus, the value of thymosin will only be evaluable in a
much larger multi-institutional trial.

In summary, there appears to be little data supporting a role for immunotherapy in small-cell bronchogenic carcinoma. Early reports of efficacy of
BCG and C parvum have not withstood the test of longer followup or larger
trials. The encouraging report by Cohen *et al.* of activity of thymosin is based
on early data and controversial statistical methods. If additional followup of
these patients, however, demonstrates significant actuarial survival benefit for
patients treated with thymosin then a larger trial is needed. Otherwise,
aggressive combination chemotherapy or chemotherapy plus radiotherapy
seems to hold more promise for this disease.

REVIEW OF CLINICAL TRIALS IN NON SMALL-CELL CARCINOMA

Since the report by McKneally [44] of survival benefit in Stage I patients
treated with intrapleural BCG there have been a plethora of trials using
various strains of this organism or its components.

The most recent report by McKneally [45] summarized the experience in 66
patients with surgical Stage I disease. 30 patients received a single intrapleural
injection of 10^7 organisms of Tice BCG. 36 controls received no immunotherapy after surgery. Actuarial survival curves to 3 years showed a significant
survival difference (p < 0.01) between the two groups in favor of BCG. Critics
of this study have pointed to the inferior survival of the control population as
the cause of the difference and have postulated that the INH administered to

the controls may have had an adverse effect on survival. Survival analysis on 100 historical controls not given INH, however, shows the two control curves to be identical. Another factor which may have influenced the results of this trial was the TN status of patients on the arms. Patients with $T_1 N_0$ lesions have a superior survival to patients with $T_2 N_0$ or $T_1 N_1$ lesions and uneven entry of more advanced Stage I patients may have skewed the results. McKneally found no benefit for BCG in patients with Stage II or Stage III tumors which were completely resected.

Wright *et al.* [46] recently reported on a randomized double-blind trial in which 136 patients with all stages of resectable lung cancer were randomized to no further therapy vs. intrapleural BCG with or without Levamisole. With a median followup in excess of one year, there was no apparent benefit for patients treated with BCG and even a hint of poorer survival in those patients who also received levamisole. These results were independent of TN stage which was controlled for in the trial by stratification. In the group receiving BCG alone, however, there was a suggestion of better recurrence-free survival and overall survival in comparison to placebo although the results were not statistically significant. Unfortunately the data were not broken down by stage of disease so that effects in Stage I could be ascertained.

Of extreme interest in this report was the finding that recurrence was possibly related to lack of conversion of the PPD skin test following BCG treatment. Of those patients who received BCG and had skin test conversion there was only a 26% recurrence rate while those patients who remained skin test negative had a 60% incidence of recurrence. These data were independent of surgical stage, performance status and skin test reactivity to other recall antigens. Thus it may be only patients who maintain some immune competence that are benefitted by non-specific immunostimulation.

Because of the promising results of the McKneally trial, the NCI started a multi-institutional double-blind trial of intrapleural BCG in surgical Stage I patients. Early results of this trial [47] showed some benefit with respect to recurrence rate for one of the two arms, however, the results remain coded as accrual continues. There are now approximately 375 patients on this study which at maturity should definitively answer the question of efficacy of regional BCG in Stage I disease and in addition provide further data on the prognostic implications of skin test conversion in this group of patients.

A French group [48] reported on 43 patients with surgically resected Stage I and II squamous cell carcinoma. Half the patients had no additional therapy and half received 75 mg of Pasteur BCG by scarification at weekly intervals. Actuarial curves in this small population showed a trend ($p = 0.07$) in relapse-free survival for the BCG group although projections suggest the difference will disappear at 3 years. Sequential data on skin test reactivity were not reported. This study was recently updated and included a total of 55 patients [49]. The results were essentially the same with actuarial survival better in the BCG group at 18 months but not at 42 months. This difference was due mainly to Stage I patients where BCG was significantly superior to no BCG.

Roscoe [50] reported on 92 patients who were randomized to no further therapy, Glaxo BCG by multiple puncture or Glaxo BCG intradermally. There was no benefit for BCG in this study but patients were not surgically staged and complete resection was not carried out in all so the results are not evaluable.

Perlin *et al.* [51] reported on 31 patients with resected Stage I and II disease who were randomized postoperatively to no further therapy, intradermal Pasteur BCG or BCG plus irradiated tumor cells. With short followup (4 recurrences only) there were no differences among the three arms. Additional entry and longer followup are necessary in this study.

A large Canadian trial was recently reported in which 308 patients with all stages of resected disease were allocated to no further therapy or 120 mg Connaught BCG orally at variable intervals for 18 months. The vast majority of the patients were Stage I and the treatment balance for all prognostic factors was good. There were no differences in the survivals between the two groups and conversion of PPD skin test had no bearing on prognosis. This study would suggest no beneficial effect of oral BCG in survival of resected non-small cell lung cancer, however, the relatively poor survival in both groups (50% alive at 3 years) is different from that observed by others using surgery alone in a population of patients who for the most part had Stage I disease [53]. Thus one must wonder in this study whether surgical staging was accurate, a common problem in multicenter trials.

Another method for using BCG has been reported by investigators from Los Angeles where BCG is injected directly into the tumor via the bronchoscope or chest wall [54]. Toxicity was minimal and antitumor response was noted as was macrophage infiltration into regional nodes. A random trial using this technique has been suggested, however, trial design would be difficult since the preoperative use of BCG precludes accurate surgical staging.

Many other studies have employed BCG and its components in the treatment of lung cancer but are hampered by analysis of small patients numbers, non-randomized study design and entry of patients with advanced or inoperable disease where immunotherapy has less chance for success. These studies do not in fact constitute surgical adjuvant studies since surgical resection was not carried out in most and are not, therefore, within the scope of this review. Interested readers are referred to a review by Mikulski [55] for data from these trials.

Thus of the trials reported to date which use BCG in resected lung cancer, which have sufficient patient numbers, and which have proper randomization and stratification, there remains a suggestion of benefit for both time to recurrence and survival in patients treated with BCG following surgery. This seems especially to be the case in patients with Stage I disease and in patients who convert their PPD skin test following BCG administration. If data from these trials or current ongoing trials confirms this benefit, future studies should consider continuous, intermittent BCG stimulation in Stage I patients to either effect or maintain skin test conversion. New studies with BCG should probably await more mature data from the above trials.

C parvum has been used in a number of trials which are all hampered by small numbers or use of the C parvum in conjunction with radiation and/or chemotherapy without use of concurrent controls so that the effect of the immune adjuvant is totally non-evaluable. These trials by Dimitrov, Bjornsson and others have been reviewed by Mikulski[55].

A single trial, however, carried out under the auspices of the Ludwig Institute in Europe is a large, well controlled trial that should provide useful data at maturity. 475 patients with completely resected Stage I and II disease were randomized to no further therapy or a single intrapleural injection of 7 mg of C parvum. Accession to the trial is complete but the median followup is less than 1 year. No differences were seen between the two groups who were well balanced for prognostic factors. The 3 year followup of this large, well designed trial will be of interest[56].

Another study from the early decade of the 70's which has been very highly publicized and has generated many of the current adjuvant trials in non-small cell bronchogenic carcinoma was that by Amery[57] using Levamisole. This trial purported to show a beneficial effect of orally administered Levamisole for time to recurrence and survival in patients who had an on-study weight of 70 kg. This trial, unfortunately, has several serious flaws which detract or even make unbelievable the published results. Some of the Levamisole-treated patients were excluded because they were 'underdosed', the patients were not staged by any current system such that treatment balance by TN status is impossible, and the study could not have been strictly randomized since there was an excess of 19 patients on the control arm. These flaws together with hints of actual adverse effects of Levamisole in the study by Wright[46] leave this author with no choice but to say the study is non-evaluable.

Levamisole is also being used in a study by the Lung Cancer Study Group in one arm of a three arm trial. Patients with completely resected Stage II and III squamous carcinoma are randomized to no additional therapy vs. postoperative radiation therapy with or without Levamisole. The feeling was that if Levamisole is an immune restorative agent, it may block the immune suppression of radiation and improve the relapse-free survival. Only 70 patients to date are on that study which is still coded but no single arm appears to be superior [47].

Further, the Southwest Oncology Group has completed a study in limited squamous cell disease which was not completely resected (a group similar to those patients in the Amery study with large tumors who did the best) and found no benefit for Levamisole when added to radiation therapy [58].

In reality, then, there is no data to support further studies of Levamisole as a postoperative adjuvant in lung cancer. Some may point to its relative lack of toxicity and thus its ease of incorporation into regimens with more profound side effects. Investigators who have used this drug, however, know well its causation of an 'influenza-like' syndrome and poor patient compliance with long-term usage.

Several other non-specific immune stimulants have been used in various stages of non-small cell lung cancer. The Japanese have been using the cell wall skeleton of BCG, nocardium rubrum and a streptococcal agent OK-432. Because the Japanese use a staging system at variance with the system adopted by the WHO and because most of their studies are in advanced, unresectable disease without concurrent controls, their highly significant results from immunotherapy cannot be accepted by most investigators.

MER-BCG has been extensively used by Israeli investigators with claims of success. Again the studies are faulted by small numbers and lack of concurrent controls and in no way give conclusive evidence for any benefit from immunotherapy.

Of all the non-specific immune stimulators, the only one which has even a hint of activity is BCG and even then in a small population of patients who have Stage I disease and who convert their PPD skin test from negative to positive.

Of the specific immune stimulators, the most well known is the Hollinshead antigen, used in a small study of 55 patients with Stage I and II resected lung cancer [59]. There was an unbalanced assignment postoperatively to high dose methotrexate with citrovorum (10 patients), no therapy (16 patients), specific active immunotherapy with Freund's complete adjuvant (16 patients) or chemoimmunotherapy with methotrexate and antigen (13 patients). Staging in this study was probably suboptimal with status of mediastinal nodes determined only by mediastinoscopy and not at thoracotomy. Thus there remains a big question in this small patient sample of balance among the four arms for extent of disease. Patients receiving immunotherapy were given monthly intradermal injections of approximately $1,500\,\mu g$ antigen. Comparison was made between the first two groups who received no immunotherapy and the second two groups who did. They report highly significant survival results in favor of those patients receiving specific active immunotherapy with or without chemotherapy. The small patient numbers, however, and the poor staging and possible imbalance among the arms for stage differences make this claim unwarranted. There is however, a Canadian-wide trial underway at the current time which anticipates a large accrual of resected Stage I and II patients to a three arm study of no further therapy vs. Freund's complete adjuvant with or without tumor specific antigen. Results will not be available for several years.

Another study by Takita [60] prospectively randomized 30 patients with resected Stage III disease to no further therapy or active specific immunotherapy. He reported a significantly longer survival for the group treated with lung vaccine but the populations are small and the control group had many more patients requiring pneumonectomy which is a negative prognostic factor for survival. This represents yet another study where results are confused by small patient numbers and study design characteristics.

SUMMARY AND CONCLUSIONS

After an extensive albeit incomplete review of the status of adjuvant immunotherapy in patients with bronchogenic carcinoma, this author is left with an overall feeling that 1) specific or non-specific immune stimulation as a therapeutic modality in this disease has as yet no proven efficacy over surgical treatment alone; 2) past studies have for the most part been poorly designed with respect to adequate staging, proper balance for known prognostic factors, and accrual of large enough patient numbers; 3) clinical studies have not included concomitant studies of *in vivo* or *in vitro* immune function in a sequential fashion during the trial such that the effect on cell mediated immunity by the biologic response modifiers can be ascertained, nor can correlations be made between alterations in these immune parameters and the course of the disease; and 4) the actual mechanisms of action of all the immune adjuvants are poorly understood and thus clinical application of these agents could await a better understanding of their effects on the immune system.

Of course clinical utilization of agents which are theoretically and potentially useful against cancer rarely awaits the time-consuming basic research necessary to elucidate the often complex description of basic mechanisms. A case in point is the usage of methotrexate for some 25 years before the pharmacology and antineoplastic mechanism of action were delineated. Surely clinical studies of BCG, C parvum, thymosin, specific tumor antigens and a host of newly developed biologic response modifiers will continue in lung cancer and other tumors over the next decade. It is hoped that these studies will be conducted in such a way that the results, either positive or negative, can be interpreted adequately and reproduced by others. There is no need or place for clinical trials of biologic response modifiers in lung cancer which are not prospectively randomized and balanced for known prognostic factors, which make any statement based on small patient numbers or which do not explore to some extent the effects of the modifier on host immunity.

With the ever increasing number of patients developing bronchogenic carcinoma and the apparent inability of surgery, radiation therapy and chemotherapy to alter the survival significantly in the past two decades, immunotherapy still offers some promise. This promise will be recognized only if clinicians and basic immunobiologists join forces to design large, well controlled trials which clearly show a survival benefit for patients treated with agents which affect the immune system and can at the same time prove that this survival advantage has an immunologic basis.

REFERENCES

1. Murray JL and Axtell LM: Impact of cancer: Years of life lost due to cancer mortality. J Natl Cancer Inst 52:3-7, 1974.
2. Levin DL, DeVesa SS, Godwin JD and Silverman DT: Cancer rates and risks. DHEW Publication No (NIH) 75-691, 1974.
3. Selawry OS and Hansen HH: Lung cancer. In: Cancer Medicine, Holland JF and Frei E (eds), Philadelphia, Lea and Febiger, 1973, p 1473-1518.
4. Legha SS, Muggia FM and Carter SK: Adjuvant chemotherapy in lung cancer: review and prospects. Cancer 39: 1415-1424, 1977.
5. Krant MJ, Manskopf G, Brandrup CS and Madoff MA: Immunologic alterations in bronchogenic cancer. Cancer 21:623-631, 1968.
6. Holmes CE: Immunology and lung cancer. Ann Thorac Surg 21:250-258, 1976.
7. Wells SA, Burdick JF, Joseph WL, Christianson C, Wolfe WG and Adkins PC: Delayed cutaneous hypersensitivity reactions to tumor cell antigens and to non-specific antigens. J Thorac Cardiovasc Surg 66:557-572, 1973.
8. Wanebo HJ, Rao B, Miyazawa N, Martini N, Middleman MP, Oettgen HF and Beattie EJ: Immune reactivity in primary carcinoma of the lung and its relation to prognosis, J Thorac Cardiovasc Surg 72:339-350, 1976.
9. Hellstrom I, Sjogren HO, Warner G and Hellstrom, KE: Blocking of cell mediated immunity by sera from patients with growing neoplasms. Int J Cancer 7:226-237, 1971.
10. Inoue H, Ishihara T, Kobayashi K and Fukai S: Sequential evaluation of DNCB reactivity in patients with primary lung cancer. J Thorac Cardiovasc Surg 76:479-482, 1978.
11. Israel L, Mugica J and Chaminian P: Prognosis of early bronchogenic carcinoma: Survival of 451 patients after resection of lung cancer in relation to the results of a preoperative tuberculin skin test. Biomedicine 19:68-72, 1973.
12. Brugarolas A and Takita H: Immunologic status in lung cancer. Chest 64:427-430, 1973.
13. Hughes LE and Mackay WD: Suppression of the tuberculin response in malignant disease. Br Med J 2:1346-1348, 1965.
14. Gross RL, Latty A, Williams EA and Newberne PM: Abnormal spontaneous rosette formation and rosette inhibition in lung carcinoma. NEJM 292:439-443, 1975.
15. Ducos J, Migueres J, Colombies P, Kessous A and Poujoulet N: Lymphocyte response to PHA in patients with lung cancer. Lancet 1:1111-1112, 1970.

16. Han T and Takita H: Impaired lymphocyte response to allogenic cultured lymphoid cells in patients with lung cancer. NEJM 286:605-606, 1972.
17. Herberman RB: Existence of tumor immunity in man. In: Mechanisms of tumor immunity, Green I, Cohen S, McCluskey RT (eds), New York, John Wiley and Sons, 1977, p 175-191.
18. Stewart THM: The presence of delayed hypersensitivity reactions in patients toward cellular extracts of their malignant tumors. Cancer 23:1380-1387, 1970.
19. Hollinshead AC, Stewart THM and Herberman RB: Delayed hypersensitivity reactions to soluble membrane antigens of human malignant lung cells. J Natl Cancer Inst 52:327-338, 1974.
20. Wells SA, Burdick JF, Christiansen C, Ketcham AS and Adkins PC: Demonstration of tumor — associated delayed cutaneous hypersensitivity reactions in patients with lung cancer and in patients with carcinoma of the cervix. Natl Cancer Inst Monogr 37:197-203, 1973.
21. Mavligit GM, Gutterman JU, McBride CM and Hersh EM: Cell mediated immunity to human solid tumors in vitro. Detection by lymphocyte blastogenic response to cell associated and solubilized tumor antigens. Natl Cancer Inst Monogr 37:167-176, 1973.
22. Dean JH, Jerrels TR, Cannon GB, Kibrite, A, Baumgardner B, Wesse JL, Silva J and Herberman RB: Demonstration of specific cell-mediated anti-tumor immunity in lung cancer to autologous tissue extracts. Int J Cancer 22:367-377, 1978.
23. Henney CS: Mechanisms of tumor cell destruction. In: Mechanisms of tumor immunity, Green I, Cohen S, McCluskey RT (eds), New York, John Wiley and Sons, 1977, p 55-86.
24. Jubert AV, Lee ET, Hersh EM and McBride CM: Effects of surgery, anesthesia and intraoperative blood loss on immunocompetence. J Surg Res 15:399-403, 1973.
25. Wingard DW, Lang R and Humphrey LJ: Effect of anesthesia on immunity. J Surg Res 7:430-432, 1967.
26. Cochran AJ, Spilg WGS, Mackie RM and Thomas CE: Postoperative depression of tumor-directed cell-mediated immunity in patients with malignant disease. Br Med J 4:67-70, 1972.
27. Silverman NA, Alexander JC, Potvin C and Chretien PB: Effect of nonthymic irradiation on cellular immunocompetence. Surg Forum 26:345-346, 1975.
28. Wheeler GP: Alkylating agents. In: Cancer medicine, Holland JF, Frei E (eds), Philadelphia, Lea and Febiger, 1974, p 791-805.
29. Bast RC, Zbar B, Borsos T and Rapp HJ: BCG and cancer. NEJM 290: 1413-1418, 1974.
30. Bast RC, Zbar B, Borsos T and Rapp HJ: BCG and cancer. NEJM 290: 1458-1468, 1974.
31. Mitchell MS: Studies on the immunologic effects of BCG and its components: Theoretical and therapeutic implications. Biomedicine 24: 209-213, 1976.
32. Fisher B, Rubin H, Sartiano G, Ennis L and Wolmark N: Observations following corynebacterium parvum administration to patients with advanced malignancy. Cancer 38: 119-130, 1976.
33. Baum M and Breese M: Antitumor effect of corynebacterium parvum. Br J Cancer 33:468-473, 1976.
34. Greco FA, Einhorn LH, Richardson RL and Oldham RK: Small cell lung cancer: Progress and perspectives. Sem Oncol 3:323-335, 1978.
35. Holoye PY: Chemoimmunotherapy of small cell bronchogenic carcinoma. Proc Am Assoc Cancer Res 18:278, 1977.
36. Holoye PY, Samuels ML, Smith T and Sinkovics JG: Chemoimmunotherapy of small cell bronchogenic carcinoma. Cancer 42: 34-40, 1978.
37. Einhorn LH, Hornback NB and Bond WH: Combination chemotherapy, radiotherapy and immunotherapy in small cell undifferentiated lung cancer. Proc Am Soc Clin Oncol 18:267, 1977.

38. McCracken J, White J, Reed R, Livingston R and Hoogstraten B: Combination chemotherapy, radiotherapy, and immunotherapy for oat cell carcinoma of the lung. Proc Am Soc Clin Oncol 19:395, 1978.

39. Aisner J, Esterhay RJ and Wiernick PH: Chemotherapy vs. chemoimmunotherapy for small carcinoma of the lung. Proc Am Assoc Cancer Res 18:310, 1977.

40. Jackson DV, Richards F, Muss HB, Cooper MR, White DR and Spurr CL: Immunotherapy of small cell carcinoma of the lung: A randomized study. Proc Am Soc Clin Oncol 20:367, 1979.

41. Israel L, Depierre A, Choffel C, Milleron B and Edelstein R: Immunochemotherapy in 34 cases of oat cell carcinoma of the lung with 19 complete responses. Cancer Treat Rep 61:343-347, 1977.

42. Tenczynski TF, Valdivieso M, Hersh EM, Khalil KG, Mountain CF and Bodey GP: Chemoimmunotherapy of small cell bronchogenic carcinoma. Proc Am Soc Clin Oncol 19:376, 1978.

43. Cohen MH, Chretien PB, Ihde DC, Fossieck BE, Makuch R, Bunn PA, Johnston AV, Shackney SE, Matthews MJ, Lipson SD, Kenady DE and Minna JD: Thymosin fraction V, and intensive combination chemotherapy. Prolonging the survival of patients with small-cell lung cancer. JAMA 241:1813-1815, 1979.

44. McKneally MF, Maver C and Kausel HW: Regional immunotherapy of lung cancer with intrapleural BCG. Lancet 1:377-379, 1976.

45. McKneally MF, Maver CM, ALLey RD, Kausel HW, Older TM, Foster ED and Lininger L: Regional immunotherapy of lung cancer using intrapleural BCG: Summary of a four year randomized study. In: Lung cancer: Progress in therapeutic research, Muggia, F and Rozencweig M (eds), New York, Raven Press, 1979, p 471-476.

46. Wright P, Hill L, Peterson A, Anderson R, Bagley C, Berstein I, Ivey T, Johnson L, Morgan E, Ostenson R and Pinkham R: Adjuvant immunotherapy for lung cancer. In: Adjuvant therapy of cancer II, Jones, SE and Salmon, SE (eds), New York, Grune and Stratton, 1979, p 545-552.

47. McGuire WP: Clinical trials of the lung cancer study group. In: Adjuvant therapy of cancer II, Jones, SE and Salmon, SE (eds), New York, Grune and Stratton, 1979, p 561-569.

48. Pouillart P, Palangie T, Huguenin P, Morin P, Gautier H, Lededente A, Baron A and Mathe G: Adjuvant nonintrapleural BCG. In: Lung cancer: Progress in therapeutic research, Muggia, F and Rozencweig, M (eds), New York, Raven Press, 1979, p 477-481.

49. Pouillart P, Palangie T, Jouve M and Garcia-Giralt E: Systemic BCG in squamous lung cancer. In: Adjuvant therapy of cancer II, Jones, SE and Salmon, SE (eds), New York, Grune and Stratton, 1979, p 553-560.

50. Roscoe P, Pearce S, Ludgate S and Horne NW: A controlled trial of BCG immunotherapy in bronchogenic carcinoma treated by surgical resection. Cancer Immunol Immunother 3:115-118, 1977.

51. Perlin E, Weese JL, Heim W, Reid J, Oldham R, Mills M, Miller C, Blom H, Green D, Bellinger S, Law I, Cannon G, Herberman R and Connor R: Immunotherapy of carcinoma of the lung with BCG and allogenic tumor cells. In: Neoplasm immunity: Solid tumor therapy, Crispen, RG (ed), Chicago, The Franklin Institute Press, 1977, p 9-21.

52. Miller AB, Taylor HE, Baker MA, Dodds DJ, Falk R, Frappier A, Hill DP, Jindani A, Landi S, MacDonald AS, Thomas JW and Wall C: Oral administration of BCG as an adjuvant to surgical treatment of carcinoma of the bronchus. Can Med Assoc J 121:45-54, 1979.

53. Martini N and Beattie EJ: Results of surgical treatment in stage I lung cancer. J Thorac Cardiovasc surg 74:499-505, 1977.

54. Holmes EC, Ramming KP, Bein ME, Coulson WF and Callery CD: Intralesional BCG immunotherapy of pulmonary tumors. J Thorac Cardiovasc Surg 77:362-368, 1979.

55. Mikulski SM, McGuire WP, Louie A, Chirigos MA and Muggia FM: Immunotherapy of non-small cell lung carcinoma: Brief review of past experience and present ongoing trials in man. Cancer Treat Rev, 1980 (in press).
56. Zelen M: The Ludwig cancer study. Personal communication, February, 1979.
57. Amery WK: Final results of a multicenter placebocontrolled levamisole study of resectable lung cancer. Cancer Treat Rep 62: 1677-1683, 1978.
58. Livingston RB: Personal communication, February, 1979.
59. Stewart THM, Hollinshead AC, Harris JE, Raman S, Belanger R, Crepeau A, Crook AF, Hirte WE, Hooper D, Klaassen DJ, Rapp EF and Sachs HJ: Survival study of immunochemotherapy in lung cancer. In: Immunotherapy of cancer: Present status of trials in man, Terry, WD and Windhorst, D (eds), New York, Raven Press, 1978, p. 203-216.
60. Takita H, Takada M, Minowada J, Han T and Edgerton F: Adjuvant immunotherapy of stage III lung carcinoma. In: Immunotherapy of cancer: Present status of trials in man, Terry WD and Windhorst D (eds), New York, Raven Press, 1978, p 217-223.

3. The Immunotherapy of Lung Cancer

E. CARMACK HOLMES

INTRODUCTION

The importance of immunologic factors in the progression of cancer is well-recognized, and the relationship between host immunocompetence and prognosis has been well-defined. In addition, there is evidence that suggests that lung tumors as well as other human tumors contain antigens which are capable of evoking an immune response in the host. Therefore, while human tumors may contain tumor antigens, cancer is associated with immunosuppression and a diminished capacity of the host to respond to these antigens.

Patients with lung cancer are among the most profoundly immunosuppressed of all patients with solid neoplasms. Delayed cutaneous hypersensitivity reactions are impaired in many patients with lung cancer, and the more profound the impairment, the worse the prognosis and the more likely it is that the patient will be unresectable[1]. The functional activity of lymphocytes obtained from patients with lung cancer is severely suppressed. This *in vitro* suppression is also associated with a poor prognosis and more advanced disease. The mechanism of this immunosuppression in patients with lung cancer is not clear. However it has been shown that serum from patients with lung cancer is capable of suppressing normal lymphocyte function[2]. This suggests the possibility that the tumor elaborates a humoral substance which is responsible for the suppression of cell-mediated immunity. More recent studies have indicated that lung cancer patients have suppressor cells which may play a role in the immunosuppression of patients with lung cancer[3]. In view of these immurological findings, it seemed reasonable to assume that manipulations of the immune response may improve prognosis. However our current understanding of the mechanism of immunosuppression in patients with lung cancer is poor, and it is difficult to manipulate a poorly understood mechanism. Therefore, while there have been many clinical trials evaluating

R.B. Livingston (ed.), Lung cancer 1, 51–62. All rights reserved.
Copyright © 1981 Martinus Nijhoff Publishers bv, The Hague/Boston/London.

immunotherapy in patients with lung cancer, the agents which have been used have largely been selected empirically and not on the basis of a thorough understanding of the immunologic relationship between the host and the tumor and an understanding of the mechanism of action of the immunotherapeutic agents. A variety of agents have been evaluated (Table 1). These include bacillus Calmette-Guerin (BCG), Corynebacterium parvum, BCG cell wall skeleton, Levamisole, and a tumor antigen combined with Freund's adjuvant. The mechanism of action of all of these agents is poorly understood, and many of the details of their administration such as dose, timing and route have not been studied. However in spite of these many disadvan-

Table 1. Adjuvant immunotherapy in lung cancer.

Intrapleural BCG	*Reference*
McKneally *et al.*	15
Wright *et al.*	16
Lowe *et al.*	17
Intradermal BCG	
Perlin *et al.*	10
Pouillart *et al.*	11
Edward and Whitwall	12
Roscoe	13
Miyazawa *et al.*	14
Sarna *et al.*	23
Intralesional BCG	
Holmes *et al.*	29
BCG-Cell wall	
Yasumoto *et al.*	18
Levamisole	
Amery	25
Anthony *et al.*	26
Tumor antigens	
Stewart *et al.*	27
Taikita	28
C parvum	
Israel	21

tages, some clinical trials have yielded clearly detectable benefits of immunotherapy in patients with lung cancer. Primarily the clinical trials reported to
date have used nonspecific immunotherapy, although a few studies evaluating
so-called specific immunotherapy with tumor cell vaccine or tumor antigens
have been reported.

I. BACILLUS CALMETTE-GUERIN (BCG)

BCG is an attenuated viable bovine tubercule bacillus and is prepared and
supplied in a variety of ways [4]. This agent has been evaluated extensively in
animal tumor systems and also in clinical trials [5–9]. BCG is capable of
non-specifically stimulating the immune response in animals. However there
is no evidence that BCG is capable of correcting immunosuppression. Indeed
suppression of the immune response by radiation therapy or corticosteroids
abrogates the non-specific immune stimulation by BCG. In animal models as
well as in clinical studies, the most effective way of using BCG to induce
systemic tumor resistance is by direct injection of BCG into the tumor [5–8].
Intralesional injection of BCG is capable of controlling cutaneous malignancy
in most patients so treated, and BCG is currently undergoing extensive
evaluation as a non-specific immune stimulator in a variety of solid
tumors.

As Table 1 indicates, a number of investigators have evaluated intradermal
BCG as an adjunct to surgery in patients following surgical resection of lung
cancer. Perlin [10] and his associates randomized 51 patients to receive either
BCG intradermally, BCG and a whole tumor cell vaccine or no further
treatment following surgical resection of stage I and II patients. In this study
Pasteur BCG was used. The BCG treatment resulted in a statistically significant prolongation of the disease-free interval in patients with stage I resected
lung cancer. In this study there was no advantage with the addition of the
whole tumor cell vaccine. In another study Pouillart and his associates evaluated Pasteur BCG given weekly, intradermally following surgery [11]. Fifty-
six patients were randomized postoperatively to receive BCG or no further
treatment. The median followup in this study was 36 months, and there was
a significant difference in survival in favor of the BCG treated group at 24
months (66% vs. 38%). In stage I patients the difference in survival is
statistically significant in favor of the BCG treated group. Edwards and
Whitwell performed a study using a single dose of glaxo BCG given intradermally ten days after resection of the lung cancer [12]. Sixty consecutive
patients received BCG postoperatively, and their survival was compared with
that of 60 consecutive patients who were used as historical controls. The
differences between the two treatment groups did not reach statistical signif-

Table 2. Survival results of surgical adjuvant BCG therapy in lung cancer (Edwards and Whitwell).

Treatment	2 years	3 years	4 years	5 years
BCG	52%	38%	32%	30%
Control	38%	28%	22%	20%

icance, however, there was a difference in favor of the BCG treated group in each of the five followup years (Table 2). In addition, in those patients in this study in whom the lymph nodes were negative for tumor, there was a 47% five year survival in the BCG treated group and a 33% five year survival in the historical control group. This suggests that BCG may have been effective in those patients in this study who had stage I resectable disease. Roscoe *et al.* studied 92 patients with bronchogenic carcinoma who were treated by surgical resection followed by immunotherapy with glaxo BCG[13]. Patients were randomized into three groups: 1) Those receiving BCG by the multipuncture technique, 2) Those receiving BCG by the intradermal technique, and 3) Those patients receiving no further therapy. The median survival for the control group was 24 months, for the multipuncture BCG group 24 months, and for those receiving BCG by the intradermal group the median survival was in excess of 33 months. These differences did not reach statistical significance. Unfortunately in this study, 37% of the patients had positive mediastinal nodes, but the patients were not stratified for this variable. Miyazawa and colleagues evaluated BCG obtained from the Japan BCG Institute in a prospective randomized study in which BCG was given once before surgery and four times following surgery by the intradermal route[14]. All patients were given Cytoxan following surgery, and the pleural cavity was routinely irrigated by Mitomycin C. The patients were observed from ten to 28 months, and there was an 81% survival in the BCG treated group and a 58% survival in the control group (p < 0.05).

BCG has also been evaluated by the intrapleural route by several investigators. McKneally *et al.* randomized 110 patients to receive intrapleural BCG postoperatively or no further treatment. Both groups of patients received Isoniazid (INH) therapy in order to minimize the risk of systemic BCG infection. Intrapleural BCG appeared to have no effect on patients with stage II and III resected lung cancer. However intrapleural BCG significantly prolonged the survival of patients with stage I disease[15]. Wright *et al.* randomized patients postoperatively to receive either intrapleural BCG plus Levamisole or intrapleural BCG plus a Levamisole placebo or a placebo control group[16]. One hundred and fifty patients have been randomized into this study with a median followup of approximately 12 months. There is a trend toward better survival in the intrapleural BCG only group but the differences are not yet significant. These investigators did note, however, that those patients who were PPD negative and converted to PPD positive following BCG treatment had a significantly lower response rate than the non-converters. Only 12% of the PPD converters relapsed whereas 42% of the PPD non-converters relapsed. This suggests that a subgroup of patients who are PPD converters may benefit most from BCG treatment. A similar observation was made by Pouillart and McKneally in their studies. Recently Lowe and colleagues have reported a study in which 92 patients were randomized to receive postoperative intrapleural Glaxo BCG or no further treatment [17]. Control patients were given an isoniazid placebo, and the BCG treated patients were placed on Isoniazid beginning 14 days after surgery and continuing for two months. Unfortunately, the patients were not stratified for histologic type or stage of disease prior to randomization and treatment. In addition, there were 14 patients in this series with anaplastic carcinoma. There was no difference in survival when all the patients randomized were considered, and there was no difference in survival when patients with stage I disease were analyzed. These results have not confirmed McKneally's findings; however, it should be pointed out that McKneally employed Tice strain BCG, these investigators employed Glaxo, and the stratification parameters were not similar.

In Japan BCG cell wall skeleton (CWS) has been evaluated extensively in patients with lung cancer. This BCG product is a non-viable chemical extract which contains as its major component the cell wall skeleton of BCG. Using this agent Yasumoto *et al.* has reported a statistically significant increase in survival in patients with stage I and stage II resectable lung cancer treated with BCG CWS [18].

A review of the completed trials evaluating BCG as a surgical adjunct in lung cancer indicates that there have been few entirely negative studies. While not all of the studies have reached statistical significance, most show a definite trend in favor of the BCG treatment. However all of these studies have suffered from a lack of proper definition of prognostic factors, and because careful surgical and pathological staging was not performed, the patients were not properly stratified. There are several ongoing clinical trials in which these prognostic factors are being carefully documented, and the patients have been stratified accordingly. The studies performed to date suggest that certain subgroups may benefit from immunotherapy more than others. Patients with Stage I disease appear to benefit most. Pouillart, McKneally and Wright have all indicated that patients who convert from a PPD negative status to a PPD positive status after BCG treatment benefit most from immunotherapy. This important observation needs to be further evaluated. Although the studies to date suggest a biological affect of BCG, our understanding of the mechanisms of action of BCG immunotherapy are very rudimentary, and this lack of information makes it difficult to determine the proper dose, the proper timing and the proper route of administration of this agent.

Non-specific immunotherapy as an adjunct to chemotherapy and radiation therapy in lung cancer has also been evaluated. Kerman and Stefani randomized patients with locally advanced lung cancer to receive radiation therapy or radiation therapy plus BCG given intradermally[19]. The median survival in the immunotherapy group was significantly longer than the radiotherapy alone group (P<.01). Pines has also evaluated BCG in conjunction with radiation therapy[20]. He did observe a significant difference in survival at 12 months, however, the survival differences following 12 months were not significantly different. Israel evaluated the results of C-Parvum in advanced lung cancer[21, 22]. Seventy-five patients received chemotherapy alone, and 68 patients received the same chemotherapy plus C-parvum. All patients had squamous carcinoma of the lung, and both groups had approximately a 50% response rate. However the survival was significantly prolonged in the C-parvum treated patients. Sarna evaluated BCG and Corynebacterium parvum in combination with chemotherapy in lung cancer patients and found no benefit from the addition of BCG or C-parvum to this chemotherapeutic regimen[23].

II. LEVAMISOLE

Levamisole (L-tetramisole) has been widely used as an anti-helminthic in animals and in man. In contrast to BCG, Levamisole is a chemical that can be taken orally in the form of a tablet. This agent is felt to be an immuno-potentiator or an anti-anergic agent. Some studies suggest that Levamisole is capable of stimulating the immune response in immunosuppressed patients and in some patients with lung cancer. Levamisole appears to be capable of reversing the suppression of lymphocyte function[24]. Therefore, Levamisole is an attractive agent for the treatment of this disease. Levamisole has been evaluated in at least two prospective randomized trials in resected lung cancer patients. In these double-blind studies, patients who were candidates for thoracotomy were randomized to receive Levamisole preoperatively and post-operatively. In the study coordinated by Amery, more than 200 patients were randomized and prolonged followup was obtained[25]. When the two populations are considered as a whole, there is a slight trend in favor of the Levamisole treated group. However the results were not consistently statistically significant. When the patients were evaluated on the basis of body weight, there was a striking difference in favor of Levamisole in patients who weighed less than 70 kg. The investigators felt that a fixed dose of 150 mg of

Levamisole daily for three days every two weeks was an insufficient amount for patients weighing greater than 70 kg and therefore, have recommended that Levamisole be administered in a dose of 2.5 mgs/kg. However a second study evaluating Levamisole [26] in which the dose was adjusted to the body weight indicated that the Levamisole treated patients did significantly worse than the control group. The excessive deaths in the Levamisole treated group were non-cancer related. When the non-cancer related deaths are excluded, there was no difference between the placebo and the Levamisole treated group. These investigators felt that the increase in deaths in the Levamisole treated patients was due to cardiorespiratory failure. This has not been reported previously in Levamisole treated patients and a close analysis of this data indicates that it is very unlikely that Levamisole has any cardiorespiratory toxic effects. The value of Levamisole as a surgical adjuvant in lung cancer remains very much an open question.

III. SPECIFIC IMMUNOTHERAPY

The evaluation of specific immunotherapy in lung cancer has not been as extensive as with non-specific immune stimulators. Specific immunotherapy requires the use of tumor cells in various degrees of purification, hopefully containing tumor-associated antigens. Tumor cells are difficult to propagate in tissue culture, and the precise subfraction of the cell which contains the antigens which are presumably important in inducing an anti-tumor immune response in the host is not at all well-delineated. For these reasons, specific immunotherapy is much more difficult to apply and is certainly much more expensive than other forms of therapy.

Concomitant but Non-Randomized Control Groups:

Stewart *et al.* has evaluated specific immunotherapy in patients with lung cancer [27]. In this study, partially purified tumor antigens derived from lung cancer were mixed with complete Freund's adjuvant and used as an immune stimulating agent. Patients were randomized following surgical resection to receive postoperative methotrexate alone, tumor antigen with Freund's adjuvant or methotrexate as well as tumor antigen with Freund's adjuvant. A concomitant but not randomized surgery only control group was employed. Since these trials have not employed the appropriate control group, that is a group receiving Freund's adjuvant alone, it is difficult to separate the effect of the Freund's adjuvant from the effects of the tumor antigen. These studies are being repeated in an appropriately randomized phase III trial. Takita has reported another trial involving specific immunotherapy of patients with stage III lung cancer [28]. In this study patients with extensive stage III lung cancer who underwent complete resection of the tumor were randomized to a group receiving no further immunotherapy and a group receiving an autologous tumor vaccine treated with Vibrio cholerae neuraminidase. Some of the patients were also treated with radiation therapy. The median survival in the control group was 12 months, and the median survival in the treated group was 34 months. The encouraging results of this phase II study have led to a phase III trial to more accurately assess the effectiveness of this form of therapy.

IV. INTRALESIONAL BCG

Studies in animal tumor models as well as previous experience with BCG immunotherapy in man have indicated that one of the most effective ways to induce tumor immunity with BCG is by direct intratumor injection [5–9]. In animal models the intratumor injection of BCG gives rise not only to complete regression of the injected tumor, but also to regression of regional lymph node metastases and the establishment of systemic antitumor immunity. In view of these findings, it seemed reasonable to evaluate this therapeutic modality in patients with lung cancer [29]. The direct intralesional injection of BCG has been evaluated in a phase II trial in 50 patients with pulmonary tumors. Ten patients have received BCG administered directly into the tumor by way of the bronchoscope. All of these patients had endobronchial disease which was either obstructing the bronchus or bleeding. In eight of these ten patients a response was obtained resulting in decreased size of the tumor and/or cessation of the bleeding. Forty patients received direct intratumor injection of BCG by percutanous needle injection under fluoroscopic control.

Table 3. Mixed lymphocyte culture (MLC) cell-mediated lympholysis (CML) in tumor infiltrating lymphocytes (TIL), peripheral blood lymphocytes (PBL) and regional lymph node lymphocytes (LNL) in BCG injected and noninjected patients.

Cells	BCG	Number tested	MLC[1]		CML[2]	
			Unstimulated	Stimulated	4 : 1	32 : 1
TIL	Yes	7	851	15488	12%	17%
	No	14	961	3642	2%	5%
LNL	Yes	4	3162	15399	22%	36%
	No	6	2113	51487	46%	58%
PBL	Yes	7	990	44524	41%	57%
	No	13	771	37153	36%	51%
Control PBL		20	551	56040	40%	55%

[1] Average CPM.
[2] Average percent cytotoxicity.

Table 4. Natural killer cell activity (% to release) of tumor infiltrating lymphocytes (TIL) regional lymph node lymphocytes (LNL) and peripheral blood lymphocytes (PBL) and BCG injected and uninjected patients.

(1) BCG uninjected patients.

Patient	TIL BCG (−)	LNL	PBL	Control PBL
1	1		23	23
2	1		12	23
3	5	11	7	20
4	2		42	29
5	2		12	26
6	7		38	18
7	5		56	14
8	2		30	19
9	0	37	9	19
Mean ± SE	2.8 ± 0.8	24.0 ± 13.0	25.4 ± 5.7	21.2 ± 1.5

(2) BCG injected patients

Patient	TIL BCG (+)	TIL BCG (−)	LNL	PBL	Control PBL
1	13		21	16	27
2	41	0	11	34	10
3	37	15	33	53	34
4	8	2	28	43	26
Mean ± SE	24.8 ± 8.3	5.7 ± 4.7	23.3 ± 4.8	36.5 ± 7.9	24.3 ± 5.1

TIL BCG (−) in BCG uninjected patients vs. TIL BCG (+) in BCG injected patients	$p < .05$
TIL BCG (−) vs. PBL in BCG uninjected patients	$p < .005$
TIL BCG (+) vs. BCG (−) in BCG injected patients	$p < .1$

Thirty-nine of these 40 patients subsequently underwent surgical resection two weeks after the intratumor BCG injection. The toxicity was directly related to the preinjection PPD reaction. Patients with positive PPD reactions had a febrile response occasionally associated with chills. Most patients who were PPD negative had no detectable toxicity following injection of BCG. At the time of thoracotomy there was little intrapleural reaction. In two instances the BCG was inadvertently not completely injected into the tumor, and there was spillage into the pleural space. In these two patients there was extensive pleural effusions and intrapleural reactions. The BCG organisms could be

Table 5. Intralesional BCG followed by resection. Disease free survival — Median followup 14 months.

Bronchogenic carcinoma	85% (14 patients)
Metastatic tumors*	
1) BCG injected	55% (25 patients)
2) Concomitant, non-randomized, uninjected controls	37% (40 patients)

* Considered candidates for metastasectomy because of evident disease confined to the lung.

demonstrated by culture and by staining techniques in the injected tumor as well as the regional lymph nodes.

Histologic examination of the resected tumors revealed an intense granulomatous inflammatory reaction which is similar to that described in animal models. There was an intense mononuclear infiltrate in all of the injected tumors. In vitro functional assays of the lymphocytes infiltrating the BCG injected tumors indicate that there was a marked increase in the functional activity of the lymphocytes infiltrating the tumor as well as a marked increase in the NK cell content of these BCG injected tumors (Tables 3 and 4). The postoperative survival of these 39 resected patients was compared to a concomitant but nonrandomized group of patients. The survival of the intralesional BCG injected patients was considerably better than the control group at a median followup of 15 months (Table 4). These results indicate that intralesional BCG in the treatment of pulmonary tumors is safe, and the preliminary findings indicate that this treatment prolongs survival and increases the functional activity of the lymphocytes infiltrating the injected tumor.

REFERENCES

1. Holmes EC and Golub SH: Immunological defects in lung cancer patients. J Thor Cardiovasc Surg 71:161-168, 1976.
2. Giuliano AE, Rangel DM, Golub SH, Holmes EC and Morton DL: Serum mediated immunosuppression in lung cancer. Cancer 43:971-924, 1979.
3. Jerrells TR, Dean JH, Richardson GL, Vadlamudi S and Herberman RB: Supressor cell activity in immunodepressed lung and breast cancer patients (Abstract). Proc Am Assoc Cancer Res 19:73, 1978.
4. Bast RC, Zbar B, Borsos T and Rapp HJ: BCG in cancer. New Eng J Med 290:13-20, 1974.
5. Holmes EC: Immunotherapy of solid tumors. Surg Clin North Am 59:371-380, 1979.
6. Morton DL, Eilber FR, Holmes EC, Hunt JS, Ketcham AS, Silverstein MJ and Sparks FC: BCG immunotherapy of malignant melanoma. Ann Surg 180:635-643, 1974.
7. Nathanson L: Use of BCG in treatment of human neoplasms: A review. Sem in Oncol 1:337-350, 1974.

8. Hanna MG, Jr: Immunological aspects of BCG mediated regression of established tumors and metastases in Guinea pigs. Sem in Oncol 1:319-335, 1974.

9. Zbar B, Canti G, Rapp HJ, Ashley MP, Sukumar S and Bast RC: Immunoprophylaxis of syngeneic methylcholanthrene induced Ewing's sarcomas with bacillus calmette guerin and tumor cells. Cancer Res 40:1036-1042, 1980.

10. Perlin E, Weese JL, Heim W, Reid J, Oldham R, Mills M, Miller C, Bloom H, Green D, Bellinger S Jr, Law I, Cannon G, Herberman R and Connor R: Immunotherapy of carcinoma of the lung with BCG and allogeneic tumor cells In Neoplasms immunity: Solid tumor therapy. (Crispen RG, ed) Proc of a Sympos pp 9-21, 1977.

11. Pouillart P, Mathe G, Palangie T, Schwarzenberg, L, Huguenin P, Morin P, Gautier H, Parrot R: Trials of BCG immunotherapy in the treatment of resectable squamous cell carcinoma of the bronchus (Stages I and II). Cancer Immunol. & Immunother 1:271-273, 1976.

12. Edwards FR and Whitwell F: Use of BCG as an immunostimulant in the surgical treatment of carcinoma of the lung: A five year followup report. Thorax 33:250-252, 1978.

13. Roscoe P, Pearce S, Ludgate S, Horn NW: A control trial of BCG immunotherapy in bronchogenic carcinoma treated by surgical resection. Cancer Immunol Immunother 3:115-118, 1977.

14. Miyazawa N, Suemasu K, Ogeta T, Yoneyama T, Tsuguo N, Tsuchiya R: BCG immunotherapy as an adjunct to surgery in lung cancer: A randomized prospective trial. Jap J Clin Oncol 9:19-26, 1979.

15. McKneally MF, Maver CM, Kausel HW: Regional immunotherapy of lung cancer using postoperative intrapleural BCG In Terry and Windhorst Immunotherapy of cancer: Present status of trials of man (Raven Press), PP 161-171, 1978.

16. Wright PW, Hill LD, Peterson AV, Anderson RP, Hammer SP, Johnson LP, Morgan EH and Pinkham RD: Adjuvant immunotherapy with intrapleural BCG and levamisole in patients with resected non-small cell lung cancer (abstract). 2nd International Conference on Immunotherapy of Cancer.

17. Lowe J, Iles PB, Shore DF, Langman MJS, Baldwin RW: Intrapleural BCG in operable lung cancer. Lancet 11-13, January 5, 1980.

18. Yasumoto K, Manade H, Yanagawae Nagano N, Ueda H, Hirota N, Ohta M, Nomoto K, Azuma I, Yamamura Y: Nonspecific adjuvant immunotherapy of lung cancer with cell wall skeleton of mycobacterium bovis, bacillus calmette-guerin. Cancer Res., 38:3262-3267, 1979.

19. Kerman R and Stefani S: Radiotherapy and immunotherapy of lung cancer: A preliminary report In Neoplasms immunity: Solid tumor therapy (Crispen RG, ed), Proc of Symposium, 29-35, 1977.

20. Pines A: A five year control study of BCG and radiotherapy for inoperable lung cancer. Lancet 1:380-381, 1976.

21. Israel L: Preliminary results of nonspecific immunotherapy for lung cancer. Cancer Chemotherapy Reports 4:283-287, 1973.

22. Israel L: Nonspecific immune stimulation with corynebacterium in lung cancer In Lung Cancer: Natural history, prognosis and therapy (Israel L and Chahinian P eds), Academic Press, New York, 273-280, 1976.

23. Sarna GP, Lowitz BB, Haskell CM, Cline MJ: Chemoimmunotherapy of bronchogenic carcinoma. Proc Am Assoc Cancer Res 18:89, 1977 (abstract).

24. Golub SH and Holmes EC: In vitro assays of immunocompetence in patients with lung cancer treated with Levamisole. Cancer Immunol Immunother 7:143-149, 1979.

25. Amery WK: A placebo-controlled Levamisole study in resectable lung cancer In Immunotherapy of cancer: Present status of trials in man. (Terry WD and Windhorst D eds), Raven Press, New York, 191-200, 1978.

26. Anthony HM, Mearns AJ, Mason MK, Scott DG, Moghissi K, Deverall PB, Rozycki ZJ and Watson DA: Levamisole in surgery in bronchial carcinoma patients: Increase in deaths from cardiorespiratory failure. Thorax 34:4-12, 1979.

27. Stewart THM, Hollinshead A, Harris J, Raman S, Blanger R, Crepeau A, Crook A, Hooper D, Klaassen D, Rapp E, Sachs H: A survival study of specific active immunotherapy in lung cancer In Neoplasms immunity solid tumor therapy (Crispen RG ed), Proc of Symp 37-48, 1977.

28. Takita H, Takaada M, Minowada J, Hahn T, Edgerton F: Adjuvant immunotherapy of Stage III lung carcinoma In Immunotherapy of Cancer: Present status of trials in man. (Terry WD and Windhorst D eds), Raven Press, New York, 217-223, 1978.

29. Holmes EC Ramming KP, Bein ME, Coulson WF and Callery CD: Intralesional BCG immunotherapy of pulmonary tumors. J Thorac Cardiovasc Surg 77:362-368, 1979.

4. The Use of Pre-operative Radiation Therapy in the Treatment of Lung Carcinoma

DAVID M. SHERMAN and RALPH R. WEICHSELBAUM

INTRODUCTION

The natural history of lung cancer precludes curative therapy in a majority of cases. For example, fifty to sixty percent of patients who present with upper lobe lesions have bilateral mediastinal lymph node metastasis as do 30% of patients with lower lobe lesions[1, 2]. Hematogenous spread with multiple organ involvement has been reported in 30% of all patients at the time of diagnosis with oat cell carcinoma having the highest incidence of distant metastasis[3–5].

Based upon the poor ultimate survivals with surgery, except for early limited disease and the autopsy findings of residual disease following surgery[6], a rationale can be made for adding radiation therapy to surgery in an attempt to salvage a subset of patients who might have failed with local or regional disease only. Unfortunately, this potential subset of patients who might benefit from this combined modality approach is a small portion of the total group of patients who are seen with lung cancer.

Matthews[6] has reported on autopsy data from 202 patients from the Veteran's Administration Surgical Adjuvant Group (VASAG) and the Surgical Collaborative Study for Roswell Park and Memorial Hospital. These patients died one month following curative surgical procedures and the incidence of residual disease was assessed. For the group of patients with epidermoid carcinoma, residual disease was found at autopsy in 33% of the patients (44/131). In 50% of those patients[22], disease was local or regional only. For other histologies, only 2/29 had local disease only with most of those patients having distant metastasis at the time of death.

The rationale for the use of preoperative radiation, in an attempt to enhance survival, was expressed by Bloedorn[7] and included 1) the ability of radiation therapy to convert unresectable cancer to resectable lesions, 2) the known ability of radiation to sterilize the mediastinum in 30% to 40% of patients with biopsy proven mediastinal disease and 3) the possible reduction of the number of cells capable of implantation at the time of thoracotomy to local or distant sites. Thus, it was hoped that the subset of patients with local and/or regional disease could have their survival enhanced by adjuvant radiotherapy.

The first preoperative trial of radiotherapy in lung cancer was reported by Bromley and Szur[8] in 1955. Sixty-six patients were selected to receive preoperative radiation of 4500 rad in 5 to 6 weeks, utilizing orthovoltage radiation followed in 4 weeks by surgical resection, if possible. The patients were categorized by extent of disease although only 11 patients were initially inoperable. The survival of the total group of patients showed no improvement in the overall survival when compared to surgery alone. However, of greater interest was the observation that 44% of the irradiated patients had no tumor histologically in the surgical specimen. This initial observation led to the subsequent investigation of the use of preoperative radiation in an attempt to improve survivals in lung cancer.

Large scale randomized studies in the use of preoperative radiation have been disappointing to date. The National Collaborative Study[9], in which 17 medical centers cooperated, randomized patients with operable lung cancer at the time of diagnosis to receive either immediate surgery or preoperative radiation followed by curative surgical resection. Most patients received a minimum of 4000 rad over 4 weeks duration. The 5 year survivals of the two groups were identical: 14% in the group receiving radiation versus 16% in the group receiving immediate surgery. When patients were analyzed with respect to local control, no statistical benefit was ascribed to preoperative radiation with 20% (32/162) showing no evidence of recurrent thoracic carcinoma versus 26% (36/140) in the surgery only group. There were 425 patients who were considered inoperable initially who received high dose radiation and were not included in the above study. Of those 425 patients, 152 were considered resectable following radiation and were subsequently randomized to undergo a curative thoracotomy or no further therapy. The survival was, again, statistically equivalent for both groups, 8% and 6% respectively.

The V.A. Surgical Adjuvant Center conducted a similar randomized trial comparing preoperative radiation with surgery alone[10]. Patients were randomly assigned to preoperative radiation (170 patients), or surgery alone (169 patients). Patients in the preoperative group received 4000 rad to 6000 rad over 4 to 6 weeks with most patients receiving less that 5000 rad. This was followed in 12 weeks by thoractomy. Survival and postoperative complications were similar in both groups with no advantage noted for patients receiving preoperative radiation.

Bloedorn et al. reported[7] on a series of patients with advanced lung carcinoma receiving preoperative radiation followed by surgical resection, if possible. There were 83 patients who were initially operable and 109 patients who were inoperable, 46 by clinical criteria and 63 proven unresectable at thoractomy. Patients received high dose radiation – 4500 rad to an initial large volume followed by a boost of 1000 to 1500 rad by reduced fields for a total of 6000 rad. The resectability rate for the patients who finished the prescribed course of radiation was greater than 80% (82/98). The expected incidence of positive lymph nodes was also diminished in patients completing radiation and undergoing surgery. Despite the high resectability rate and the sterilization of primary disease as well as mediastinal lymph nodes, the overall survival was not improved. A high complication rate was observed in 82 patients who underwent curative resection following high dose radiation. A mortality of 29% was reported with the most common complications being bronchopleural fistula and empyema.

Saxena et al. [11] reported on a smaller series of patients in which preoperative radiation was followed by limited surgical resection in an attempt to conserve as much normal pulmonary tissue as possible. These patients were selected from an initial population of 182 referred for primary surgery. Patients received 4500 rad to 5000 rad over a one month period. There were 4 deaths, 4/42 (9%) who died of treatment related complications and one patient who died an immediate postoperative death. It is difficult to relate the excellent survival in this series to the others reviewed in that they were probably earlier stage patients who were potential candidates for limited surgery. It is of interest to note that local recurrence was low in this group – 2/31 patients.

A smaller series was also reported by Widow [12] from Germany, 122 patients received 3000 rad to 4000 rad preoperatively followed in 6 weeks by thoractomy. Of 85 patients who were operable following radiation [72], 85% were resectable and 13 unresectable. Again, a high complication rate was observed (15%) mostly as a result of fistula development. The 5 year survivals were equivalent, 19% for surgery only and 20% for patients receiving preoperative radiation and were found to be resectable. A high complication rate was, again, associated with preoperative radiation and surgical resection.

Based on the above data as well as the analysis of failure presented (Matthews), only a small subset of patients benefit from preoperative or postoperative radiotherapy and in a large clinical trial, these patients may not be identified since a majority will die of distant metastasis. We will highlight the group of patients who may benefit from adjunctive radiotherapy.

SUPERIOR SULCUS TUMORS

Pancoast in 1932 [13] described tumors as occurring 'at a definite location at the thoracic inlet producing a constant and characteristic clinical phenomenon of pain in the 8th cervical and 1st and 2nd thoracic trunk distribution and Horner's Syndrome.' These tumors were frequently associated with local rib and vertebral involvement. He also noted the infrequent involvement of the scalene or mediastinal lymph nodes with superior sulcus tumors.

Bronchogenic carcinomas [14] developing peripherally in the upper lobe in either lung and invading the superior sulcus of the chest are usually low grade epidermoid carcinomas which grow slowly and metastasize late. These lesions frequently invade the lymphatics of the endothoracic fascia and involve the lower roots of the brachial plexus, the intercostal nerves, stellate ganglion, sympathetic chain, adjacent ribs, and vertebrae producing pain and Horner's syndrome. The average expected time of survival reported in the literature, prior to preoperative radiation and surgery, was 10 to 14 months. The longest survival in patients receiving no treatment was 10 months [15]. Paulson et al. [14–16], described 48 such patients with superior sulcus tumors who were treated with a planned course of preoperative radiation followed by an aggressive en block surgical resection in 36 patients. Twenty-six patients had a minimum follow-up of two years. Of those patients completing surgical resection, 9 are alive without evidence of disease 3 to 9 years post surgery. The 2 year survival was 39% and the 4 year survival was 35%. The surgical technique involved radical en bloc resection of the involved chest wall with frequent resection of the first three ribs and transverse processes, portions of the thoracic vertebrae, intercostal nerves, lower trunk of the brachial plexus, stellate ganglion and associated sympathetic chain as well as the involved lung. Surgery followed radiation by 4 to 6 weeks.

Pre-treatment proof of malignancy by a biopsy was felt not to be necessary to proceed with the planned course of radiation and subsequent surgery in Paulson's series because of the inaccessibility of the lesion and its potential for local or distant spread with surgical manipulation within the operative site. The potential for disturbance of the vascular bed was also felt to have a potential adverse effect on the radiation response on the tumor.

The benign causes of superior sulcus syndrome such as inflammatory lesions, tuberculosis and fibrosing mediastinitis, were minimized by careful pre-treatment evaluation and appropriate radiographs. In Paulson's series, there were 5 patients without primary lung carcinoma, 2 patients with metastatic disease and 3 patients with tuberculosis.

The results of preoperative radiation in this selective series with superior sulcus tumors, has resulted in a superior survival when compared to either surgery or radiation alone [17, 18]. The surgical technique described by Paulson must be adhered to in order to yield reproducible results with this combined modality.

Hilaris *et al.* [18, 19], have presented an extensive experience in the combined use of external beam radiation, surgery and the intra-operative use of radioactive materials in superior sulcus tumors. Patients were initially treated with external radiation followed by an en block resection described by Paulson. In patients who had a complete resection, the survivals were comparable to Paulson's experience, 34%. The combination of resection of the primary lesion and implantation of the chest wall also yielded a 5 year survival of 30%.

Patients who had incomplete resections were implanted with radioactive material; Radon 222, Gold 198, Iridium 192, and most recently, Iodine 125, with supplemental external radiation when the dose distribution was not satisfactory. The 5 year survival was 16% in such patients who were found unresectable at thoracotomy and might have otherwise been unsalvageable. Patients who received external radiation alone for inoperable lung carcinoma, had a 5 year survival of 5%.

These results would suggest that while the preferred treatment of superior sulcus tumors is preoperative radiation followed by an en bloc resection, some of these patients can still be salvaged if found to be inoperable, or have incomplete resection by interstitial implantation. Superior sulcus tumors represent a small subset of lung carcinoma which benefits by aggressive local treatment because its pattern of metastasis is relatively late in its natural history.

JOINT CENTER FOR RADIATION THERAPY EXPERIENCE

We [20] reported a series of patients with locally advanced marginally resectable lung cancer who were treated with preoperative and postoperative radiation at the Harvard Joint Center for Radiation Therapy and the New England Deaconess Hospital, Department of Radiation Therapy and Surgery, Harvard Medical School. This study was designed to treat patients with advanced localized Stage III disease, utilizing the rational of Bloedorn for the effect of preoperative radiation on resectability and on the sterilization of the mediastinum and a technique of a short course of large radiation fractions to increase tumor cell kill and shortened treatment time, allowing for an earlier surgical resection. A lower dose than reported by Bloedorn [7], and others [9, 12] was utilized in an attempt to reduce post-surgical morbidity and mortality. A dose of 3000 rad was selected because of excellent results previously reported by Paulson *et al.* [14–16].

From July, 1968 to December, 1974, 53 patients with advanced localized

Table 1. TNM Staging — All Patients (53).

	T_1	T_2	T_3	Total
N_0	0	0	12	12
N_1	0	4	11	15
N_2	1	15	9	25
M_1		1		1
Total	1	20	32	53

lung cancer were selected to undergo a course of preoperative radiation followed by an aggressive surgical attempt at resection. Table 1 lists the patients by the TMN Staging Classification. There were 4 patients with Stage II disease, T_2N_1, the remaining patients were all Stage III. The Stage II patients were included because of marginal pulmonary function studies and the desire to treat them with less than a pneumonectomy. All patients completed the prescribed course of radiation, however, 7 did not go on to thoracotomy because of the demonstration of distant metastasis or refusal to undergo surgery. Of 46 patients who underwent thoracotomy, 38 patients were resectable (83%). A pneumonectomy was performed in 25 patients and lobectomy in 13. Half of the patients who underwent lobectomy had superior sulcus tumors. Table 2 shows the histologic types subdivided by resectable and unresectable patients.

The structures included in the preoperative radiation field included the hilum, mediastinum, and a generous margin around the carina to incude the subcarinal lymph nodes using opposed anterior and posterior fields. Forty-six of the patients received 3000 rad in 10 treatments over 2 1/2 weeks, 6 were given 3600 rad and 1 patient received 4200 rad. There were 10 patients who received postoperative radiation for additional doses of 2100 rad to 3200 rad by small volume conedown fields utilizing an oblique opposed arrangement to avoid the spinal cord. Radiation was given because of the findings of tumors at the surgical margin or gross mediastinal disease at thoracotomy.

The actuarial survival is shown in Fig. 1. The 5 year actuarial survival for the total of 53 patients was 18%. For the 38 resectable patients, the survival

Table 2. Histologic type.

	Epi.	Adeno.	Oat	Large cell	Undiff.
Resectable (38)	20	4	1	6	7
Non-resectable (8)	1	1	2	0	2*

* 2 patients with unspecified type of tumor.

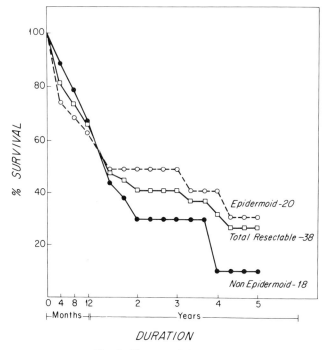

Fig. 1. The actuarial survival.

was 27% and for the 20 resectable patients with epidermoid carcinoma, 31%. Eighteen patients with other histologies had a 5 year survival of only 10%. There were no survivors in the group of the 7 patients who were not explored with the longest survival of 6 months. Of 8 patients who were explored and found unresectable, the longest survival was 18 months and 7 of those patients died within 8 months. There were 12 survivors of the 38 resectable patients with a median survival of 48 months. Table 3 indicates the extent of disease for all the resectable patients, subdivided by the 12 survivors and the 26 non-survivors. Six of the 12 surviving patients were Stage III because of T_3 disease and hilar involvement (T_3N_1). Five of the 6 T_3 patients were staged accordingly because of pulmonary artery involvement and 1 with pericardial involvement. There were 3 surviving patients with both hilar and mediastinum involvement and 2 with superior sulcus tumors. The additional patient indicated with Stage III, T_3 was on the basis of collapse of the entire left lung. Table 4 indicates the extent of surgery subdivided according to survivors and non-survivors in the 38 resectable patients. Of the 12 survivors, 11 underwent pneumonectomy and 1 had a lobectomy. The survival of patients who had a pneumonectomy (44%), was significantly better (p < .05) than the patients who had a lobectomy, 8%.

Table 3. Extent of disease in resectable patients.

	Hilar	Med.	H + H	S. Sulcus	Other
Survivors (12)	6	0	3	2	1
Non-survivors (26)	5	5	3	7	6
Total (38)	11	5	6	9	7

Table 4. Extent of surgery in resectable patients.

	Pneumonectomy	Lobectomy
Survivors (12)	11 (1)*	1
Non-survivors (26)	14 (2)*	12 (7)*

* ( ) with chest wall resection.

Survival was analyzed on the basis of histologic type. Of the long term survivors, a majority (8 patients) had epidermoid carcinoma, as has also been shown with survival in patients who undergo either surgery [21–23] or radiation primarily [24]. A correlation, but not statistically significant, was noted between patients who had a complete response to radiation and ultimate survival. Table 5 compares tumor response and survival in the resectable group of 38 patients. Six of 14 patients (45%), who had a complete response, survived. The mortality was comparable to other series and less than that reported by Bloedorn. There was one fatal radiation complication secondary to hemoptysis. There were 6 patients with surgically related complications, 2 with bronchopleural fistula, and 2 with empyemia. These complications resulted in 2 surgical deaths, 1 three days postoperatively and the second patient, 6 days postoperatively secondary to pulmonary emboli. The survival in our series was superior to that of unresectable lung carcinoma in general, and similar to the survival of all patients with initially resectable

Table 5. Response and survival in resectable patients.

	Complete response	Partial response
Survivors (12)	6/12 (1)*	6/12
Non-survivors (26)	8/26 (3)*	18/26
Total	14/38 (4)*	24/38

* ( ) with chest wall involvement.

lesions [21, 22, 25]. With the exception of superior sulcus tumors, in most series, chest wall involvement has predicted a low survival probability and this was also noted in this series.

While patients with tumor involvement of the pulmonary artery are generally thought to have an ominous outlook, 5 of the 12 long-term survivors had tumor spread to this vessel. This observation might suggest that such patients who are suspected to have major vessel involvement should undergo a course of preoperative radiation followed by an aggressive surgical resection, if possible.

Patients who underwent a pneumonectomy had a superior survival to that of patients undergoing lesser surgical procedures. This is in contrast to the reported surgical literature [17, 23, 25, 26] which suggests an improved survival in patients undergoing a lesser surgical procedure, i.e., lobectomy versus pneumonectomy (75% vs. 39%) [5]. The explanation in the surgical literature supporting improved survival in patients able to undergo a lobectomy rather than a pneumonectomy, proposes that patients who must undergo a pneumonectomy are usually patients with more advanced local or regional disease. In addition, there is an increased operative mortality and morbidity associated with the more extensive surgical procedure. The results of improved survival in patients undergoing pneumonectomy versus lobectomy (44% vs 8%) would support the conclusion that patients in this series had advanced local disease which was only encompassable with the more extensive surgical procedure. This would also support the general principle that both surgical and radiotherapeutic procedures must encompass the original volume of tumor and the regions of potential spread. The predilection for greater survival of patients with squamous cell carcinoma, has been demonstrated in surgically treated patients [8, 21, 23], patients treated with radiotherapy alone [24], and of combinations of the two mortalities [27]. Patients with squamous cell carcinoma in the present series also did better than patients with other histologies (31% versus 10%, 5 year survival).

These results indicate in this group of selected patients with marginally resectable lung carcinoma but without distant disease, a course of preoperative radiation of approximately 3000 rad over 2 1/2 weeks followed by aggressive surgery, has an enhanced survival comparable to that of patients with less advanced lesions treated with surgery alone. In addition, these data also suggested that a radical pneumonectomy was the surgical procedure of choice. It should be emphasized that these patients represent a selected subgroup and emphasize the necessity of cooperation between the radiotherapist and surgeon.

POSTOPERATIVE RADIOTHERAPY

Green *et al.* [17] reviewed 219 patients who were treated with postoperative radiation. Most patients received full dose radiation, 5000 to 6000 rad. Patients with negative lymph nodes showed no improvement in survival. Patients with involvement of either hilar or mediastinal nodes, post resection, showed an improved 5 year survival (23/66 surviving) versus 1/30 patients surviving at 5 years who did not receive postoperative radiation. Kirsh [28] confirmed improved survival in patients treated with postoperative radiation with involved mediastinal nodes with squamous cell carcinoma, although not in the subset of adenocarcinoma.

CONCLUSION

Routine preoperative radiation of operable lung carcinoma is not indicated. Clinical circumstances, such as superior sulcus tumors, selected patients with marginally resectable lesions, and postoperative treatment of patients with resected lesions and positive nodes, hilar or mediastinal, warrant local adjuvant radiotherapy.

REFERENCES

1. Hinson KRW: The spread of carcinoma of the lung, carcinoma of the lung, ed by Bignell JR, Williams and Wilkins Co, p 130, 1938.
2. Bloedorn F, Crowley A, Cuccia C, Mercado R Jr: Combined Therapy: Irradiation and surgery in the treatment of bronchogenic carcinoma. Am J Roentgenol 85:875-885, 1961.
3. Line DH, Dealy DJ: The necropsy findings in carcinoma of the bronchus. Br J Dis Chest 65:238-242, 1971.
4. Wilkins EW Jr, Scannell JG, Carver JG: Four decades of experience with bronchogenic carcinoma at the Massachusetts General Hospital. J Thorac Cardiovas Surg 76:364, 1978.
5. Overholt RH, Neptune WB, Ashraf MM: Primary cancer of the lung: A 42-year experience. Ann Thorac Surg 20:511, 1975.
6. Matthews MJ, Kanthouwa S, Picken J *et al.*: Frequency of residual tumor in patients undergoing curative resection of lung cancer. Ca Chem Rep 4:63-67, 1973.
7. Bloedorn FG, Crowley RA, Cuccian CA *et al.*: Preoperative irradiation in bronchogenic carcinoma. Am J Roentgenol Radium Ther Nucl Med 92:77-78, 1964.
8. Bromley LL, Szur L: Combined radiotherapy and resection for carcinoma of the bronchus. Lancet 2:937-941, 1955.
9. Preoperative irradiation of cancer of the lung: Final report of a therapeutic trial. A collaborative study. Cancer 36:914-925, 1975.
10. Roswit B, Higgins GA, Shields W *et al.*: Preoperative radiation therapy for carcinoma of the lung: Report of a national VA controlled studies. In: Frontiers of Radiation Therapy and Oncology, Vol 5, JM Veath, Ed Muchhen, Skarger, pp 163-176, 1970.

11. Saxena V, Hendrickson FR, Jensik RJ *et al.*: Conservative surgery following preoperative radiation for lung cancer. Am J Roentgenol Radium Ther Nucl Med 114:93-98, 1972.
12. Widow W: Preoperative irradiation of bronchial carcinoma. Cancer 28:798-800, 1971.
13. Pancost HK: Superior pulmonary sulcus tumors. JAMA 99:1391, 1932.
14. Paulson DL: The survival rate in superior sulcus tumors treated by presurgical irradiation. JAMA 196, No. 4:342, 1966.
15. Paulson DL, Shaw RR, Kee J *et al.*: Combined preoperative radiation and resection for bronchogenic carcinoma. J Thorac Cardiovas Surg 44:281-294, 1962.
16. Paulson DL: Treatment of superior sulcus tumors. In Rush BF Jr and Greenlaw RH, eds, Cancer Therapy by Integrated Radiation and Operation, Springfield, Illinois, Chas C Thomas, 1968, pp 74-82.
17. Boyd DP: Current Cancer Concepts: Is extended radical resection superior to lobectomy in treating resectable bronchial cancer. JAMA 195:157, 1966.
18. Hilaris S, Luomanen RK, Beattle EJ: Integrated irradiation and surgery in the treatment of apical lung cancer. Cancer 27:1369-1373, 1971.
19. Hilaris BS, Martini N, Luomanen RKJ *et al.*: The value of preoperative radiation therapy in apical lung cancer. Surgical Clinics of North America 54:831-840, 1964.
20. Sherman DM, Neptune W, Weiselbaum RR *et al.*: An aggressive approach to marginally resectable lung cancer. Cancer 41:2040-2045, 1978.
21. Bignall JR, Moon AJ: Survival after lung resection for bronchial carcinoma. Thorax 10:183-190.
22. Mountain C: The relationship of prognosis of morphology and anatomic extent of disease: Studies of a new clinical staging system. In: Lung Cancer natural History Prognosis and Therapy, Academic Press, NY, New York, 107-139, 1976.
23. Shimkin MB, Connelly RR, Marcus SC, Cutler SJ: Pneumonectomy and lobectomy in bronchogenic carcinoma. J. Thorac. Cardiovasc Surg. 44:503-520, 1962.
24. Hellman S, Kligerman MM, Von Essen CF, Scibetta PM: Sequelae of radical radiotherapy of carcinoma of the lung. Radiology 82:1055-1061, 1964.
25. Lawrence GH, Walker JH, Pinkers L: Extended resection of bronchogenic carcinoma. NEJM 263:615-620, 1960.
26. Thompson DT: Conservative resection in surgery for bronchogenic carcinoma. J Thorac Cardiovasc Surg 53:159-162, 1967.
27. Green N, Kurohara SS, George FW, III: Post-resection irradiation for primary lung cancer. Radiology 116:405-507, 1975.
28. Kirsh MM, Rotman H, Argenta L, Bove E, Cimmio V, Tashian J, Sloan H: Carcinoma of lung: results of treatment over ten years. Ann Thorac Surg 21:371, 1976.

5. Lung Cancer – Post Resection Irradiation

NATHAN GREEN

INTRODUCTION

Over the past ten years there has been a marked increase in the number of patients afflicted with bronchogenic carcinoma. 100 000 new cases are predicted for next year. Less than 10 000 of these patients can be expected to survive five years. Bronchogenic carcinoma causes 33% of all male cancer deaths and 11% of all female cancer deaths. With the exception of small cell carcinoma, resection remains the mainstay in definitive treatment. Unfortunately, more than 70% of lung cancers are not detected early enough to be eligible for resection. At the time of diagnosis, localized carcinoma is found in 15%, regional spread in 30% and distant metastasis in 55% [1–3].

Although strict indications for surgical procedures have evolved since the early 1940's, post operative survival has not substantially increased [4]. Following resection, approximately 75% of patients die of recurrent cancer. Survival rates are influenced by the stage of tumor development and the biologic behavior of the tumor [4]. However, extreme variations in biologic behavior can exist with apparently early disease being biologically late [5]. It has been generally held that surgical failure occurs from occult distant metastasis present at the time of diagnosis [6]. Autopsy studies have supported this impression. Following a resection of curative design, more than two thirds of patients have developed extra thoracic metastasis [7]. Logically, in recent years, the investigative thrust has been to explore the use of adjunct chemotherapy and immunotherapy. Each modality offers the potential for irradicating occult thoracic as well as extra thoracic residual disease. Regrettably, with rare exception, neither single nor combination drug chemotherapy nor immunotherapy has been effective [8–15]. Selawry reviewed eight clinical trials employing adjuvant chemotherapy and showed no survival advantage [9]. Although carefully controlled studies employing adjuvant immunotherapy have for the most part failed to show a significant impact on survival, some

R.B. Livingston (ed.), Lung cancer 1, 75–111. All rights reserved.

reports have been promising [12, 16, 17]. Higher survival rates have been observed in patients when the post operative course has been complicated by empyema [17]. Levamisole has been reported to improve survival perhaps by enhancing immunity that has been depressed by surgery [16, 17]. Following resection of cancer limited to the lung, instillation of BCG into the pleural space may improve survival. It has been speculated that survival benefit may be from the effect of BCG on systemic immunity. However, the survival benefit may be solely a local effect. Survival benefit was not observed in patients with lymph node metastasis [18]. Following instillation of BCG, a marked inflammatory reaction occurs. Macrophages become larger and more phagocytic. Residual cancer cells could be destroyed in a specific or nonspecific way. Lymph nodes do not show the specific and maximum pathologic changes.

In recent years, clinical and investigative interest has reached out for alternatives. There has been a resurgence of interest in the use of adjuvant radiation therapy [19–21]. The intent of this report is to explore the rationale for post operative irradiation and comments will be confined to an evaluation of patients with squamous cell carcinomas, adenocarcinoma, and large cell poorly differentiated carcinoma. Patients with small cell carcinoma are not included as a great preponderance have systemic disease present at the time of diagnosis [22].

RATIONALE

Prognostic factors known to exert an influence on survival are age, performance status, associated pulmonary disease, histology and stage of disease [23]. When one tries to identify and give proportional weight to the prognostic factors which reliably predict survival, it becomes apparent that the most important determinant is the stage of disease [23, 24]. Once cancer has spread locally beyond surgically removed tissues, recurrence is inevitable and can become the dominant factor causing a patient's demise. The adverse effects from local recurrence can be distressing and morbid or local recurrence can become a source for distant metastasis [25–27]. Adjunct post operative irradiation should be considered. The justification for treatment is the presumption that malignant cells may be present following resection and may be ablated before becoming clinically evident. Radiation is thus extended to the areas where recurrence is most likely and where there is a chance of enhancing cure.

RATIONALE

Background – Surgery

The initial step in the evaluation of a combined modality approach employing surgery and radiation therapy is the identification of patients that are candidates for resection and the segregation of these patients into comparatively homogeneous subsets with respect to morphology, anatomic extent of the cancer and biologic behavior[28]. Mountain described a system of clinical staging that has become adaptable for international use. The accuracy of clinical staging has been related to the thoroughness of the pre-operative evaluation. Despite exhaustive diagnostic procedures, micrometastasis have been difficult to detect in the asymptomatic patient[29]. There is an increasing rate of validity to the staging process as one moves from clinical staging to surgical staging. This relates to the increased amount of data available from the gross and microscopic examination. Pathologic findings indicating the size of the primary tumor, the extent of tumor spread and the presence of regional lymph node involvement form the basis for surgical staging of lung cancer[30, 31]. Unfortunately, even surgical staging has limitations. The diagnosis of lymph node metastasis is subject to the sampling procedures of the surgeon and the pathologist. Multiple sectioning of each lymph node and examination of all of the lymph nodes are rarely performed. Still, survival data and patterns of failure according to the surgical stage do provide a logical basis for assessing the indication and merit of adjuvant post operative irradiation.

Patients with cancer truly confined to the lung may be cured by surgery alone. Martini *et al.* reported 115 patients who underwent resection for non-oat cell carcinoma of the lung. Each patient was carefully evaluated and classified as stage I disease after the resected specimens were reviewed histologically and the regional and mediastinum lymph nodes examined and found free of cancer. After three years, 77% of the patients were alive and free of disease. No patient had local recurrence[32]. Carr reported a 65% five year survival rate for surgical stage I disease in patients with squamous cell carcinoma of the lung. About half of the patients who did not survive, died of intercurrent disease. Carr concluded that adjunct therapy has limited potential for stage I disease as only 15% to 20% of all patients die from recurrent cancer[33].

Approximately half of all patients who come to resection have lymph node metastasis. The frequency is related to the individual surgeon's criteria for resectability[37]. The surgical experience in the management of patients with lymph node metastasis has shown that patients with regional disease do not invariably develop distant metastasis. The probabilities of cure have been related to the location of lymph node involvement, the number of lymph nodes involved and the extent of metastasis within the nodes, i.e.: internodal or perinodal [24, 26, 30, 34]. The frequency and patterns of failure following surgical resection indicate the population that might potentially benefit from adjunct irradiation. Spread to the segmental lymph nodes has not exerted a significant adverse impact on survival, whereas spread to the interlobar, hilar or mediastinal lymph nodes has exerted an increasingly negative impact on survival. With increasing magnitude of lymph node involvement, there is less certainity as to the adequacy of the surgical resection and a greater probability for the presence of occult distant metastasis [35–38]. Distinctions in survival according to the location of the lymph node metastasis become somewhat blurred by the lack of a clear anatomic separation between the hilum and mediastinum [35–38]. Borrie believed a solitary intralobar or hilar lymph node metastasis was compatible with survival. However, if three or more intrapulmonary lymph nodes contained metastasis, the patient was unlikely to survive [24]. Shields *et al.* analyzed 1,216 patients with lymph node metastasis. Following a potentially curative resection, the five year survival was 93/464, (20.1%) for interlobar lymph node metastasis; 84/484 (17.4%) for hilar lymph node metastasis and 24/268 (8.9%) for mediastinal lymph node metastasis [26, 30, 38]. Vincent *et al.* noted 0/60 (0%) five year survival for hilar lymph node metastasis and 3/52 (6%) five year survival for mediastinal lymph node metastasis [39]. Smith *et al.* reported 16/56 (28.5%) five year survival for mediastinal lymph node metastasis [40]. Confusion regarding the cause for the marked variation in survival rates of patients with mediastinal lymph node metastasis has arisen because most studies have not analyzed survival according to the exact location of the lymph node metastasis; the number of nodes involved and the extent of involvement within each lymph node. Naruke *et al.* excellent study has resolved some of the confusion. 468 patients underwent a lobectomy or pneumonectomy in conjunction with a complete dissection of the hilar and mediastinal lymph nodes. The site of lymph node metastasis was carefully mapped out and correlated with survival. 12/64 (18.8%) patients with mediastinal lymph node metastasis survived five years; 3/33 (9.1%) with subcarinal lymph node metastasis as compared to 9/31 (29%) with ipsilateral tracheobraonchial lymph node metastasis. Naruki suggested the presence of subcarinal lymph node metastasis indicated a high probability of contralateral mediastinal spread [41, 42]. Bergh *et al.*, observed that metastasis confined to the lymph nodes conferred a better prognosis than perinodal spread. Ninety-nine patients with lymph node metastasis underwent curative resection. 15/99 (15%) remained free of disease from two and one half to ten years. The metastasis of fifteen patients showed intranodal growth. 13/15 patients with intranodal growth survived whereas only 2/84 patients with perinodal growth survived. Bergh did not correlate the characteristics of the primary tumor with the degree of lymph node involvement. He did report that all patients with regional tumor spread beyond the lung died of their disease [34]. Paulson's report gives additional credence to the ominous implications of perinodal spread. 417 patients underwent exploration; 173 had lymph node metastasis. Mediastinal lymph node involvement was found in 56/147 (13.4%). 16/56 patients survived five years (28.5%). Perinodal involvement predominated in all histologic types. Only one patient with perinodal involvement lived over two years after resection. Almost all the survivors were found in the subset in whom the lymph node metastasis was in the low ipsilateral mediastinum. This subset comprised 12% of the total. 15/16 survivors had intranodal invasion and were managed by pneumonectomy. Four survivors had poorly differentiated carcinoma [3, 43].

In the United States, 50% of all primary lung cancers are classified as squamous cell carcinoma, 20% adenocarcinoma, 10% undifferentiated large cell carcinoma and 20% undifferentiated small cell carcinoma [44]. Patients with squamous cell carcinoma have the best overall prognosis with an accumulated five year survival of 25%. Theirs is a more favorable outlook as there is a lower incidence of lymph node metastasis. Vincent reported lymph node metastasis in approximately 40% of epidermoid carcinoma, 50% of adenocarcinoma and 70% of large cell carcinoma [39]. When there has been spread to the mediastinum, there is a higher incidence of unilateral involvement in patients with squamous cell carcinoma. Consequently a greater proportion of patients with squamous cell carcinoma have tumors amenable to resection. Patients with adenocarcinoma and undifferentiated large cell carcinoma have a lower five year survival of approximately 13%. Distinctions in survival become less obvious with progression of the clinical stage. The accumulative five year survival of clinical stage T2 squamous cell carcinoma is 28%, adenocarcinoma 11%, and large cell carcinoma 16%. The accumulative five year survival of clinical stage T3 squamous cell carcinoma is 8%, adenocarcinoma 2% and large cell carcinoma 8%. In the presence of clinically determined ipsilateral hilar lymph node metastasis the five year survival for squamous cell carcinoma is 19%, adenocarcinoma 7% and large cell carcinoma 5% [27–29].

Distinctions in survival according to cell type are much less apparent in patients who were surgically staged. In Shields' experience, variations in survival rates between squamous cell carcinoma, adenocarcinoma and undifferentiated large cell carcinoma remained insignificant when lymph nodes were uninvolved, and were of borderline significance when they contained metastasis. The overall five year survival for patients without lymph node metastasis was 50% for squamous cell carcinoma, 56% for adenocarcinoma and 41% for large cell carcinoma. Intrapulmonary or hilar lymph node metastasis lowered the survival to 40% for squamous cell carcinoma, 24% for adenocarcinoma and 26% for undifferentiated large cell carcinoma. Once the mediastinal lymph nodes were involved, a much poorer outcome was observed with five year survivals of 13% for squamous cell carcinoma, 11% for large cell carcinoma and only 2% for adenocarcinoma [26, 30, 38].

Any description of the biological behavior of lung cancer by cell type has been limited by problems arising from the interpretation and classification of lung cancer. The limitations are the faithfulness by which any one sample represents the total tumor characteristics, the bias imposed by the source material used for interpretation, the differences in criteria used by each pathologist for classification and the inconsistencies of interpretation by different pathologists or by the same pathologist at different times [45–48]. Although increasing numbers of pathologists have adhered to the classifications of lung cancer recommended by the World Health Organization, some pathologists believe that a tumor should be named by its most mature element, whereas others feel that a tumor should be named by its dominent component. In 1968, the World Health Organization proposed a revision in the criteria used to classify squamous cell carcinoma. When the original material was reviewed and reclassified there was a lower frequency of squamous cell carcinoma. A panel of experts reviewed the same slides. Agreement on the diagnosis of poorly differentiated adenocarcinoma was reached in less than 50% of the cases and on the diagnosis of large cell carcinoma in less than 10% of the cases [49]. Kern reported agreement of the final histologic classification was noted in only 43% of patients when the same slide material was reviewed by three pathologists. One pathologist studied the same slide material several weeks later. He disagreed with the original diagnosis 7% of the time. Disagreement was common even in the recognition of squamous cell carcinoma [50].

Insight into the potential value of adjunct post-operative irradiation can be gleaned from an appreciation of the patterns of surgical failure. The incidence and sites of recurrence have been analyzed from clinical experience and autopsy studies. Green et al. reported that approximately 10% of patients who undergo curative resection developed local recurrence without distant metastasis. Of forty-six patients who presented with post-resection local recurrence, twenty-one patients had squamous cell carcinoma, thirteen patients adenocarcinoma, ten patients large cell poorly differentiated carcinoma and two patients small cell carcinoma. The site of tumor recurrence could not be predicted from the location of the primary tumor or the presence of lymph node metastasis. 17/21 (81%) patients with lymph node metastasis at original surgery developed hilar or mediastinal lymph node recurrence whereas 12/23 (52%) patients without lymph node metastasis developed hilar or mediastinal lymph node recurrence. 3/8 (37%) patients with invasion of tumor into the parietal pleural developed chest wall recurrence. Eight recurrences were

Table 1. Comparison of extent of disease at surgery to site of local recurrence*.

Disease at surgery	Incision	Chest wall	Paren-chymal	Bronchial stump	Main stem	Hilar	Media-stinal
No lymph nodes (23)**	2/23	5/23	2/23	4/23	1/23	6/23	8/23
Hilar lymph nodes (15)	1/15		1/15	1/15		4/15	8/15
Mediastinal lymph nodes (6)	2/6	1/6	1/16	1/6		1/6	4/6
Unknown (2)	1/2			1/2			

* Green N., Kern W. The clinical course and treatment results of patients with postresection locally recurrent cancer. Cancer 42 : 2478-2479, 1978.
** Total patients.

located in the bronchial stump or main stem bronchus (Table 1). Distant metastasis developed in less than half the patients and often was not the major cause of death[25]. Patients usually died from dysphagia, pulmonary consolidation, respiratory insufficiency and tracheoesophageal fistula. The implication is that in spite of aggressive surgical management, microscopic residual in unresected lymph nodes were a frequent occurrence in patients with all cell types. One could assume that adjunct post-operative irradiation would have been of value for these patients. Tumor recurrence might have been delayed or prevented and survival thereby improved.

Information obtained from autopsy studies is a great deal more accurate than the information obtained from clinical studies. However, autopsies can also underestimate or overestimate the incidence and sites of recurrence. If there has been a short time interval between surgery and death, there is little opportunity for occult tumor to increase in size and become visible. A tumor must become visible or palpable to the prosector to be reliably sampled. Occult disease may not be appreciated [7, 51–53]. The patterns of surgical failure determined from autopsy studies have been shown to be related to the extent of disease at surgery, the histologic cell type and the time interval between surgery and autopsy. A surprisingly large percentage of patients who had early and inadvertent death following an apparently curative resection have been found to have residual local, regional disease without distant metastasis. Local regional recurrences were most prevalent in patients with tumors confined within the lung, whereas local regional recurrences and distant metastasis were of equal frequency in patients who had contiguous tumor spread to adjacent structures. In patients with squamous cell carcinoma the preponderance of recurrences were local and regional. However, in patients with adenocarcinoma and large cell carcinoma, distant metastases were more common.

Matthews *et al.* reported an autopsy study of 235 patients who died within thirty days of a pulmonary resection. Nineteen patients had small cell carcinoma and are excluded from this analysis. At surgery, 186 patients had tumor confined to the lung or hilar lymph node metastases. Resection was considered curative. Autopsy showed residual disease in forty-six patients. Twenty-two patients had regional disease and twenty-four patients distant metastasis. The high rate of residual disease indicated that carcinoma assumed to be totally resected in many instances was not. At the time of surgery, the mediastinum was visualized and tumor was either unrecognized or not confirmed. Matthews observed the patterns of failure to be different for each cell type. Of 131 patients with epidermoid carcinoma, twenty-one were found to have residual local regional disease and fifteen distant metastasis. No patient with adenocarcinoma or large cell carcinoma was found to have residual local regional disease, whereas 7/21 (33%) and 2/21 (15%) respectively had distant metastasis. These findings suggest that patients with adenocarcinoma and large cell carcinoma are at risk for distant metastasis rather than local regional recurrence. However, the total number of autopsies with these cell types are too few to be confident of this impression [52].

Rasmussen reported sixty-four autopsies performed two months or longer after a pulmonary resection. Local recurrence was the dominant feature of fifty-four patients dying from lung cancer and was usually found to be the primary cause of death. 20/64 (31%) had local recurrence alone; 30/64 (47%) local recurrence and distant metastasis and 10/64 (16%) distant metastasis alone. At resection, nineteen patients had hilar and mediastinal lymph node metastasis. Of these 7/19 (37%) had local recurrence alone, 9/19 (47%) had both local and distant metastasis and 3/19 (16%) only distant metastasis. Rasmussen also observed the patterns of failure to be related to the histologic cell type. Patients with squamous cell carcinoma had predominately local recurrences, whereas patients with undifferentiated large cell carcinoma and adenocarcinoma had a high incidence of distant metastasis [54].

Spjut *et al.* reported seventy-two autopsies performed one month or longer after resection. 5/15 (33%) patients who died within one month had mediastinal lymph node metastasis. In two patients this was the only site of residual disease. The relative proportion of autopsies showing recurrent tumors in the hemithorax increased as the duration from surgery to death increased and reached a peak of 59% in patients surviving six months or longer after resection [51].

Matthews *et al.* reported an autopsy study of 418 patients with inoperable lung cancer. Hilar and mediastinal lymph node metastasis were found in 77% of patients with epidermoid carcinoma, 80% of patients with adenocarcinoma and 84% of patients with large cell carcinoma. 89/418 (21%) autopsies showed the cancer localized solely in the chest, involving the mediastinal lymph nodes, pleural, chest wall, diaphragm, heart or pericardium. This pattern was noted for all cell types but more commonly in patients with squamous cell carcinoma. In total, 46% of patients with epidermoid carcinoma, 20% of patients with adenocarcinoma and 14% of patients with large cell carcinoma had local regional disease without distant metastasis [52]. Line and Deeley's autopsy review of 680 patients showed comparable findings [53].

RATIONALE

Background – Radiation Therapy

The promise of adjunct post-operative radiation therapy can be appreciated by a review of the application of irradiation in the treatment of the primary tumor. Radiation therapy is the most effective cytoreductive agent known for treating lung cancer short of a surgeon's knife. Radiation response has been evaluated in terms of tumor response, tumor sterilization and survival [55–57]. Tumor response has been estimated by the percentage disappearance of the tumor shadow on chest X-rays taken prior to, during, and following completion of radiation therapy. Tumor sterilization has been evaluated from the operative specimens of patients who have received pre-operative irradiation and from the autopsies of patients treated definitively with irradiation [58, 59].

A favorable tumor response to irradiation has been observed in up to 70% of patients. Approximately 20% of patients develop complete tumor regression [60–62]. The response rate and degree of response has been related to the total tumor dose, timedose fractionation and cell type. Perez reported the optimal total tumor dose is in the range of 5000 to 6000 rads [62]. Rubin noted increasing local tumor control and survival rates at one year in patients treated to 5000 rads or more as compared to patients treated to a lower dose [63]. Phillips reported local tumor control was a function of radiation dose. Optimal tumor control occurred in patients treated to 6600 rads, 200 rads per fraction. Complete tumor regression was observed in 32% of patients receiving 5000 to 6000 rads and 63% of patients receiving 6600 rads [56]. A greater rate of complete regression occurs with large cell carcinomas than squamous cell carcinoma or adenocarcinoma. However, because regression rates can be slow, analysis of tumor response early after completion of irradiation may lead to erroneous conclusions.

Radiation therapy has been delivered by either a continuous or a split course. A continuous course is uninterrupted therapy delivered four or five days a week. A split course is the scheduled and deliberate interruption of radiation therapy for a one or two week duration, one or more times before completion of the entire course. Theoretical arguments suggest an advantage to split course therapy. Tumor oxygenation can be enhanced during the rest period. There is less radiation toxicity because of the interrupted therapy. However little difference in tumor response or survival has been observed between the two methods of therapy [64–69].

Pre-operative irradiation has been locally effective. Unfortunately, there has not been a concomitant improvement in survival. Bloedorn reported a prospective study of 192 patients that underwent an exploratory thoracotomy with biopsy of the primary tumor and palpable mediastinal lymph nodes. All patients subsequently received irradiation to the primary tumor and mediastinum. The planned dose was 6000 rads. Following radiation therapy, ninety-eight patients came to re-exploration. Sixteen patients were found to be unresectable. 23/80 (27%) of those resected had no demonstrable tumor in the resected specimen. 9/17 (53%) found to have mediastinal lymph node metastasis at exploration had a negative re-exploration [72]. A cooperative study organized by the committee for radiation therapy established by the National Cancer Institute, the United States Public Health Service, reported 568 patients randomly assigned to receive pre-operative irradiation or immediate surgery. The five year survival rate was 14% and 16% respectively. Shields *et al.* also reported a randomized study comparing pre-operative irradiation to surgery alone. No improvement in survival was observed. The pre-operative radiation group had more frequent major complications. Bronchopleural fistulae were noted to be three times more common. Survival rates could not be analyzed according to the presence or absence of lymph node metastasis as pre-operative irradiation obscured the pathologic detection of lymph node metastasis. The frequency of local recurrence was reported to be comparable. However, the criteria used to diagnose local recurrence precluded a true analysis of the local effectiveness of irradiation. Local recurrence was defined as disease developing anywhere in the thorax, including tumors that developed within or outside the irradiated volume [71–73].

Autopsy studies have confirmed the efficacy of irradiation. Rissanen *et al.* reviewed the autopsies of sixty patients with inoperable lung cancer treated by megavoltage irradiation. 4000 to 7000 rads was delivered over five to seven weeks. 18/60 (30%) showed no residual carcinoma and 14/60 (23%) had extensive fibrosis with islets of carcinoma cells within the treatment volume. The latter finding implied that tumor growth may have been retarded [59]. Abadir *et al.* reviewed the autopsies of forty-eight patients who had undergone irradiation therapy for localized carcinoma of the lung. No lethal tumor effect was noted when dosages of less than 4000 rads were delivered. 8/48 (35%) were sterilized at dosages of greater than 4000 [74].

Emami *et al.* showed the value of elective irradiation in controlling occult lymph node metastasis. 241 patients with inoperable lung cancer were treated with radiation therapy. Seventy-nine patients received elective irradiation to the supra-clavicular lymph nodes and 153 patients did not. A total of 5000 rads was delivered. Clinically detectable supraclavicular disease developed in 1/79 (1.3%) electively irradiated and 21/153 (14%) not electively irradiated [75].

Cure has been realized in those patients in whom radiation therapy was effective. Smart treated forty select patients in whom the primary lesion was localized and there was no clinical evidence of lymph node metastasis. A total dose of 4000 to 5500 rads was delivered in seven to eight weeks. 9/40 (23%) survived five years [76]. Smart's results raised the conjecture that radiation therapy might be as effective as surgery in the management of lung cancer. Morrison *et al.* did a controlled clinical trial that laid this hope to rest. Fifty-eight patients with operable cancer of the lung were treated by surgery or radical supervoltage irradiation. The four year survival rates for the surgery group was 23% and radiation therapy group 7%. The results of surgery were significantly better in patients with squamous cell carcinoma. There was no appreciable difference in the results of surgery or irradiation in patients with anaplastic tumors [68]. Overall, the five year survival rates in patients with localized unresectable lung cancer managed by definitive megavoltage irradiation has ranged from 1–8% [57].

POST OPERATIVE IRRADIATION

Through the years, interest in post operative radiation therapy has been generated by knowledge of the radiation responsiveness of lung cancer and the impression that some patients might benefit from adjunct irradiation. Post-operative radiation therapy has had theoretical appeal when compared to pre-operative radiation therapy. Surgery is not delayed. A higher dose can be delivered without increasing the operative morbidity or mortality. The extent of disease can be determined from the surgical findings. Patients can be segregated into groups that might benefit. Until recently, interest in post-operative irradiation has been dampened by the conclusions of two randomized studies [77, 78]. In each study, patients underwent curative resection and received post-operative irradiation to treatment fields that encompassed the hilum and adjacent mediastinum. Both studies failed to show improved survival. However, treatment techniques were inadequate by current standards. The treatment fields did not encompass all of the regional area at risk. The total dosage delivered was suboptimal. Patients with extensive disease or gross residual disease were included in each study. Such patients cannot be expected to benefit from adjunct irradiation. The end results were not analyzed according to the extent of the primary tumor spread or the status of the lymph nodes.

The study reported by Patterson and Russell randomized 202 patients to pneumonectomy or pneumonectomy and post-operative irradiation. A mediastinal lymph node dissection was not done. Patients with massive mediastinal disease were excluded on the basis of the chest X-ray findings. Undoubtedly some patients with gross mediastinal lymph node metastasis were inadvertently included in this study. Radiation was delivered with three 10×5 cm fields directed toward the hilum and adjacent mediastinum. A total dose of 4500 rads was delivered. The three year survival rates were comparable for surgery (36.4%) and surgery with post-operative irradiation (33%)[77]. Bangma reported seventy-three patients randomized to resection or resection and post-operative irradiation. Forty-six patients had a lobectomy and twenty-seven patients a pneumonectomy. Fifty-five patients were characterized as having either a peripheral or a central tumor without lymph node metastasis. Eighteen patients had invasive tumor or lymph node metastasis. Radiation therapy was given by a variety of techniques including rotation therapy and multiple fixed fields. 4500 rads was delivered to the hilum and homolateral mediastinum. Forty-four patients had squamous cell carcinoma without lymph node metastasis. The one year survival was 17/23 (74%) for surgery and 13/21 (62%) for surgery with post-operative irradiation. The reported end results did not segregate the patients according to the degree of primary tumor spread. Inclusion of patients with tumor invasion beyond the visceral pleural creates a negative bias in the end results that can obscure the potential benefit of post-operative irradiation for patients with a more favorable primary tumor presentation. The survival rate of patients with lymph node metastasis was not reported. It was noted that intrathoracic recurrences were less common in patients who received post-operative irradiation. However, the sites of recurrence and anatomic relationship to the treatment volume were not described[79].

In recent years, there has been a resurgence of interest in post-operative irradiation based on two non-randomized studies suggesting survival benefit in patients with lymph node metastasis. These studies must be accepted with some reservations as the survival of patients managed by surgery combined with post-operative irradiation was not too dissimilar from the best survival figures that have been achieved by surgery alone[20, 21, 80].

Kirsch et al. reported 437 patients who underwent a thorough mediastinal lymph node dissection in conjunction with a pulmonary resection. The homolateral paratracheal, para-esophageal, anterior mediastinal, and subcarinal nodes were completely removed. On the left side the subaortic nodes were also resected. The presence of high ipsilateral lymph nodes was not a contraindication to surgery. Kirsch felt the prognosis in that situation may not be hopeless. A lobectomy was the preferred procedure when technically feasible. A pneumonectomy was performed for tumors that could not be removed with the lesser procedure. A total of 367 patients had a 'curative' resection. Post-operative irradiation was given only to patients with mediastinal lymph node metastasis. A total dose of 5000 to 5500 rads was delivered to the entire mediastinum. Kirsch noted 2/34 (6%) developed local recurrence. The incidences of local recurrence in patients managed by surgery alone was not described. Survival was analyzed according to histologic cell type and lymph node status. Patients with tumor extension to the diaphragm, pericardium and chest wall were not analyzed separately. The five year survival of 193 patients with squamous cell carcinoma without lymph node metastasis was 53%; with hilar lymph node metastasis 47.5%, and with mediastinal lymph node metastasis 34.4%. The five year survival of 127 patients with adenocarcinoma without lymph node metastasis was 44%. There were no survivors with hilar lymph node metastasis. 11.8% survived with mediastinal lymph node metastasis. The authors did not analyze the five year survival of the nineteen patients with large cell poorly differentiated carcinomas as the numbers were too small. Kirsch concluded that post-operative irradiation was of value for patients with squamous cell carcinoma and mediastinal lymph node metastasis but not indicated for patients with adenocarcinoma and mediastinal lymph node metastasis. However, one should bear in mind that the patients with adenocarcinoma and hilar lymph node metastasis had not received post-operative irradiation and there were no survivors whereas patients with mediastinal spread were treated with post-operative irradiation and 11% survived [20, 80].

Green *et al.* reported 219 patients who underwent a lymph node dissection in conjunction with a pulmonary resection. Patients with tumor spread beyond the visceral pleura were excluded. Usually only the grossly involved lymph nodes were excised. No consistent or extensive surgical dissection was performed on the mediastinal lymph nodes. 123 patients had no detectable lymph node metastasis. Ninety-six patients had hilar or mediastinal lymph node metastasis. 125 patients received post-operative irradiation, fifty-nine patients without lymph node metastasis and sixty-six patients with lymph node metastasis. Radiation treatment fields included the hilum, mediastinum and bilateral paraclavicular nodes in patients who underwent a lobectomy and included the mediastinum and homolateral paraclavicular nodes in patients who underwent a pneumonectomy. An average midline dose of 4400 rads in five and one half weeks was delivered. Patients without lymph node metastasis had a comparable survival when managed by surgery alone or surgery and post-operative irradiation (Table 2). Important differences in five year survival were observed in patients with lymph node metastasis; 1/30 (3.0%) patients treated by surgery alone, and 23/66 (35%) treated by surgery and

Table 2. Patients without node metastases

Five year survival.

Histological type	Treatment	
	Surgery alone	Surgery plus irradiation
Squamous-cell carcinoma	10/37 (27%)	12/43 (28%)
Adenocarcinoma	3/16 (19%)	2/8 (25%)
Anaplastic carcinoma	1/11 (9%)	2/8 (25%)
Total	14/64 (22%)	16/59 (27%)

post-operative irradiation. Survival benefit was noted for patients with hilar as well as mediastinal lymph node metastasis and for all cell types (Table 3). Survival was not specifically documented according to the number of lymph nodes involved nor the extent of involvement of each lymph node. Green concluded that adequate excision of the primary tumor and grossly involved lymph nodes combined with vigorous post-operative irradiation can be advantageous. Surgery has a better prospect of controlling bulky tumor than does radiation. Patients with lymph node metastasis are at an increased risk for local regional failure. Undoubtedly some patients with hilar lymph node metastasis have unappreciated mediastinal metastasis. Resection of all mediastinal lymph node is not possible [21, 81]. It is rational to employ post-operative irradiation for patients with hilar or mediastinal lymph node metastasis.

There are important differences in the reports of Kirsch and Green. Kirsch felt it was the presence, not the number, size, or location of lymph node metastasis that determined survival rates, provided patients underwent vigor-

Table 3. Patient with lymph node metastases*

Five year survival.

Histological type	Treatment	
	Surgery alone	Surgery plus irradiation
Squamous-cell carcinoma	1/16 (6%)	6/28 (21%)
Adenocarcinoma	0/6 (0%)	10/16 (62%)
Anaplastic carcinoma	0/8 (0%)	7/22 (32%)
Total	1/30 (3%)	23/66 (35%)

* Green N., Kurohara S.S., George F.W., et al. Postresection irradiation for primary lung cancer. Radiology 116 : 405-407, 1975.

ous resection and post-operative irradiation. Post-operative irradiation was limited to the mediastinum. He concluded that post-operative irradiation was of value only for patients with squamous cell carcinoma and mediastinal lymph node metastasis. Green felt the most important determinents of survival were the degree of primary tumor spread and the extent of lymph node metastasis. A vigorous lymph node dissection was not essential. Rather the resection could be limited to removal of gross lymph node metastasis provided patients receive post-operative irradiation. The implication is that a less extensive lymph node resection might be more applicable and be associated with a lower surgical mortality. However, there is an approximate 10% error in assessment of mediastinal lymph nodes if they are not removed surgically and studied histologically [32]. The involved lymph nodes may not be selected for analysis or sampled properly. The occasional skipping of metastasis makes all lymph nodes suspect [81]. Green employed post-operative irradiation to patients with hilar as well as mediastinal lymph node metastasis with apparent benefit for all cell types [21].

Kirsch and Green's reports have appeal on the basis of reason. There are reservations. Rubin has taken a less optimistic position, believing that less than 20% of patients who undergo a resection can be expected to benefit from post-operative irradiation. It was his conviction that at the time of detection, lung cancer is pathologically disseminated in the vast majority of patients. Post-operative irradiation would not influence survival in patients who already have distant metastasis nor prevent the dissemination of disease at the time of surgery [82, 83]. Therefore, in considering adjunct post-operative radiation therapy, it must be shown that neither extensive surgery nor vigorous irradiation is as curative as the combination of both modalities. It also must be shown that the combination of the two modalities does not greatly increase the morbidity or mortality for this would counterbalance any gain. The true value of post-operative irradiation will be determined only by a carefully designed prospective randomized study. In such a study, it is suggested that the precise anatomic location of the lymph node metastasis, the number of nodes involved and the presence or absence of pericapsular invasion be recorded. Patients should also be studied according to the important prognostic factors of tumor size, regional extent of tumor spread, age and general medical condition.

POST OPERATIVE IRRADIATION

Surgical Considerations

The capabilities and limitations of surgery and radiation therapy should be well understood in order to optimally integrate the two therapeutic regimens.

An appreciation of the lymphatics of the lung is essential to an understanding of the therapeutic options. The spread of lung cancer to regional lymph nodes usually proceeds in an orderly fashion with involvement of segmental, intralobar and hilar lymph nodes. The hilar lymph nodes are located in the angle between the bronchial bifurcation and are closely related to the pulmonary arteries and veins. There is frequent failure of complete anatomic division of the lobes. Some lymph nodes within one lobe are fed by lymph vessels from neighboring lobes. Heavily involved lymph nodes may fail to act as a filter resulting in capricious local and distant lymphatic spread. Carcinomas of the right upper lobe do not drain below the level of the intermediate bronchus. A right upper lobectomy and regional lymph node dissection may be an adequate procedure. Carcinomas of the right lower lobe drain into the lymph nodes inferior and posterior to the right lower lobe bronchus and around the right intermediate bronchus. In order to resect all involved lymph nodes draining the right lower lobe, the middle lobe and its regional lymph nodes should also be removed. Carcinomas of the left lung drain to a constant group of lymph nodes lying in a fissure between the upper and lower lobes. Removal of all lymph nodes in the performance of a left upper or left lower lobectomy is most difficult. Shields doubted whether it was truly possible to do an adequate lymph node dissection in combination with a lobectomy. Many lymph nodes are not visualized or excised [35, 36, 81]. There is no precise anatomic delineation between the hilum and mediastinum. Initially mediastinal spread is to the low tracheobronchial and subcarinal lymph nodes. With progression there is involvement of the periesophageal, high paratracheal, anterior, posterior, and contralateral mediastinal lymph nodes [35, 36, 81, 84–86]. Approximately 5% of carcinomas of the right lung spread to the contralateral mediastinum. There is a higher incidence of contralateral mediastinum lymph node metastasis from carcinoma of the left lung. Consequently, carcinomas of the left lung have a poorer prognosis [81, 85, 86].

Most surgeons have relied upon mediastinoscopy and parasternal mediastinotomy to determine the site and extent of lymph node metastasis prior to considering definitive resection. These tests are good indicators for resectability since 85% of patients who have a negative study had resectable tumors according to the criteria used for resectability [4, 85–87]. Other investigators have felt that mediastinotomy and mediastinoscopy are not of value. They recommend patients be offered an exploratory thoracotomy before a final decision is reached [41, 80, 88]. Conversely, some physicians feel mediastinal lymph node biopsy is not indicated, and assess all patients by chest X-ray. If the chest X-ray indicates gross lymph node metastasis, the patients are excluded from surgery [89].

A curative resection should remove all feasible tumor and the surgical margin should be free by gross and microscopic examination [4]. It is generally agreed that candidates for curative resection are patients in whom the primary tumor is technically resectable and the extent of the lymph node involvement is limited to the ipsilateral tracheobronchial, paratracheal lymph nodes or subcarinal lymph nodes. In such cases, the outcome will be highly conditioned by whether the lymph nodes are intact and whether the most peripheral lymph nodes are microscopically free of metastatic disease. Resection is usually futile if the most distant lymph nodes are microscopically involved or if the tumor has spread through the lymph node capsule [43]. Contralateral mediastinal spread is an absolute contra indication to resection. At best, less than 50% of patients with mediastinal lymph node metastasis present with disease so limited that resection is feasible [86]. The technique and thoroughness of the hilar and mediastinal lymph node dissection differs from surgeon to surgeon and from center to center. Fishman expressed concern that once mediastinal lymph nodes have been involved by cancer, the five year survival rates from surgery alone may be lower than the operative mortality [4]. Martini and Shields have questioned whether a pulmonary resection should be performed in patients with adenocarcinoma or large cell carcinoma if patients have mediastinal lymph node metastasis. In their experience, the survival rates were 2.9% and 6.1% respectively [26, 30, 32, 38].

If the options are present to choose between a lobectomy and a pneumonectomy, an increasing number of surgeons have elected a lobectomy. The absolute disease free survival rate has been thought to be equal when the topography of the tumors are equivalent and when lobectomy is technically feasible [31, 37]. The more limited resection has been associated with less morbidity and mortality and has the advantage of conserving lung tissue [90]. A pneumonectomy is usually performed when the disease is too extensive to be handled by a more limited resection [90]. As the magnitude of the surgical procedure increases, the operative mortality rate increases. Vincent noted an operative mortality rate of 1.9% for a lobectomy, 11.9% for a pneumonectomy and 20% for an extended pneumonectomy [39]. The average surgical mortality has been 5% for a lobectomy and 12% for a pneumonectomy. The operative mortality rate in patients under the age of 40, in good general health who undergo a lobectomy has been 1% whereas the operative mortality rate in patients over the age of seventy in poor general health who undergo a pneumonectomy has been 40% [24]. In the final analysis, the ultimate decision regarding resectability and the optimal procedure to use is a matter of surgical judgment based on the findings at operation and an estimation of the patients ability to withstand the proposed resection.

It is essential that the radiation therapist and surgeon be in close communication to appreciate the extent of disease resected and the potential sites for persistent disease. If it has been elected to do a lobectomy, and lymph node metastasis are found, it is logical to offer these patients post-operative irradiation. Treatment fields should be generous and include the hilum, entire mediastinum and bilateral paraclavicular lymph nodes with adequate margins. In patients with mediastinal lymph node metastasis one is left with concern that unresected lymph nodes may contain microscopic deposits. Cahan *et al.* advocated a radical pneumonectomy with an 'enbloc' removal of the mediastinal lymph nodes feeling that this procedure would ensure a more satisfactory removal of the lymph node metastasis [81]. Shields doubted that a true 'en bloc' dissection of the mediastinum can be performed [90]. It is logical to offer these patients post-operative irradiation. Treatment fields should include the mediastinum and homolateral paraclavicular lymph nodes and when feasible the hemithorax.

The cardiopulmonary status of the patient can influence the decision with regard to operability, type resection and use of post-operative irradiation. Close melding of the disciplines offers the opportunity to design a coordinated program which could improve tumor control with the least compromise of pulmonary function. Considerations should be given to the impact of the reduced respiratory function subsequent to a pulmonary resection. The severity of any observed impairment must be matched to the anticipated extent of the resection. The criteria for resection tends to be liberal in view of the seriousness of the disease. The loss of respiratory function correlates with the number of pulmonary segments removed. Surgeons agree that one should sacrifice as small an amount of pulmonary parenchyma as is consistent with complete removal of the tumor. Pulmonary insufficiency is less frequent after a lobectomy but does occur [92–95]. In patients who undergo a pneumonectomy, the mortality rates rise sharply as the maximum breathing capacity falls below 55% of normal and the FEV is less than 1 liter. No one set of pulmonary function studies can be used to determine at what level impaired function makes a pneumonectomy too hazardous. The laboratory results must be reviewed in light of the patients age, the amount of functioning lung loss due to the tumor and the degree of cooperation of the patient in performing the study [37]. If post-operative radiation therapy is potentially indicated, the pulmonary function following resection must be matched against the potential benefit of post-operative irradiation and the possible additional loss of pulmonary function caused by the radiation therapy [96]. In marginal situations, it is important for both the surgeon and radiation therapist to participate in the decision regarding the type of resection. If a radical lobectomy rather than a pneumonectomy has been performed in order to conserve pulmonary function, the surgeon should appreciate that additional loss of pulmonary function may occur as radiation treatment portals usually encompass the hilum and thereby unavoidably include functioning lung. If, on the other hand, the surgeon performs a radical pneumonectomy and leaves the patient with a marginal pulmonary reserve, it may not be possible to deliver post-operative irradiation. Mediastinal radiation treatment portals might unavoidably include portions of the remaining lung.

POST OPERATIVE IRRADIATION

Radiation Therapy Considerations

The goal of radiation therapy is to deliver a sterilizing dose to the anatomic region at risk with minimal adverse effect on the contiguous normal structures. Radiation therapy techniques should be standardized insofar as the optimal total dose, time dose fractionation, and treatment field; yet individualized according to an estimate of the patient's ability to withstand the treatment regimen. Recent advances have permitted the delivery of higher dosages to achieve a greater degree of local control. These advances include accurate simulation techniques which permit precise beam positioning, computerized axial tomography which provides more information about the anatomic relationships of the tumor to critical normal structures and increased knowledge of the tolerance of the lungs, heart and spinal cord to irradiation. Field size and beam angles are designed to include the volume of interest and spare normal organs. With the help of chest X-rays and computerized axial tomograms, the volume of interest is drawn into an anatomic cross section of the patient. The irradiated volume is individually defined with tailor made blocks. Localization films are taken on the treatment unit with the patient in the proper treatment position. The localization films assure that the size and position of the treatment fields corresponds to the areas of intended irradiation.

In patients who have undergone a simple or radical lobectomy, the homolateral hilum, entire mediastinum and the bilateral supraclavicular lymph nodes should be treated. The mediastinal portion of the treatment field should be of sufficient width and length to include the entire mediastinum. By this measure the mediastinum can receive the full therapeutic dose. The hemithorax is not treated as large volumes of irradiated lung result in significant morbidity (Figs. 1, 2). In patients who have undergone a simple or radical pneumonectomy, the entire mediastinum and homolateral paraclavicular nodes should be treated. The hemithorax should also be treated in patients with good performance status as they can be expected to tolerate large field therapy. The high percentage of patients who have residual disease in the hemithorax after an apparently curative resection provides ample rationale for treating the hemithorax. Careful attention should be given to sparing the contralateral lung. Following pneumonectomy air is absorbed from the thoracic space causing a progressive shift of the mediastinum towards the ipsilateral

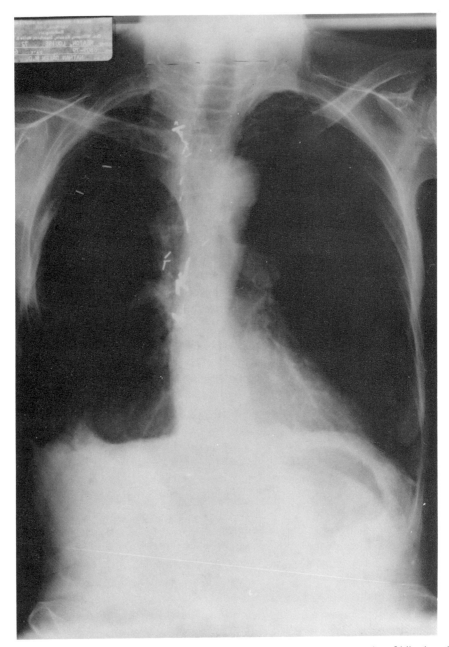

Fig. 1. Chest x-ray following a right upper lobectomy. Surgical clips delineate site of hilar lymph node metastasis.

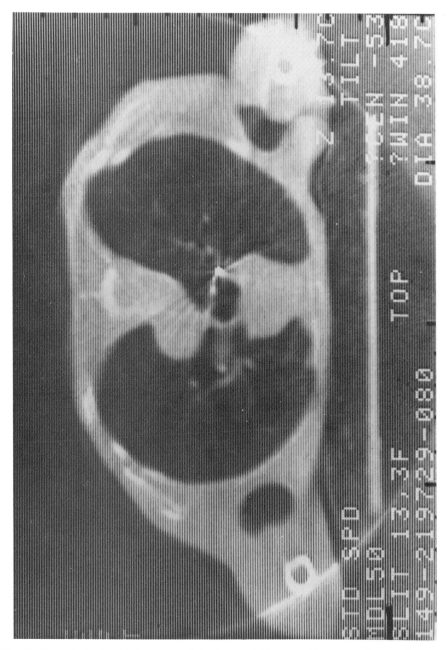

Fig. 2. Computerized axial tomogram following a right upper lobectomy. The mediastinum remains central. The surgical clips in the right hilum cast a shadow artifact.

side. The shift usually begins several weeks after surgery. The remaining lung expands and partially herniates into the post pneumonectomy site to fill the residual thoracic volume [36]. Treatment portals need to be individualized taking into special regard the patient's cardiopulmonary reserve. It may be necessary to exclude portions of the contralateral mediastinum, to avoid inclusion of inordinate portions of the herniated lung (Figs. 3, 4, 5). The risk for geometric miss can, in part, be circumvented by starting irradiation soon after surgery. An added dividend to early initiation of adjunct irradiation is to minimize the time frame during which gross tumor recurrence can develop. The dose used for adjunct irradiation is not adequate to manage gross tumor recurrence.

The biologic effect of a given dose of irradiation is related to the time dose fractionation [1]. A daily tumor dose of 180 rads each day, five fractions per week, to a total tumor dose of 5000 rads in five and one half weeks delivered to the mid portion of the thorax at the level of the carina is optimal [62, 75]. 5000 rads is assumed to be effective to diminish the incidence of recurrence in the resected hermithorax, hilum, and mediastinum. This dosage has been shown to be effective for minimal metastasis in patients with breast and head and neck cancer and has also been effective in reducing the incidence of supraclavicular recurrence in patients with inoperable lung cancer [44, 75]. Megavoltage irradiation should be used with a minimal source skin distance of 80 cm. Parallel opposed fields and treatment of both fields each day are recommended [64]. Most patients can be irradiated with continuous therapy, interrupted only for significant complaints. A split course regimen offers no theoretical advantage in adjunct irradiation.

Radiation complications are not readily justified in patients that may have been cured by surgery. Therefore it is pertinent to briefly review the radiation tolerance of critical intrathoracic structures. Radiation injury of the lung impairs ventilatory and diffusion capacity. The severity of the injury is related to the volume of lung irradiated and the total dose delivered. The magnitude of the injury varies greatly from patient to patient. Physiologic changes in the lung have been observed at 600 rads and radiation pneumonitis at 2000 rads or more [98]. Fibrosis of the lung occurs with increasing frequency as higher dosages are delivered and when sufficient time has been available for follow-up [99–101]. There are considerable differences in the degree of patient adaptation to the progressive restriction of respiratory capacity. If there is adequate pulmonary reserve, the recommended dose can usually be given to the volume of interest with acceptable sequelae. The remaining lung may show compensatory changes with resultant stability of lung function. When there has been a significant reduction in pulmonary reserve, as observed in patients with pre-existent chronic pulmonary disease or following a pneumonectomy, one has to be very cautious in the delivery of irradiation. Less loss of

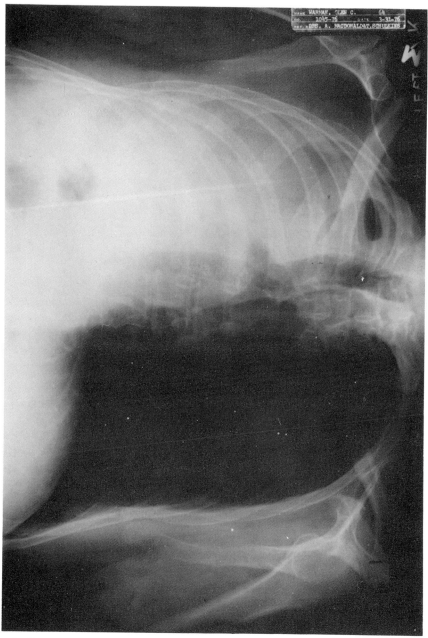

Fig. 3. Chest x-ray one week following a left pneumonectomy. The trachea and mediastinum have shifted to the left. Portions of the right lung have expanded across the midline into the left hemithorax.

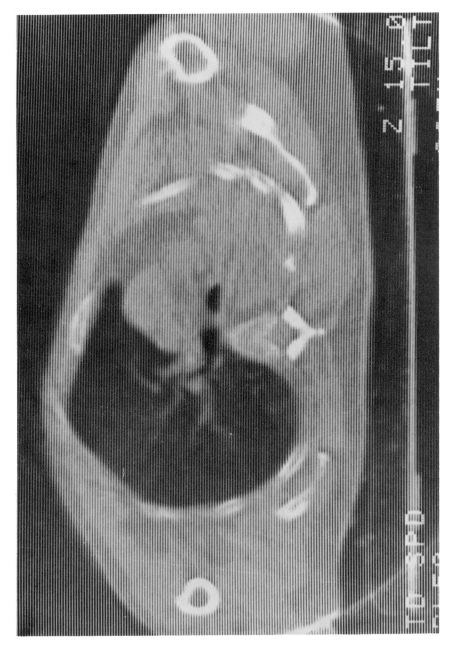

Fig. 4. Chest; Computerized axial tomography six weeks following a left pneumonectomy. The mediastinum has shifted to the left. The right lung has expanded into the left hemithorax.

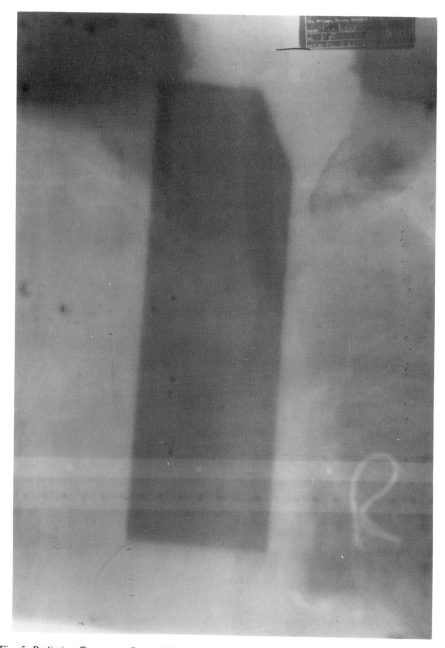

Fig. 5. Radiation Treatment Portal. The treatment portal includes the mediastinum and homolateral supraclavicular nodes. A small portion of the contralateral mediastinum is excluded in order to spare pulmonary reserve.

pulmonary function can be tolerated. Careful attention to the radiation therapy details are necessary. Treatment regimens may need to be individualized according to the clinical estimate of cure versus complications. When the probabilities of long term survival or cure are low, treatment fields must be designed to avoid excessive irradiation of uninvolved lung. It may not be possible to deliver full dosage to the entire volume at risk. Modifications in irradiation techniques include the use of shrinking fields, exclusion of the contralateral supraclavicular fossa or exclusion of portions of the contralateral mediastinum. Post-operative irradiation should not be used if a significant degree of pulmonary function is from the area of lung to be included in the treatment field [98, 98, 101].

Irradiation can affect the heart in a variety of ways leading to a spectrum of pathologic changes. Serous and fibrotic reactions of the pericardium, myocardium and endocardium occur. Radiation induced pericarditis is a significant risk of high dose radiation therapy. Constrictive pericarditis may be an end sequel and require a pericardiectomy [102, 103]. On rare occasion, the development of coronary artery disease can be accelerated [104]. Injury has rately been observed at radiation doses of less than 4000 rads. The probabilities of injury increase in proportion to the volume of heart included in the treatment field and the total dose delivered. The entire heart should receive not more than 4500 rads. Less than 50% of the heart may receive 5000 rads in six weeks [102].

One of the most tragic complications is radiation injury to the spinal cord. This complication is irreversible. The incidence of radiation myelopathy increases with higher dose fractions, shorter treatment time, higher total dosage and increased length of the spinal cord treated. Lambert et al. observed that patients do not develop radiation myelitis if the total dose does not exceed 5000 rads in twenty-five fractions. 3/61 (4.9%) patients receiving more than 5000 rads developed thoracic myelopathy [105]. Patients who developed thoracic cord myelopathy were treated to the upper thorax where the slope of the chest was greater and hence the dose to the upper thoracic spinal cord may have been higher than the central or lower segments of the thoracic spinal cord. In order to circumvent injury, angled fields or midline blocks have been advocated to exclude the spinal cord at 4000 or more [1, 83]. However, angled fields require precise reproduction of patient positioning on a daily basis in order to consistently treat the volume of interest. While precise patient positioning is strived for in every radiation therapy department, it has not been readily achieved in practice. Therefore, these complex treatment regimens may deliver less than an optimal dose to the posterior mediastinum. Opposing anterior and posterior portals offer the virture of simplicity in reproduction, and adequately encompasses the entire mediastinum. Homogeneous dosages can be delivered throughout the volume of interest. A midline block is not necessary as thoracic spinal cord injuries are extremely rare when a total dose of 5000 rads is delivered at 180 rads per increment.

MARGINALLY RESECTABLE LUNG CANCER

An additional segment of the lung cancer population deserving of consideration for post operative irradiation is the population with marginally resectable, locally advanced lung cancer that invades adjacent structures. This includes tumors that invade the pericardium, parietal pleurae and chest wall, involve the pulmonary artery or are located in the main stem bronchus. Included in the category of marginally resectable lung cancers are tumors that might require a compromised resection because of poor pulmonary function rather than because of local tumor spread.

There are substantial differences in the criteria used by major centers for operability and resectability of marginally resectable lung cancer. The differences are based on considerations of the probability of cure and the anticipated operative morbidity or mortality. At operation, it becomes readily evident whether resectability is technically feasible or should not be attempted. There are certain local manifestations which preclude resection. Local extension of neoplasm resulting in laryngeal or phrenic nerve paresis almost always suggests non-resectability because of extensive mediastinal disease. With rare exception, a solitary lymph node metastasis may be the cause and can be resected [90]. There may be occasion in which resection of the pericardium and the phrenic nerve can offer a chance for cure. Tumors that involve the main stem bronchus and carina, or encroach upon the tracheal wall are usually considered unresectable. An adequate length of proximal bronchus cannot be obtained for safe closure of the stump. If resection is attempted and it becomes essential to transect tumor, primary closure of the bronchus may not be secure. These patients are at much greater risk for surgical complications and mortality [106, 107]. Resections could be considered when it is possible to get beyond the tumor and secure primary closure of the bronchus and trachea or closure by a bronchoplastic procedure. Selected cases involving the chest wall lend themselves to curative resection [108, 109]. The extent of the resection has been a matter of surgical judgment. Following resection the surgeon is often left in doubt that there has been total removal of the tumor. Survival rates have varied from low in patients with main stem bronchus lesions, to encouraging in patients with chest wall involvement [106, 110].

When the primary tumor is central, arising in or extending to the main stem bronchus, the minimal procedure for total removal is a pneumonectomy [106]. Ideally, the proximal margin of the proposed resection should be identified as being clear of cancer by appropriate frozen section biopsy. Submucosal spread may be present, but is rarely greater than 2 cm [44]. Under all circumstances, the surgical margin would be extremely close. Shields et al. reported 15/124 (12%) patients had positive biopsies from the carina when the gross appearance of the carina was normal [36]. Green et al. reported 8/46 local recurrences in the bronchial stump or main stem bronchus after an apparently curative resection [25]. Ashor et al. reported four patients with tumors at the margin of the bronchial resection who survived ten years or more [111]. Weiss et al. reviewed the historical experience of patients with main stem bonchial tumors. The overall five-year survival was 2%. In his experience with 125 patients, twenty underwent resection. Almost all were dead within two years. Review of the tumor registry records of a group of 111 patients with operable main stem bronchus carcinoma found 23/111 patients (21%) to be alive at four years [106]. Naef et al. reported forty-six patients who underwent a tracheobronchial reconstruction. 1/46 (2%) was alive at five years. Naef concluded this procedure was usually a palliative venture to alleviate bronchial airway obstruction [107]. Bergh et al. reported sixty-six patients who underwent an extended resection. Thirty-one patients had a pericardiotomy with intrapericardial dissection of the major pulmonary vessels, seventeen had a pericardial resection, eight patients had an atrial resection and eight patients resection of the aortic wall. Pulsations from the pulmonary artery or heart may act as an inhibitory force to tumor invasion. Bergh observed that microscopic removal of all the malignant tissues did not guarantee cure. No patient survived five years [34].

A peripheral carcinoma can grow through the visceral pleurae into the thoracic wall or diaphragm. The intercostal muscle bundles and ribs may become involved. Beneath the parietal pleura there is a profuse network of lymphatics and great vascularity. Local and distant pathways of dissemination are facilitated [112]. In 1956, Gronqvist et al. reviewed the literature and reported a total of 2/23 (10%) patients with tumor extending into the thoracic wall were alive and well after resection. In his own experience 5/16 (31%) patients that underwent resection of carcinoma involving the thoracic wall were alive and well. 3/5 patients with tumor involvement of the parietal pleural and no deep invasion survived, whereas 2/13 patients with tumor involvement of the intercostal muscle and nerves survived [108]. Grillo et al. reported 3/19 (16%) with resected chest wall involvement survived five years [112]. Bergh noted no survivors in eight patients who underwent resection of portions of thoracic wall and diaphragm [34]. Ashor et al. reported fourteen patients with pleural invasion survived ten or more years following resection [111]. Geha et al. reviewed the experience of 2,013 patients who underwent surgical exploration. 158 patients had chest wall invasion. A low incidence of lymph node metastasis was noted. In forty patients, the primary tumor could be excised and the surgical procedure considered curative. 11/40

(27%) survived five years. Once lymph node metastasis were present, surgical resection rarely resulted in cure [110, 113]. Rees *et al.* reviewed the experience of forty-six patients who had poor pulmonary function due to associated pulmonary disease. As an alternative to a pneumonectomy, all patients were managed by lobectomy with a sleeve resection. Surgical mortality was 2.2% as compared to the 6% for a pneumonectomy performed on all other patients at the same center. Five year survival rates were 35%. Of nineteen patients with mediastinal lymph node metastasis, none survived five years. Only one patient developed recurrence at the site of the anastomosis [95].

Autopsy studies of patients who underwent a marginal resection for locally advanced tumors showed a great likelihood for persistent regional as well as distant disease. Matthews reported forty-three patients who underwent an extended resection and had inadvertent death within one month of surgery. Six patients were considered to have had a curative resection and thirty-seven patients, a palliative resection. Thirty patients were found to have persistent disease. 15/30 (50%) had regional disease and 15/30 (50%) distant metastasis. The incidence of regional and distant failures were comparable for each cell type [52].

The experience with adjunct radiation therapy for patients with marginally resectable lung cancer has been predominantly with pre-operative irradiation. An important study reported by Sherman *et al.* indicated that radiation therapy followed by agressive surgery appears to have an advantage over surgery alone. Irradiation therapy techniques were carefully designed to include the primary tumor, hilum and mediastinum. Generous clearance around the carina was usually attempted. A dosage of 3000 to 4200 rads in two and one half to four weeks was delivered. Ten patients received additional post operative irradiation because of microscopic findings of tumor at the margin of the resection or because of gross lymph node spread. Of fifty-three patients who received pre-operative irradiation, thirty-eight came to resection. Twenty-five had a pneumonectomy and thirteen a lobectomy. Survival was related to the tumor response to irradiation. 6/14 (43%) patients with a complete tumor response survived five years and 6/24 (25%) patients without a complete tumor response survived five years. Of the twelve survivors, eleven had a pneumonectomy and one a lobectomy. The more favorable results observed in patients undergoing a pneumonectomy lends support to the author's conclusion that a more extensive procedure is required to adequately encompass locally advanced disease. Included in the survivors were six patients with hilar lymph node metastasis, five patients with pulmonary artery involvement, one patient with pericardial disease, one patient with pleural involvement and one patient with disease within one cm of the carina. 2/9 patients who presented with superior sulcus tumors were long-term survivors [114]. Paulson *et al.* reported the experience of patients with superior sulcus tumor treated by pre-operative irradiation and surgery. 16/46 (35%) of them who came to survived five or more years. Patients with complete tumor sterilization did well, whereas patients with viable tumor or lymph node metastasis did poorly. No patient with hilar and mediastinal lymph node metastasis survived more than one year. Paulson did not describe the radiation therapy details. One infers from the report that treatment portals might have been limited to the primary tumor and did not include the hilum or mediastinum [109]. Jensick *et al.* used pre-operative irradiation in twenty-five patients in whom the pathologic situation permitted a sleeve resection or bronchoplastic procedure and in whom poor cardiac or poor pulmonary reserve demanded a compromised surgical procedure. 14/25 (56%) were reported alive and without tumor from five months to three years. Jensick concluded adjunct irradiation might be of value in that it allows conservation of pulmonary function. However, he questioned whether survival might not be just as good with surgery alone [94]. The final report of the cooperative study organized by the National Cancer Institute reviewed the experience of patients initially considered inoperable because of mediastinal or supraclavicular lymph node involvement, chest wall invasion or involvement of the main stem bronchus. There was great hope that radiation therapy followed by surgery would lead to greater containment of disease and prolong survival. 152/425 (36%) patients were considered resectable after radiation therapy. Following irradiation, the 152 patients were randomized to receive surgery or no additional treatment. The survival of patients who received radiation therapy alone was comparable to the survival of patients treated by pre-operative irradiation and surgery. There was no clear demonstration that radiation therapy could convert a nonresectable lesion to a resectable one and thereby improve survival. The authors concluded that, with the exception of select patients, efforts to increase the usefulness of surgery in the treatment of bronchogenic carcinoma through an extended operation alone or with pre-operative irradiation might result in higher morbidity or mortality and perhaps shorten survival. Radiation therapy alone may be the treatment of choice [71].

Post-operative radiation therapy for marginally resectable lung cancer has not been subject to critical clinical analysis. The clinical experience has been scanty. Conclusions of most authors cannot be substantiated by careful review of the data. With rare exception, treatment techniques have not been well documented. The end results have not been analyzed according to the location or extent of the tumor. Survival rates following combined therapy have varied from 0–35%. The wide range of reported results can be ascribed to the manner in which the various authors selected the patients for post operative irradiation and the small number of patients so treated. Comparisons to the results of patients managed by surgery alone or radiation therapy alone cannot be made. There was no long-term survival when post-operative irradiation was used as a palliative procedure [108, 110, 113]. The outlook did not improve when post operative irradiation was used after an attempt to remove the bulk of the tumor. Guttmann reported twenty patients who had incomplete resection and were treated post-operatively with full course radiation. All patients died within thirteen months of generalized metastasis [97]. Deeley *et al.* reported a three year survival rate of 12% in a group of patients when surgical excision was incomplete and post operative irradiation was delivered to the local area and mediastinum [115]. Gronqvist *et al.* noted 2/3 patients who received post-operative irradiation survived five years or more following resection of a tumor that involved the parietal pleurae [108].

At present, the justification for post operative irradiation in patients with marginally resected lung cancer is the chance for enhancing cure when radiation is delivered to areas where recurrence is most likely. However, in terms of five-year survival, there may be no advantage to subjecting patients with locally advanced cancer to the operative morbidity and mortality incurred with a surgical resection. These patients may be as well off treated by high dose definitive radiation therapy.

SUMMARY

Adjunct post-operative radiation therapy has been a logical modality to explore in patients with lung cancer who have undergone curative resection and in whom there exists a reasonable risk for developing local or regional recurrence. Patients that might benefit can be identified from an evaluation of patterns of failure following resection. The potential to enhance survival with adjunct radiation therapy in patients with disease confined to the lung is very small, as cure rates from surgery alone are high. Surgical cure rates decline significantly in patients when there has been extension of the primary tumor beyond the visceral pleura or spread to the lymph nodes. Clinical and autopsy studies suggest that following resection many patients have residual regional disease without concomitant distant metastasis. Unanswered is the question of whether post-operative irradiation to the hemithorax, hilum and mediastinum can sterilize residual microscopic disease and salvage more patients. Two randomized studies have failed to show benefit. The results of these studies can be challenged. The radiation therapy techniques were suboptimal by current standards. Patients were not evaluated according to the presence or absence of lymph node metastasis. Recent nonrandomized studies suggest survival can be improved for all cell types by the use of post-operative irradiation in patients with hilar or mediastinal lymph node metastasis. The radiation therapy techniques employed should take into account the surgical procedure employed. Sophisticated radiation treatment regimens use modern localization techniques and megavoltage irradiation. Careful attention should be given to encompass the area of interest and preserve pulmonary function.

The promise of post-operative irradiation remains to be determined by a carefully controlled randomized study. In such a study, patients should be analyzed according to age, performance status, cell type, type resection, location and extent of the primary tumor and lymph node metastasis.

I wish to thank Thomas Comer, M.D. and Thomas Schulkins, M.D. for their advice and support.

REFERENCES

1. Johnson RRJ: Radiotherapy Primary and/or Adjuvant Modality. In: Perspectives in Lung Cancer. Frederick E Jones Memorial Symposium in Thoracic Surgery, Columbus, Ohio, 1976, Williams TE, Wilson HE, Yohn DS (eds) Basel, S Karger, 1977, pp 74-81.
2. Vicent RG: Lung Cancer – An Overview. In: Perspectives in Lung Cancer. Frederick E. Jones Memorial Symposium in Thoracic Surgery, Columbus, Ohio, 1976, Williams TE, Wilson HE, Yohn DS, (eds). Basel, S. Karger, 1977, pp 1-8.
3. Paulson DL: Editorial Operability Versus Resectability in Bronchogenic Carcinoma. Ann Thorac Surg 3-4:177-178, 1967.
4. Fishman NH, Bronstein MH: Is Mediastinoscopy Necessary in the Evaluation of Lung Cancer: Ann Thorac Surg 20:678-686, 1975.
5. MacDonald I: Biological Predeterminism in Human Cancer. Surg Gyn Necol Obstet 92:443-452, 1951.
6. Cohen MH: Diagnosis, Staging, and Therapy. In: Pathogenesis and Therapy of Lung Cancer, Harris CC. (ed) New York, Marcel Dekker, Inc. 1978, pp. 653-700.
7. Matthews MJ, Kanhouwa S, Pickren J et al.: Frequency of Residual and Metastatic Tumor in Patients Undergoing Curative Surgical Resection for Lung Cancer. Cancer Chemother Rep 4:63-67, 1963.
8. Legha SS, Muggia FM, Carter SK: Adjuvant Chemotherapy in Lung Cancer. Cancer 39:1415-1424, 1977.
9. Selawry OS: On Chemotherapy of Lung Cancer. In: Lung Cancer – Natural History, Prognosis, and Therapy, Isreal L, Chahinian AP, (eds). New York, Academic Press. 1976, pp 205-239.
10. Brunner KW, Marthaler T, Muller W: Effects of Long-Term Adjuvant Chemotherapy With Cyclophosphamide (NSC-26271) for Radically Resected Bronchogenic Carcinoma. Cancer Chemother Rep 4:125-132, 1973.
11. Swierenga J, Gooszen HC, Vanderschueren RG et al.: Immunopotentiation with Levamisole in Resectable Bronchogenic Carcinoma: A Double-blind Controlled Trial. Br Med J 3:461-464, 1975.
12. Isreal L. Problems in Designing Postoperative Strategies With Respect to Immune Status, Kinetics, and Resistance. In: Lung Cancer – Natural History, Prognosis, and Therapy, Isreal L Chahinian AP, (eds) New York Academic Press, 1976, pp 285-294.
13. Wilson HE: Chemotherapy of Lung Carcinoma – Current Picture. In: Perspectives in Lung Cancer. Frederick E. Jones Memorial Symposium in Thoracic Surgery, Columbus, Ohio, 1976, Williams TE, Wilson HE, Yohn DS, (eds) Basel, S. Karger, 1977, pp 66-73.

14. Laing AH, Berry RJ, Newman CR et al.: Treatment of Inoperable Carcinoma of Bronchus. Lancet pp 1161-1164, 1975.

15. Pavlov A, Pirogov A, Trachtenberg A et al.: Results of Combination Treatment of Lung Cancer Patients: Surgery Plus Radiotherapy and Surgery Plus Chemotherapy. Cancer Chemother Rep 4:133-135, 1973.

16. Ritts RE, Jacobsen DA, Caron JA et al.: Is the Lung Cancer Patient Immunologically Competent? In: Perspectives in Lung Cancer. Frederick E Jones Memorial Sumposium in Thoracic Surgery, Columbus, Ohio, 1976, Williams TE, Wilson HE, Yohn DS, (eds) Basel, S. Karger, 1977, pp 47-56.

17. McKneally MF: Implications of Immunostimulation in Lung Cancer. In: Perspectives in Lung Cancer. Frederick E Jones Memorial Sumposium in Thoracic Surgery, Columbus, Ohio, 1976, Williams TE, Wilson HE, Yohn DS, (eds) Basel, S. Karger, 1977, pp 57-65.

18. Holmes EC, Ramming KP, Bein ME et al.: Intralesional BCG Immunotherapy of Pulmonary tumors. J Thorac Cardiovasc. Surg 77:362-368, 1979.

19. Kirsh MM, Prior M, Gago et al.: The Effect of Histological Cell Type on the Prognosis of Patients with Bronchogenic Carcinoma. Ann Thorac Surg 13:303-310, 1972.

20. Kirsh MM, Rotman H, Argenta L.: Carcinoma of the Lung: Results of Treatment Over Ten Years. Ann Thorac Surg 21:371-377, 1976.

21. Green N, Kurohara SS, George FW et al.: Postresection Irradiation for Primary Lung Cancer. Radiology 116:405-407, 1975.

22. Adkins PC: Neoplasms of the Lung Carcinoma of the Lung. In: Gibbon's Surgery of the Chest, Sabiston DC, Spencer FC, (eds) Philadelphia, W. B. Saunders Company, 1976, 443-472.

23. Green N, Kurohara SS, George FW: Cancer of the Lung. An in Depth Analysis of Prognostic Factors, Cancer 28:1229-1233.

24. Lee YTN: Prognostic Factors in Surgical Treatment of Bronchogenic Carcinoma. Surg Gyn Obstet 135:961-975, 1972.

25. Green N, Kern W: The Clinical Course and Treatment Results of Patients With Postresection Locally Recurrent Lung Cancer. Cancer 42:2478-2482, 1978.

26. Shields TW: Thoughts Concerning the Management of Patients With Carcinoma of the Lung. In: Perspectives in Lung Cancer. Frederick E Jones Memorial Symposium in Thoracic Surgery, Columbus, Ohio, 1976. Williams TE, Wilson HE, Yohn DS (eds) Basel, S. Karger, 1977, pp 82-93, 1977.

27. Mountain CF: A Surgeon's Insight Into Tumor Behavior. In: Perspectives in Lung Cancer. Frederick E Jones Memorial Symposium in Thoracic Surgery, Columbus, Ohio, 1976, Williams TE, Wilson HE, Yohn DS (eds), Basel, S. Karger, 1977, pp 18-29.

28. Mountain CF: The Relationship of Prognosis to Morphology and the Anatomic Extent of Disease: Studies of a New Clinical Staging System. In: Lung Cancer – Natural History, Prognosis, and Therapy, Isreal L, Chahinian AP, (eds) New York Academic Press, 1976, pp 107-140.

29. Mountain CF, Carr DT, Anderson AD: A System for the Clinical Staging of Lung Cancer. Am J Roentgen 120:130-138, 1974.

30. Shields TW, Yee J, Conn JH et al.: Relationship of Cell Type and Lymph Node Metastasis to Survival After Resection of Bronchial Carcinoma. Ann Thorac Surg 20:501-510, 1975.

31. Mountain CF: Assessment of the Role of Surgery for Control of Lung Cancer. Ann Thorac Surg 42:365-373, 1977.

32. Martini N, Beattie EJ: Results of Surgical Treatment in Stage I Lung Cancer. J Thorac Cardiovasc Surg 74:499-505, 1977.

33. Carr DT: Does Staging Help? In: Perspectives in Lung Cancer. Frederick E Jones Memorial Symposium in Thoracic Surgery, Columbus, Ohio, 1976, Williams TE, Wilson HE, Yohn DS, (eds) Basel, S. Karger, 1977, pp 41-46.

34. Bergh NP, Schersten T: Bronchogenic Carcinoma. Acta Chir Scand (Suppl) 347:1-42, 1965.
35. Shields TW: Pulmonary Resections. In: General Thoracic Surgery, Shields TW (ed) Philadelphia, Lea & Febiger, 1972, 331-350.
36. Shields TW: Carcinoma of the Lung. In: General Thoracic Surgery, Shields TW (ed) Philadelphia, Lea & Febiger, 1972, 797-844.
37. Mountain CF: Surgical Therapy In Lung Cancer: Biologic, Physiologic and Technical Determinants. Semin Oncol 1:253-258, 1974.
38. Shields TW, Higgins GA, Keehn RJ: Factors Influencing Survival After Resection for Bronchial Carcinoma. J Thorac Cardiovasc Surg 64:391-399, 1972.
39. Vincent RG, Takita H, Lane WW et al.: Surgical Therapy of Lung Cancer. J. Thorac Carciovasc. Surg. 71:581-591, 1976.
40. Smith AR: The Importance of Mediastinal Lymph Node Invasion by Pulmonary Carcinoma in Section of Patients for Resection. Ann Thorac Surg 25:5-11, 1978.
41. Naruke T, Suemasu K, Ishikawa S: Surgical Treatment for Lung Cancer With Metastasis to Mediastinal Lymph Nodes. J Thorac Cardiovasc Surg 71:279-282, 1976.
42. Naruke T, Suemasu K, Ishikawa S: Lymph Node Mapping and Curability at Various Levels of Metastasis in Resected Lung Cancer. J Thorac Cardiovasc Surg 76:832-839, 1978.
43. Paulson DL, Reisch JS: Long-term Survival After Resection for Bronchogenic Carcinoma. Ann. Surg. 184:324-332, 1976.
44. del Regato Juan, Spjut HJ: Cancer of the Respiratory System and Upper Digestive Tract. In: Cancer – Diagnosis, Treatment, and Prognosis. del Regato JA, Spjut HJ (eds) St. Louis, C V Mosby Company. 1977, pp 224-409.
45. Green N, Kurohara SS, George FW et al.: The Biologic Behavior of Lung Cancer According to Histologic Type. Radiol Clin Biol 41:160-170, 1972.
46. Rosenblatt MB, Lisa JR, Collier F: Criteria for the Histologic Diagnosis of Bronchogenic Carcinoma. Chest 51:587-595, 1967.
47. Vincent RG, Pickren JW, Lane WW et al.: The Changing Histopathyology of Lung Cancer. Cancer 39:1647-1655, 1977.
48. Whitwell F: The Histopathology of Lung Cancer in Liverpool. The Specificity of the Histological Cell Types of Lung Cancer. Brit J Cancer 15:429-439, 1961.
49. Matthews MJ: Problems in Morphology and Behavior of Bronchopulmonary Malignant Disease. In: Lung Cancer – Natural History, Prognosis, and Therapy, Isreal L, Chahinian AP, (eds) New York, Academic Press, 1976, pp 23-62.
50. Jones JC, Kern WH, Chapman ND et al.: Long-term Survival After Surgical Resection for Bronchogenic Carcinoma. J Thorac Cardiovasc Surg 54:383-392, 1967.
51. Spjut HJ, Mateo LE: Recurrent and Metastatic Carcinoma in Surgically Treated Carcinoma of Lung. Cancer 18:1462-1466, 1965.
52. Matthews MJ, Pickren J, Kanhouwa S. Who Has Occult Metastasis? In: Perspectives in Lung Cancer. Frederick E. Jones Memorial Symposium in Thoracic Surgery, Columbus, Ohio, 1976, Williams TE, Wilson HE, Yohn DS. (eds) Basel, S. Karger, 1977, pp 9-17.
53. Line DH, Deeley TJ: The Necropsy Findings in Carcinoma of the Bronchus. Br J Dis Chest 65:238-242, 1971.
54. Rasmussen PS: The Incidence of Local Recurrence and Distant Metastasis in Surgically Treated Cases of Lung Cancer. Acta Path et Microbiol Scandinav 62:145-150, 1964.
55. Hilaris BS, Martini N, Batata M: Interstitial Irradiation for Unresectable Carcinoma of the Lung. Ann Thorac Surg 20:491-510, 1975.
56. Phillips TL, Miller RJ: Editorials – Should Asymptomatic Patients With Inoperable Bronchogenic Carcinoma Receive Immediate Radiotherapy? YES. Am Rev Respir Dis 117:405-414, 1978.

57. Lee RE: Radiotherapy of Bronchogenic Carcinoma. Semin Oncol 1:245-252, 1974.
58. Salazar OM, Rubin P, Brown JC: Predictors of Radiation Response in Lung Cancer. Cancer 37:2636-2650, 1976.
59. Rissanen PM, Tikka U, Holsti LR: Autopsy Findings in Lung Cancer Treated with Megavoltage Radiotherapy. Acta Radiologica Therapy Physics Biology 7:433-442, 1968.
60. Komaki R, Cox JD, Eisert DR: Irradiation of Bronchial Carcinoma-II Pattern of Spread and Potential for Prophylactic Irradiation. Int J Radiat Oncol Biol Phys 2:441-446, 1977.
61. Eisert Dr, Cox JD, Komaki R: Irradiation for Bronchial Carcinoma Reasons for Failure. Cancer 37:2665-2670, 1976.
62. Perez CA: Radiation Therapy for Cancer of the Lung: Previous Experience and Definition of Current Issues. Cancer Chemother Rep 4:145-152, 1973.
63. Rubin P, Ciccio S, Setisarn B: The Controversial Status of Radiation Therapy in Lung Cancer. Nat Cancer Conf Proc 6th pp 855-866, 1968.
64. Perez CA: Radiation Therapy in the Management of Carcinoma of the Lung. Cancer 39:901-916, 1977.
65. Aristizabal SA, Caldwell WL: Radical Irradiation With the Split Course Technique in Carcinoma of the Lung. Cancer 37:2630-2635, 1976.
66. Chahinian AP, Isreal L: Rates and Patterns of Growth of Lung Cancer. In: Lung Cancer. National History, Prognosis and Therapy, Isreal L, Chahinian AP, (eds) New York, Academic Press, 1976, pp 63-79.
67. Chahinian AP, Isreal L: Prognostic Value of Doubling Time and Related Factors in Lung Cancer. In: Lung Cancer. National History, Prognosis, and Therapy. Isreal L, Chahinian AP, (eds) New York, Academic Press, 1976, pp 95-106.
68. Morrison R, Deeley TJ, Cleland WP: The Treatment of Carcinoma of the Bronchus. The Lancet pp 683-684, 1963.
69. Selawry OS, Hansen HH: Lung Cancer. In: Cancer Medicine, Holland JF, Frei E. (eds) Philadelphia, Lea & Febiger, 1973.
70. Bloedorn FG, Cowley RA, Cuccia CA. Preoperative Irradiation in Bronchogenic Carcinoma. Amer J Roentgenol 92:77-87, 1964.
71. Warram J: Preoperative Irradiation of Cancer of the Lung: Final Report of a Therapeutic Trial. Cancer 36:914-925, 1975.
72. Warram J: Preoperative Irradiation of Cancer of the Lung. Cancer 23:419-470, 1969.
73. Shields TW, Higgins GA, Lawton R: Preoperative X-ray Therapy as an Adjuvant in the Treatment of Bronchogenic Carcinoma. J Thorac Cardiovasc Surg 59:49-61, 1970.
74. Abadir R, Muggia FM: Irradiated Lung Cancer. An Autopsy Analysis of Spread Pattern. Radiology 114:427-430, 1975.
75. Emami B, Lee DJ, Munzenrider J: The Value of Supraclavicular Area Treatment in Radiotherapeutic Management of Lung Cancer. Cancer 41:124-129, 1978.
76. Smart J: Can Lung Cancer Be Cured By Irradiation Alone? JAMA 195:158-159, 1966.
77. Bangma PJ: Post-Operative Radiotherapy. In: Modern Radiotherapy-Carcinoma of the Bronchus, Deeley TJ, (ed) New York, Appleton-Century-Crofts, 1971, pp 163-170.
78. Paterson R, Russell MH: Clinical Trials in Malignant Disease. Clin Radiol 13:141-144, 1962.
79. Bangma PJ, Tonkes E: De Waarde Van Postoperative Rontgenbestraling Bij Bronchus-Carcinoom. Nederl T Geneesk 109:653-657, 1965.
80. Kirsh MM, Kahn DR, Gago O et al.: Treatment of Bronchogenic Carcinoma With Mediastinal Metastases. Ann Thorac Surg 12: 11-21, 1971.
81. Cahan WG, Watson WL, Pool JL: ·Radical Pneumonectomy. J Thorac Surg 22:449-473, 1951.
82. Rubin P: Comment: Combination Therapy-Irradiation, Surgery, and Chemotherapy. JAMA 196:136, 1966.

83. Rubin P, Perez CA, Keller B: The Logical Basis of Radiation Treatment Policies in the Multidisciplinary approach to Lung Cancer. In: Lung Cancer. Natural History, Prognosis, and Therapy. Isreal L, Chahinian AP. (Eds) New York, Academic Press, 1976, pp 159-197.
84. Carlens E. Mediastinoscopy: A Method for Inspection and Tissue Biopsy in the Superior Mediastinum. Chest XXXVI:343-352, 1959.
85. Foster ED, Munro DD, Dobell ARC. Mediastinoscopy. Ann Thorac Surg 13:273-286, 1972.
86. Goldberg EM, Clicksman AS, Khan FR et al.: Mediastinoscopy for Assessing Mediastinal Spread in Clinical Staging of Carcinoma of the Lung. Cancer 25:347-353, 1969.
87. Weiss W: Operative Mortality and Five-Year Survival Rates in Men With Bronchogenic Carcinoma. Chest 66:483-487, 1974.
88. Ramsey HE, Cahan WG, Beattie EJ et al.: The Importance of Radical Lobectomy in Lung Cancer. J Thorac Cardiovasc Surg 59:225-230, 1969.
89. Sherrah-Davies E: Does Postoperative Irradiation Improve Survival in Lung Cancer: JAMA 196:133-135, 1966.
90. Shields TW: Carcinoma of the Lung. In: General Thoracic Surgery, Shields TW. (ed) Philadelphia, Lea & Febiger, 1972, pp 797-845.
91. Watson WL: Radical Surgery for Lung Cancer. Cancer 9:1167-1172, 1956.
92. Cleland WP: The Place of Surgery in the Treatment of Carcinoma of the Bronchus. In: Modern Radiotherapy-Carcinoma of the Bronchus, Deeley TJ, (ed) New York, Appleton-Century-Crofts, 1971, pp 139-151.
93. Peters RM, Clausen JL, Tisi GM: Extending Resectability for Carcinoma of the Lung in Patients With Impaired Pulmonary Function. Ann Thorac Surg 26:250-260, 1968.
94. Jensik RJ: Preoperative Irradiation and Bronchopulmonary Sleeve Resection for Lung Cancer. In: The Surgical Clinics of North America, Moulder PV, (ed) Philadelphia, W B Saunders Company, 1966, pp 145-159.
95. Rees GM, Paneth M: Lobectomy With Sleeve Resection in the Treatment of Bronchial Tumours. Thorax 25:160-164, 1970.
96. Green N, Iba G, Shirley JK: The Clinical Experience of Patients With Carcinoma of the Lung and Chronic Pulmonary Disease Treated by Radiotherapy. Radiology 111:189-192, 1974.
97. Guttman RJ. Results of Radiation Therapy in Patients with Inoperable Carcinoma of the Lung Whose Status was Established at Exploratory Thoracotomy. Am J Roentgen 93:99-103, 1965.
98. Teates D, Cooper G: Some Consequences of Pulmonary Irradiation. 96:612-619, 1966.
99. Lipshitz HI, Southard ME: Complications of Radiation Therapy: The Thorax. Semin Roentgenol IX:41-49, 1974.
100. Hellman S, Kligerman MM, von Essen CF et al.: Sequelae of Radical Radiotherapy of Carcinoma of the Lung. Radiology 182:1055-1061, 1964.
101. Gross NJ: Pulmonary Effects of Radiation Therapy. Ann Intern Med 86:81-92, 1977.
102. Cohn KE, Stewart JR, Fajardo LF: Heart Disease Following Radiation. Medicine 46:281-298, 1967.
103. Westerhof PW, van der Putte SCJ: Radiation Pericarditis and Myocardial Fibrosis. Eur J Cardiol 4/2, 213-218, 1976.
104. Tracy GP, Brown DE, Johnson LW et al.: Radiation-Induced Coronary Artery Disease. JAMA 228:1660-1662, 1974.
105. Lambert PM: Radiation Myelopathy of the Thoracic Spinal Cord in Long Term Survivors Treated With Radical Radiotherapy Using Conventional Fractionation. Cancer 41:1751-1760, 1978.

106. Weiss NS, Siverman DT, Baylis PH: Should Curative Surgery Be Attempted in Patients With Cancer of the Main Stem Bronchus? Cancer 38:1013-1016, 1976.

107. Naef AP: Tracheobronchial Reconstruction. Ann Thorac Surg 15:301-312, 1973.

108. Gronqvist YKJ, Clagett OT, McDonald JR: Involvement of the Thoracic Wall in Bronchogenic Carcinoma. J Thoracic Surg 33:487-495, 1957.

109. Paulson DL: Carcinomas in the Superior Pulmonary Sulcus. J Thorac Cardiovasc Surg 70:1095-1104, 1975.

110. Geha AS, Bernatz PE, Woolner LB: Bronchogenic Carcinoma involving the Thoracic Wall. J Thorac Cardiovasc Surg 54:394-402, 1967.

111. Ashor GL, Kern WH, Meyer BW et al.: Long-Term Survival in Bronchogenic Carcinoma. J Thorac Cardiovasc Surg 70:581-589, 1975.

112. Grillo HC, Greenberg JJ, Wilkins EW: Resection of Bronchogenic Carcinoma Involving Thoracic Wall. J Thorac Cardiovasc Surg 51:417-421, 1966.

113. Watkins E, Gerard FP: Malignant Tumors Involving the Chest Wall. J Thoracic and Cardiovasc Surg 39:117-129, 1960.

114. Sherman DM, Neptune W, Weichselbaum R et al.: An Aggressive Approach to Marginally Resectable Lung Cancer. Cancer 41:2040-2045, 1978.

115. Deeley TJ: The Treatment of Carcinoma of the Bronchus. Br J Radiol 40:801-822, 1967.

6. The Role of Radiation Therapy in the Treatment of Regional Non-small(oat)-cell Carcinoma of the Lung

JOEL ELLIOT WHITE and MURRAY BOLES

1. HISTORICAL DEVELOPMENT

The first autopsy description of lung cancer in the American medical literature appeared in the *Boston Medical Journal* in 1835[1]. The patient had expired following radical treatment with cathartics and hot toddies. Postmortem examination revealed a tumor, 'probably of lung origin,' invading the pericardium, mediastinum, pleura, ribs, and vertebral column.

In the 1860's Salter delivered a series of lectures on pulmonary disease at Charing Cross Hospital in London. These lectures were subsequently published as a series beginning in July, 1869[2]. Salter concluded his series with a discussion on lung cancer. He was pessimistic and stated: 'With regards to treatment... I need not tell you that I have nothing to tell you.'

When X-rays were discovered some 26 years later, they were put to therapeutic use almost immediately. However, the limitations in the energy of X-ray that was available were soon apparent to clinicians such as Dr. Margaret Cleaves. She indicated a need for higher energy radiation when she wrote: '... if a higher, more penetrative, and a more active chemically disorganizing vibration than is obtained from an X-ray....'[3]. She indicated that radium fulfilled those requirements, but that its clinical effectiveness suffered from the limitation of having to be placed in an accessible cavity.

In 1932, Edwards alluded to the use of 'deep X-ray,' only to indicate that results had been disappointing[4]. He expressed doubt that there was even temporary improvement. He did describe the use of interstitially-placed radioactive radon seeds, as well as the use of a newly-designed special container into which radon seeds could be placed. The container was bronchoscopically placed against the tumor for a few days.

One year later Ormerod reported 'slightly more encouraging' results with deep X-ray therapy, especially some improvement in two patients with upper lobe lesions[5]. Four years later he reported primarily on the use of radon

R. B. Livingston (ed.), Lung cancer 1, 113–156. All rights reserved.
Copyright © 1981 Martinus Nijhoff Publishers bv, The Hague/Boston/London.

seed implants and container applications, while indicating that X-ray therapy was used only on hopeless cases [6].

In 1940, Leddy and Moersch compared a group of 125 untreated patients to 125 patients who had received radiation therapy [7]. Although 88 of the 125 patients (70%) in the irradiated group received totally inadequate radiation, 20% of the irradiated group survived from 1–12 years, including five patients who survived more than five years. None of the untreated patients survived one year.

In 1944, Hocker and Guttmann reported their first 3 1/2 years' experience with a 1-Mev X-ray machine, one of the first of its kind, which had been designed by Dr. G. Failla [8]. Of 93 patients with lung cancer who were treated with tumor doses of about 4000–5000 roentgens, 21 survived from 3 to 24 months, 11 of these without evidence of disease. Two of four patients followed longer than 24 months were alive without evidence of disease.

Eight years later, in 1952, Blomfield reported to the Royal Society of Medicine on his preliminary experience with a 2-Mev Van de Graff X-ray unit [9]. He noted that while this machine was of some value in some types of carcinoma, only one of 39 lung cancer patients had survived more than two years, and that patient had developed a recurrence.

The real impetus for continuing radiation therapy in inoperable patients derives from studies of preoperative radiation which have shown tumor sterilization [10, 11]. In 1955, Bromley and Szur reported on the treatment of 573 lung cancer patients 'to tolerance' [10]. After a rest period, 66 of the 573 patients were felt to have become operable. The authors found no viable residual tumor in 46% of the 66 cases, and in 22.5% degenerating tumor was found with an occasional questionably viable tumor cell. The average tumor dose was relatively low – approximately 4700 roentgens – but because kilovoltage radiation was utilized, there was a high incidence of postoperative complications, especially empyema and fistulas. In a similar study employing megavoltage radiation, Bloedorn and associates first reported on a group of 26 patients who received 60 Gy (for megavoltage radiation, 1 Gy = 100 rad) to the chest preoperatively over a six-week period [11]. Careful study of multiple sections of the operative specimens showed no recognizable tumor cells at the primary site in 54% of patients and none in the mediastinal lymph nodes of 92% of patients. Subsequent publications by Bloedorn with additional patients gave similar findings [12].

In 1956, Smart and Hilton reported a series of patients treated by radiation therapy alone [13]. They compared 531 operable patients treated by surgery to 33 similar patients treated by radiation therapy alone. The 5-year survival for the surgical group was 32%, and the 10-year survival was 21%. Of the 12 patients eligible for 5-year followup in the radiation-alone group, four survived without evidence of disease. The authors noted, however, that only patients who had undergone successful surgery were included among the surgical group. Those patients who were found to be inoperable at the time of surgery – about 1/3 of the usual surgical series – were not counted in the survival figures. On an actuarial basis the authors found that survival was higher in the radiation-therapy-alone group during the first three years, primarily because of the adverse effect of surgical mortality, but was the same as the surgical group in the 4th and 5th year.

Thus the stage was set for the controversy that was to develop during the succeeding two decades.

2. CLINICAL ISSUES INFLUENCING TREATMENT MODALITY

2.1. Controversies

In 1968, Roswit and associates published the results of a large-scale randomized study of radiation therapy versus placebo conducted through the Veterans Administration Lung Group[14]. 800 patients with loco-regionally inoperable lung cancer and no apparent distant metastasis were randomized to one of three treatment groups. 308 patients received radiation therapy alone, 246 patients received placebo tablets, and 246 patients received a variety of chemotherapeutic agents that were under test as the series progressed. 90% of the irradiated group were treated with orthovoltage radiation, and 1/3 of all the patients received doses less than 40 Gy. About half the patients received doses in the range of 40–50 Gy, and 14% received doses over 50 Gy. Although often quoted as showing no difference in the treatment groups, this study demonstrated statistically significant improved survival at the end of one year, with a p value = .05, for the patients receiving radiation therapy. Furthermore, when the 25% of patients who lived the longest in each group were compared, those who received radiation lived at least 307 days, compared to 233 days for the two control groups (p = .01).

This study has often been misquoted as justification and rationale for not giving radiation therapy to patients with regionally inoperable disease. In fact, the ensuing decade after that study is best exemplified by the title of a presentation by Rubin and associates at the Sixth National Cancer Conference: 'The Controversial Status of Radiation Therapy in Lung Cancer'[15]. Two significant facts have emerged out of this controversy. First, in many of the older reported series, patients who were considered to have loco-regional disease would probably be found to have distant metastases if evaluated with today's current methods. Secondly, a number of factors have emerged as being of prognostic significance[14, 16–19], and these will be discussed further.

2.2. Pathological Considerations

A compilation of the commonest sites of metastasis, which is based on a weighted average of several large autopsy series (Table 1) might suggest that there is no role for local therapy in regionally advanced disease, because of the probability of widespread dissemination. However, a significant problem with this conclusion is that these series analyze all stages and cell types together, including oat cell carcinoma, which has a higher incidence of distant metastasis[30]. A second problem with this conclusion is that most of these patients have died of their lung cancer. Recently, Matthews and her associates updated their earlier analysis[25], of patients dying within 30 days after 'curative' resection[25, 31]. Only 1/3 of their patients had residual disease, and of these, 40% (30/73) had regional disease only (Table 2). The implication is that the actual incidence of dissemination in patients with regionally inoperable disease may be somewhere between the widespread involvement indicated by autopsy studies of patients dying of disseminated lung cancer,

Table 1. Weighted distribution of metastasis-pooled data.

	Number of patients*	Number (percentage) of metastasis
Adrenal	5307	1378 (26)
Bone	5307	1289 (24)
Brain	5508	1527 (28)
Liver	5307	1853 (35)
Lung	4580	965 (21)
Kidney	284	20 (7)
Pancreas	284	19 (7)

Pooled data from ten autopsy series (20, 21, 22, 23, 24, 25, 26, 27, 28, 29).
* Number of patients at each site differs, as not all sites were reported in all series.

Table 2. Incidence of residual disease in 230 non-small cell lung cancer patients dying within thirty days of curative resection.

Histologic type	Number of patients	Number (percentage) persistent disease	Number (percentage) regional only
Squamous cell carcinoma	171	53 (35)	27 (16)
Adenocarcinoma	34	16 (47)	3 (9)
Large cell undifferentiated carcinoma	25	4 (16)	0
Total	230	73 (32)	30 (13)

Modified from Matthews and associates, 1973, 1977 (25, 31).

Table 3. Site of failure after definitive radiation therapy.

Author	Number of failures	Number of loco-regional initial or only site of failure*	Percentage loco-regional initial or only site of failure*
Abadir & Muggia [20]	41	13	32
Rissanen *et al.* [27] (a)	18	10	56
Bergsagel *et al.* [32] (b)	115	56	47
Cox *et al.* [33]	146	30	21
Komaki *et al.* [34] (c)	178	108	61
Ghilezan *et al.* [35]	114	41	61
	612	258	42

* The number and percentage of patients in whom loco-regional disease was the initial or only site of failure after radiation therapy.
(a) Includes only patients with "complete response" to radiation therapy.
(b) Includes 24 patients with oat cell carcinoma.
(c) Includes 23 patients with oat cell carcinoma.

and that indicated by studies of patients dying within a short time of curative resection. This possibility is supported by the fact (Table 3) that 30–60% of patients who fail after primary treatment with radiation therapy, initially fail regionally [20, 27, 32–35], and by the fact that about 1/2 to 3/4 of these patients die of their loco-regional disease [33, 34]. Squamous cell carcinomas tend to have a higher incidence of initial loco-regional failure when compared to patients with other histologies [20, 30, 31, 33]. This is primarily because adenocarcinomas and large cell undifferentiated carcinomas have earlier and more frequent distant metastasis.

Table 4. Five year survival for inoperable carcinoma of the lung treated primarily by radiation therapy-pooled data*.

Interval (months)**	Number patients**	Number surviving	Percentage surviving
6	969	584	60
12	4656	1631	35
18	471	128	27
24	3756	675	18
36	2363	267	11
48	390	31	8
60	2434	151	6

* Pooled data on over 6000 patients (13, 14, 16, 17, 19, 35, 36, 37, 38, 39, 40, 41, 42, 43, 44, 45, 46, 47, 48, 49, 50, 51, 52, 53, 54, 55, 56).
** Only intervals for which significant data was available are employed. Number of patients in each interval differs according to intervals reported by various authors.

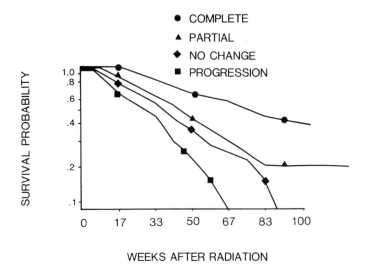

WEEKS AFTER RADIATION

Fig. 1. Survival by degree of local control. Radiation Therapy Oncology Group Protocol 73–01, preliminary analysis, January, 1979. Presented at the 21st annual meeting of the American Society of Therapeutic Radiologists, October 24, 1979, New Orleans, Louisiana. Data and graph courtesy of Dr. Carlos Perez [19].

Degree of Regression	Alive	Dead	Total	Median Survival (weeks)
Complete	27	38	65	75.3
Partial	32	90	122	44.9
No Change	55	95	150	36.5
Progression	1	17	18	29.4

Cox and associates indicated that survival was significantly shorter in those patients failing to achieve local control [17, 33, 34]. This was supported by Perez when he made his presentation of Radiation Therapy Oncology Group data (Fig. 1) in which a statistically significant difference in survival was found in favor of those who had complete or more than 50% disappearance of the primary tumor mass following radiation therapy [19]. Therefore, treatment directed at improving local control can have a significant impact on survival.

Pooled data of survival results (Table 4) from multiple series reported in the literature indicates a 5-year survival of about 6% for patients with regionally inoperable lung cancer treated by radiation alone [13, 14, 16, 17, 19, 35–56]. Despite the fact that authors report different intervals, techniques, and endpoints, the resulting average figures are remarkably close to those reported in individual series during the past two decades.

2.3. Prognostic Variables

Table 5 lists some of the factors that have emerged as being of important prognostic significance. Caldwell and Bagshaw found pain, weight loss of 10 lbs. or more, supraclavicular metastases, hemoptysis or presence of a large mass requiring treatment fields greater than 200 sq cm to be indicators of a poor prognosis [16]. Lanzotti and associates found weight loss to be the major prognostic indicator, followed by performance status, supraclavicular metastasis, and age [18]. Roswit and associates noted histology to be of importance, with well-differentiated squamous cell carcinomas and adenocarcinomas having a better prognosis with therapy [14]. Using similar criteria for purposes of analysis, Emami and associates divided patients into favorable and unfavorable categories: the favorable group had a median survival of 21 months, compared to 4 months for the unfavorable group [41]. They also noted a significantly higher rate of local control (68.3% vs. 45%) in the favorable group. In a report of Radiation Therapy Oncology Group studies, Perez and associates noted performance status and mediastinal node involvement to be important factors [19].

Table 5. Prognostic factors in regional non small cell carcinoma of the lung.

Performance status
Weight loss
Supraclavicular metastasis
Histopathology
Pain
Malignant pleural involvement
Vocal cord paralysis
Mediastinal node metastasis

Prognostic factors in regional non-small-cell lung cancer. Compiled from Caldwell and Bagshaw (16), Perez and associates (19), and Lanzotti and associates (18). Performance status is a rating of functional ability. The performance status scale employed by the Southwest Oncology Group is demonstrated in Table 6.

3. RADIATION BIOLOGY

In 1977, Gross [57] reviewed the radiation biology topics which appeared to be pertinent to treatment of pulmonary malignancies. He pointed out that the absorption of ionizing radiation in tissue results in the acceleration of orbital electrons, producing ion pairs. The ion pairs generate free radicals, and these highly reactive compounds produce the biological effects through the breakage of chemical bonds. The presence of oxygen molecules produces organic peroxides, which fix the biochemical effects of free radicals in non-restorable form. Therefore, the presence of oxygen in biological systems particularly

Table 6. Southwest Oncology Group scale of performance status.

Able to carry on normal activity; no special care is needed	10	Normal; no complaints, no evidence of disease
	9	Able to carry on normal activity; minor signs or symptoms of disease
	8	Normal activity with effort; some signs or symptoms of disease
Unable to work, able to live at home, cares for most personal needs; a varying amount of assistance is needed	7	Cares for self, unable to carry on normal activity, do active work
	6	Requires occasional assistance, but is able to care for most of his needs
	5	Requires considerable assistance and frequent medical care
Unable to care for self; requires equivalent of institutional or hospital care; disease may be progressing rapidly	4	Disabled; requires special care and assistance
	3	Severely disabled, hospitalization is indicated, although death not imminent
	2	Very sick; hospitalization necessary; active supportive treatment necessary
	1	Moribund; fatal process progressing rapidly
	0	Dead

For purposes of protocol analysis and stratification, the performance scale is usually divided into 3 groupings: 1-4, 5-7, 8-10.

enhances the effects of sparsely ionizing radiation, such as photons (X-rays and gamma rays).

3.1. Genetic and Non-genetic Damage

The biological effect of radiation on the cell expresses itself either by damage to DNA or to non-genetic macromolecules such as proteins and polysaccharides. The polymer-strand breakage produced by radiation is repairable in vivo, and it has been concluded that a single large dose of radiation is more damaging to these macromolecules than the same total dose administered in several fractions.

The effect of the genetic damage through DNA is expressed following mitosis in which non-viable daughter cells occur.

Damage to the cell by a non-genetic mechanism probably occurs through increased permeability of membranes and fragmentation of connective tissue. This results in immediate lethal effects.

With the exception of certain highly sensitive cells such as lymphocytes it generally appears that genetic damage occurs at much lower doses than lethal non-genetic damage.

3.2. Cytokinetics

Since lower doses are required for genetic damage, it is assumed that the majority of damage to tumor cells and normal tissue with clinical radiotherapy regimes occurs through the genetic mechanism. As a result, cells with a high mitotic rate, such as rapidly-dividing stem cells, manifest genetic damage earlier.

In pulmonary tissue, the cells which are more likely to suffer radiation-induced chromosomal changes are the bronchial epithelial cells, capillary endothelial cells and type II pneumocytes.

4. BEAM ENERGY

Guttmann reviewed the advantages of megavoltage radiation therapy (cobalt-60 energy or greater)[40]. These advantages include increased percentage depth dose; skin sparing; decreased backscatter, which results in increased normal tissue tolerance; and decreased absorption of radiation in bone and cartilage, which decreases the incidence of necrosis in these tissues.

One of the major criticisms of the first VA study by Roswit and associates, which demonstrated no long-term advantage of radiation therapy over untreated patients, was that orthovoltage equipment was used to treat 90% of the patients[14]. Rey and Haase reported that megavoltage therapy was more effective in terms of increased two and three-year survival results, but that the five-year survival rate was not altered[58].

CONCLUSIONS

When compared to orthovoltage, megavoltage radiation allows the delivery of a higher, more homogeneously-distributed radiation dose to the tumor, while sparing more of the normal tissues. Criticism which focuses on the lack of dramatic improvement in 'cure' rates ignores the improved tumor control rates in the chest with megavoltage modalities, and that the major problem with raising the 'cure' rates is distant dissemination. As new combined modality techniques evolve, the improved normal tissue tolerance of megavoltage radiation, as well as its more homogeneous dose distribution, will become increasingly important. Most current cooperative group protocols containing radiation therapy require megavoltage equipment for participation [59–63].

Table 7. Change in lung cancer treatment volume in 32 patients evaluated by computed tomography.

Characteristic	Number of patients (percentage change)
Altered treatment ports for more adequate tumor coverage	9 (28)
Decreased normal tissue volume irradiated	13 (40)

    Modified from Emami and associates, *AJR*, 1978 (65).

5. TREATMENT VOLUME

Both the most probable boundaries of the primary tumor and the most likely sites of potential or actual lymphatic metastasis must be considered in the design of radiation treatment ports.

The boundary between the primary tumor and normal tissue is often obscured by atelectasis and/or obstructive pneumonitis[42]. In some instances, it may be necessary to include the entirety of one lung in the initial treatment volume[64].

Invasion of mediastinal structures is difficult to detect with routine radiographic procedures. The use of computed tomography to assist in treatment planning is still investigational, but appears to be promising. Emami and associates[65], reported better tumor delineation in 75% of patients evaluated by computed tomography. There was a change in treatment ports for more adequate tumor coverage in 28% of patients evaluated (Table 7).

Deeley first described the inclusion of a 2-cm margin of normal tissue in lung cancer treatment fields[43, 44, 66, 67]. This distance has become a guideline for current United States national cooperative group studies (Southwest Oncology Group Protocols 7415, 7635, 7628; Radiation Therapy Oncology Group Protocols 78–11, 79–07, 79–14, 79–17; Eastern Cooperative Oncology Group Protocol 3578; Southeast Cooperative Oncology Group Protocol 76 LUN 308), which usually specify a minimum margin of 1 cm and a maximum margin of 2 cm of normal tissue. There is difficulty in adhering to this standard because of the large volume of normal lung that must be included

Fig. 2. Contrast-enhanced computed tomography of the chest.   ⟶

    A. Mediastinal lymph node involvement (arrows) undetected by other radiographic procedures. The treatment plan was altered to include mediastinal nodes in the boost volume.

    B. Vertebral metastasis (arrow) undetected by other radiographic and nuclear procedures. Patient considered candidate for palliative rather than definitive therapy.

    (CT scans courtesy of Steven C. Gross, M.D., Department of Diagnostic Radiology, Henry Ford Hospital, Detroit, Michigan.)

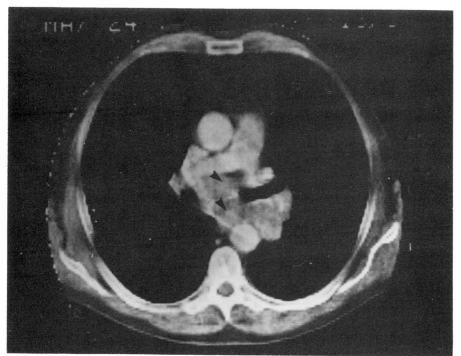

A

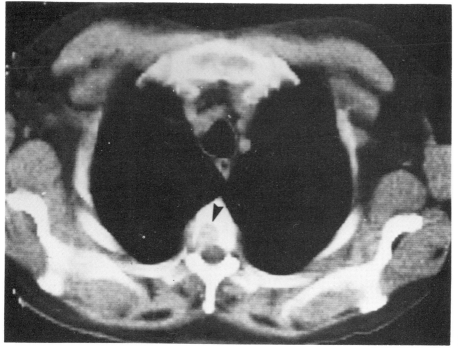

B

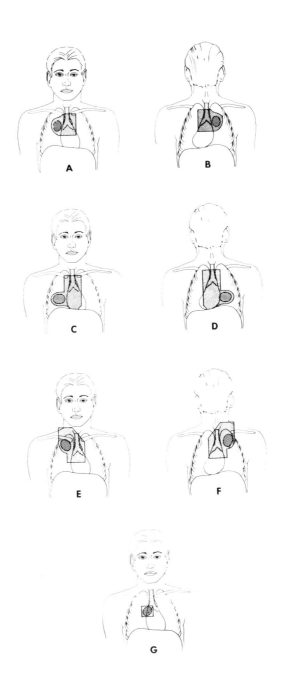

when the boundary of the tumor has not been discretely defined. Probably a majority of patients with lung cancer have compromised pulmonary function. While they can nevertheless be treated, restricting the volume of irradiated normal tissue leads to improved tolerance [42, 68]. Emami and associates reported that they were able to reduce the volume of normal tissue irradiated (Table 7) in 40% of patients they evaluated with computed tomography [65]. The authors have found CT scanning useful in both treatment planning and staging (Figure 2).

The frequency of mediastinal node involvement varies from 28–50%, even for potentially operable cases [69–72]. Upper lobe lesions frequently have mediastinal involvement without hilar metastasis [69, 70]. Bowen and associates found mediastinal node metastasis in 36% of 28 patients who had left upper lobe lesions and negative hila [69]. Goldberg and associates found mediastinal nodes and/or invasion in 48% of patients studied, 123 of whom had upper lobe tumors and 38 of whom had lower lobe tumors [70]. Well differentiated squamous cell tumors have less frequent mediastinal node metastasis [70, 71, 72], as do peripheral tumors [71, 72]. Goldberg and associates reported such involvement in 10 of 64 well differentiated squamous cell carcinomas, compared to 47 of 74 patients with poorly differentiated squamous cell or large cell undifferentiated carcinomas, and 12 of 18 patients with adenocarcinomas [70]. Whitcomb and associates reported 4 of 56 mediastinum-involved cases of squamous cell carcinoma, compared to 11 of 38 adenocarcinomas and 13 of 25 large cell undifferentiated carcinomas [72]. Regionally

←

Fig. 3. Treatment ports for well-differentiated tumors *without mediastinal invasion or mediastinal node metastasis*. For all ports it is recommended that the 90% isodose curve encompass the entire primary tumor site plus a minimum of 1 cm and maximum of 2 cm margin of normal tissue. The superior border should be 1 cm above the sternal notch. The maximum dose to the spinal cord should be limited in all cases by employment of a posterior block through the entire length of the treatment field to restrict the calculated spinal cord dose to the equivalent of a total of 50 Gy in 5 weeks or longer. In general, for co-axial opposed fields this implies insertion of the block at around 40 Gy midplane dose.

A. & B. Anterior and posterior treatment ports for central tumors without evidence of mediastinal involvement and/or mediastinal node metastasis; the inferior margin of the treatment port extends to 5 cm below the carina. The contralateral mediastinum is encompassed to its radiographic edge.

C. & D. Anterior and posterior treatment ports for lower lobe lesions without evidence of mediastinal involvement and/or mediastinal node metastasis. Note the inferior border of the mediastinal portion of the treatment port is extended down to the diaphragm.

E. & F. Anterior and posterior treatment ports for upper lobe lesions without evidence of mediastinal involvement and/or node metastasis. Note inclusion of the ipsilateral supraclavicular fossa. The inferior margin of the mediastinal port is 5 cm below the carina.

G. Primary tumor reduced 'boost' port. Portal arrangements should be such that the spinal cord receives none or only a negligible amount of the radiation delivered to the boost field. Many such treatment port arrangements are possible. An example is shown in Figure 4.

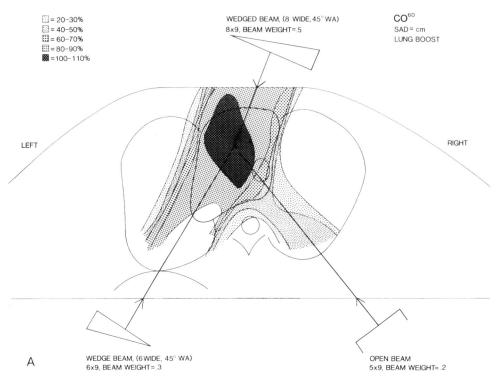

A

Fig. 4. Boost port isodose curves. A (cobalt-60) and B (6 MeV photons — Clinac 12 Linear Accelerator) are isodose distributions for boost fields designed to deliver added radiation to the gross tumor volume while sparing normal tissue, especially lung and spinal cord. In order to achieve this latter goal, it will sometimes be necessary to sacrifice perfect dosage homogeneity through the tumor volume, especially if the volume is relatively large. (Courtesy of Lenore I. Andres, R.T.T., Dosimetrist, Department of Therapeutic Radiology, Henry Ford Hospital, Detroit, Michigan.)

inoperable tumors frequently have mediastinal involvement as a cause of inoperability, or have a high risk of such involvement because they are large and/or are centrally located. Most authors include the mediastinal nodes in their treatment ports [16, 17, 35, 42–45, 66, 67].

Treatment of supraclavicular nodes is somewhat more controversial. About 20–30% of patients will be found to have scalene node involvement if routine biopsies are performed [73, 74]. Huber and associates noted more frequent involvement by adenocarcinoma (47% of 19) and large cell undifferentiated carcinoma (36% of 66) than by squamous cell carcinoma (29% of 182) [74]. Six of 140 inoperable patients (4.3%) who did not receive supraclavicular radiation therapy failed in that site [71]. Four of the six had involved mediastinal nodes. Perez and associates reported a higher incidence (33% vs. 8.7%) of supraclavicular recurrence when that area was not included in the treat-

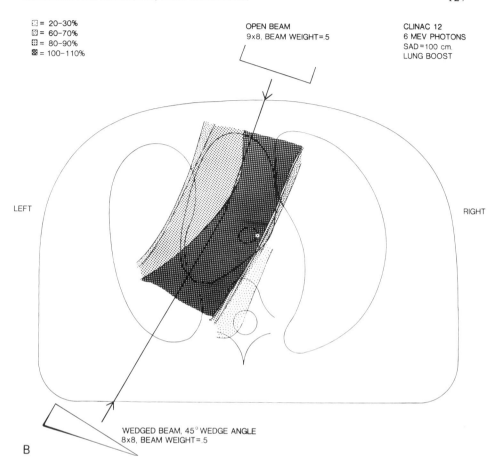

B

ment field in patients with superior vena cava syndrome (usually indicative of mediastinal involvement)[75].

Treatment field size is also controversial. Ghilezan and associates found the best 5-year survival (7.6%) in a group of patients treated with fields smaller than 150 cm², indicating smaller, earlier-stage tumors[35]. Caldwell and Bagshaw found superior survival among patients treated with fields between 100–200 cm²[16]. They felt that fields smaller than 100 cm² were inadequate to cover all potential disease, and that fields over 200 cm² indicated very bulky disease incurable by radiation alone.

CONCLUSIONS

It is the general recommendation of the authors that a minimum 1-cm margin and a maximum 2-cm margin of normal tissue be encompassed by

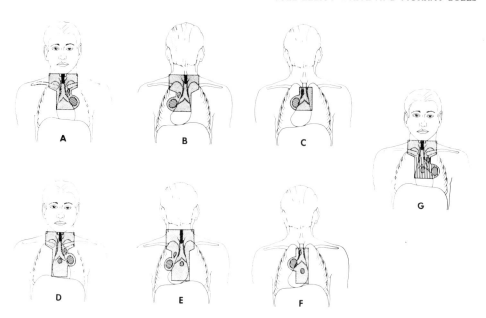

Fig. 5. Treatment ports for *mediastinal invasion and/or mediastinal node metastasis.* (Also for poorly-differentiated or undifferentiated tumors.) The primary tumor margin is as described in Figure 3. The bilateral supraclavicular regions are treated in all cases. A 1 cm wide, 5-half-value-layer block is employed anteriorly to protect the trachea and midline larynx if the field extends that high; the block extends from the superior border of the supraclavicular port to 1 cm above the suprasternal notch; care should be taken not to shield the superior mediastinum, especially if it is involved. When the supraclavicular regions are also treated from the posterior, a 2-cm wide, 5-half-value-layer block should extend from the superior margin of the treatment port to the level of the first thoracic vertebra to protect the spinal cord. A spinal cord block should be employed along the entire length of the posterior treatment port as described in Figure 2 to restrict the spinal cord dose.

   A. & B. Anterior and posterior treatment ports for patients who do not have subcarinal node involvement or lower lobe lesions. The inferior border extends to 5 cm below the carina.

   C. Alternate posterior treatment port used in conjunction with 'A.' This port does not include the supraclavicular region. When this port is used, the supraclavicular region should be boosted as in G.

   D. & E. Anterior and posterior treatment ports for patients with subcarinal and/or lower mediastinal node involvement and/or lower lobe lesions. The inferior border extends to the level of the diaphragm.

   F. Alternate posterior treatment port used in conjunction with 'D.' This port does not include the supraclavicular region. When this port is used, the supraclavicular region should be boosted as in 'G.'

   G. Supraclavicular boost port for use with posterior configuration C or F. If the supraclavicular port is treated from the anterior field only, it will receive a low dose. Therefore, the supraclavicular dose should be calculated and boosted. In order to avoid the problem of matching fields, the supraclavicular boost should be given by employing the anterior treatment port and then blocking the lower portion up to the sternal notch. (This technique was first suggested for use in Southwest Oncology Group protocols by Dr. Joaquin Mira of the Department of Radiation Oncology, University of Texas Medical Branch, San Antonio, Texas.)

the 90% isodose curve. Recommended treatment ports are outlined in Figs. 3 and 5. The mediastinum should be included to 5 cm below the carina for patients with upper lobe lesions, and down to the diaphragm for lower lobe lesions or when there is subcarinal node involvement. We recommend that· the supraclavicular regions be treated bilaterally in adenocarcinomas, poorly differentiated carcinomas, all large-cell type central carcinomas, and any cell type with mediastinal involvement. These recommendations are similar to those of Perez [76] and Logie and Kinzie [77].

6. TIME-DOSE RELATIONSHIPS

Since the clinical problem of radiation in malignancy is that doses must be limited so as to minimize normal tissue damage, a considerable number of studies have occurred documenting the factors leading to increased normal-tissue damage.

Ellis [78] was the first to attempt to demonstrate the equivalent biological effect in terms of a single unit, the relative equivalent therapy (RET). In a series of articles he expressed this unit in terms of total dose, number of fractions and time over which the total dose was given. This concept has proven to be useful in determining the probability of developing radiation complications and damage to normal tissue. It has been shown that there is increased damage to normal tissues when the total dose is increased, the number of fractions is decreased or the lapsed time in days is decreased. It has also been demonstrated that the larger the volume of lung irradiated, the higher the incidence of complications.

7. SPLIT-COURSE v. CONTINUOUS RADIATION

In 1959 Scanlon [79] reviewed the status of radiation therapy in what can be considered a classical treatise. He based his primary concept on the observed radiation biology effect of mitotic suppression. Scanlon postulated that because certain phases of mitosis are more radiosensitive, those cells in a radiosensitive phase would be eliminated initially in a course of radiation, and that as they are depleted, the radio-resistant cells become the predominant cell in the malignancy. He postulated that a rest period before resuming radiation therapy would allow recovery and resumption of mitotic activity, and permit the restoration of the radio-sensitive elements of the tumor. He postulated that this would result in increased cell kill. Scanlon's theory led to clinical trials by both himself [80, 81] and others in subsequent years (41, 48, 51–54, 56, 82, 83].

In 1969, Holsti *et al.* [53] reviewed the literature leading up to Scanlon's studies and also the studies done in the ten years thereafter. He reported his own series which included clinical trials in various malignancies. He reported a study of 322 patients with carcinoma of the lung, randomized between split-course and a continuous-irradiation technique. The split-course technique consisted of 27 to 30 Gy given at 10 Gy per week followed by a repeat course after 2 to 3 weeks rest. The continuous-irradiation course of this randomized study consisted of irradiation at the rate of 10 Gy per week to a total dose of 55 to 62 Gy. Of the 118 patients in the split-course arm, 23% were recurrence-free at the end of 1 year, and of the 90 patients receiving continuous-course irradiation, 18% were recurrence-free at the end of 1 year. The 1- and 2-year survivals did not show any significant difference between the two groups.

Evaluation of the literature regarding the efficacy of split-course radiation regimes for carcinoma of the lung is difficult because of the variety of regimes studied and the poor survival with patients with this diagnosis.

Abramson and Cavanaugh [48] reported a non-randomized series of 271 patients with disease limited to the chest and supraclavicular areas. His regime was 20 Gy in 5 days, followed after 3 weeks rest by a repeat course to the mediastinum and primary tumor. This radiation regime was also given concurrently to the supraclavicular area in patients who had a positive scalene node biopsy or palpable nodes in this area. The 1-year survival was 38.1%, but was increased to 50% if all of the primary was removed at the time of surgery.

Other authors compared different regimes of split-course. Guthrie and associates [51] randomized 97 patients between 2 variations of split-course regimes. His group A of 47 patients was treated with 30 Gy in 2 weeks, and this course was repeated after 1 month's rest. In group B, 51 patients were treated with 20 Gy in 1 week. This course was repeated after one month's rest. The mean survival time of group A was 8.5 months, and of group B was 6.8 months. There was no significant difference in survival rates at 18 months, and only 1 patient survived 24 months with no evidence of disease.

Scruggs and associates [56] reported a series of 235 patients, in which 93 patients were given a standard radiotherapy course, which consisted of 35 to 40 Gy given in 3 to 4 weeks in a continuous technique. Of the remaining 142 patients, 128 of these completed their course of treatment and were reported. These were divided into two split-course treatment groups. Group A consisted of 48 patients treated with field sizes less than 15 × 15. These patients received 20 Gy in 5 days, followed by a 2-week rest and a second course of 20 Gy in 8 days. Group B consisted of 80 patients treated with field sizes greater than 15 × 15. These patients received 20 Gy in 8 to 10 days, followed by a 2-week rest and a repeat course of 20 Gy in 5 to 10 treatments. In selected cases, a 10-Gy boost dose was given to a small field after a further 2-week rest. The 1-year survival rate was 27% for the continuous-treatment regime, and 30% for the split-course regimes combined. The 2-year survival rate was 7% for the continuous-treatment regime and 19% for the split course regimes. The 1-year survival rate was 42% for Group A, and 23% for Group B. The 2-year survival rates for these two groups were 25% and 8%, respectively.

The authors stated that the split-course cases had a less favorable prognosis when compared to the continuous-course patients, but that they had higher 1- and 2-year survival rates than the continuous-treatment group.

Hazra and associates[52] reported a series of 75 patients with inoperable bronchogenic carcinoma who were given a regime of 30 Gy in 2 weeks, followed by 15 Gy in 1 week after a 2-week rest. The survival rate at the end of 1 year was 94%, and at the end of 2 years was 43%.

Emami and associates[41] reported a series of 100 patients randomized to continuous fractionation or a split-course technique. 76 patients received 50 to 60 Gy with continuous radiation. The remaining 24 patients received split-course radiation, which consisted of 25 Gy in 10 treatments, a 3-week rest period and a repeat of the initial course. All patients were unresectable or inoperable. Approximately 8% of both groups failed to complete treatment. Local control was achieved in 58.5% of the continuous-treatment group, and in 45.4% of the split-course group. Median survival was 14 months for those patients treated continuously, and 9 months for those treated with the split course. There were no fatal complications, but it was observed that complications decreased with decreased total dose and smaller daily fractions.

Levitt and associates[82] reported on a protocol in which the split course consisted of 18 Gy in 3 treatments, which was repeated after 28 days rest. The continuous course consisted of 40 Gy in 4 weeks given by co-axial opposing fields. The dose was then carried to 60 Gy in 6 to 8 weeks by means of a 3-field technique. If the supraclavicular nodes were positive, these were given the same dose as the primary tumor. The authors reported that there was no significant difference in symptomatic response, survival or X-ray response. Complications were not reported.

Salazar and associates[83] reported a study of 160 patients. 101 were treated with 4 different continuous-therapy schedules, and 59 were treated with 3 different split-course schedules. Those treated with a split course at the higher nominal standard (RET) doses had a higher percentage of tumor resolution per histological type, milder radiation toxicity, decreased incidence of local failure and a better survival rate. The authors did determine that those patients who showed a 50% decrease in tumor shadow at the end of 1 month showed a better statistical survival. Those patients who had more than 50%

shadow regression had a mean survival of 13.3 months versus 7 months in those showing less than 50% regression. The authors explored the optimum radiation dose and concluded that 60 Gy or more of continuous radiation was more effective than 50 Gy, but it was less efficient because of the higher complication rate. The split course technique of 25 Gy in 10 treatments, repeated twice, with a 2-week rest gave the highest rate of complete tumor resolution in squamous cell cancer, and had the lowest incidence of radiation pneumonitis.

Landgren and associates [54] reported a study of 54 cases randomized to split-course radiation versus split-course radiation plus hydroxyurea. No oat cell carcinomas were included. The split-course radiation regime consisted of 30 Gy in 2 weeks in 10 fractions, followed by a 4-week rest period and a repeat of the initial course. The spinal cord was excluded for the last 15 Gy.

Of the 34 patients who completed the second course, 14 received radiation alone, and 20 received radiation plus hydroxyurea. The authors did not show any difference in survival between these two groups.

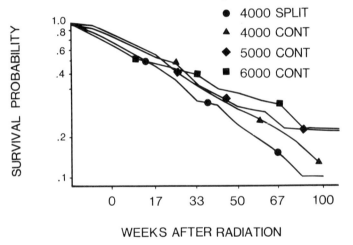

Fig. 6. Analysis of survival according to treatment arms. Radiation Therapy Oncology Group Protocol 73-01, preliminary analysis, January, 1979. Presented at the 21st annual meeting of the American Society of Therapeutic Radiologists, October 24, 1979, New Orleans, Louisiana. Data and graph courtesy of Dr. Carlos Perez [19]. Split = split course, Cont = continuous course.

Treatment Arm	Dead	Total	Median Survival (weeks)
4000 Split	68	93	36.8
4000 Cont	66	97	45.5
5000 Cont	58	91	41.0
6000 Cont	56	84	47.2

Another group of 32 patients was treated with 50 to 60 Gy in 5 to 6 weeks by means of a continuous-treatment regime. The 2-year survival for this group was 19%, compared to a 12% survival in the split-course group. 4 of the 32 patients in this group were long-term survivors (3 or more years), while there were no long-term survivors in the split-course group.

Perez and associates (Fig. 6) reported on a Radiation Therapy Oncology Group study which compared a 40-Gy, split-course regime to three continuous-radiation regimes, varying from 40 to 60 Gy [19]. Median survival of 36.8 weeks for the split-course regime was significantly worse than the continuous-radiation regimes, the median survival of which varied from 41.0 to 47.2 weeks, depending on the total dose.

CONCLUSIONS

The clinical rationale for split-course therapy is that following the initial course, the patient can be observed for a period of time and the treatment then completed only if metastasis have not intervened. Another clinical reason for the utilization of split-course techniques is their logistic advantages when using adjuvant chemotherapy regimes. It does not appear that the controversy as to whether split-course or continuous radiation is more efficacious in long-term local control has been resolved, but it does appear that complications may be greater with split-course therapy when doses are given that are high enough to achieve survival rates comparable to those of the continuous regimes. Carcinoma of the lung may not be the correct clinical model to use in attempting to resolve this clinical question, but it would seem that local control may be a critical issue, if adjuvant therapy proves to be of value in enhancing long-term survival. Because of the small number of long-term survivors in carcinoma of the lung, long-term local control cannot be adequately evaluated. At the present time it would appear that the continuous-radiation technique may have the edge in local control, and may also produce a decreased rate of severe complications.

It also appears that the initial radiation biology concepts which gave the impetus to clinical studies in split-course techniques, namely factors related to cell cycle effects, may not be the determining factors in local control. Thomlinson and Gray [84] first described hypoxic cells in human lung cancers in 1955. At the present time, available evidence seems to indicate that local control may be determined by the fact that hypoxic cells are resistant to conventional radiotherapy modalities. The ability of the malignancy to reoxygenate when fractionated regimes of radiotherapy are used thus takes on increasing significance. If reoxygenation is indeed a factor, high doses of radiation given in shorter elapsed times, as in split-course techniques, may

not give ample time for (1) recovery in normal tissue and for (2) revasculari-
zation in order to reoxygenate the hypoxic cells in malignant tissue. This
provides the rationale for the use of continuous radiation techniques in those
patients who may benefit from curative radiation.

In the opinion of the authors, a minimum of 60 Gy given at the rate of
1.8–2.0 Gy per fraction, 5 days a week, should be given to adequately control
known disease. Adjacent areas of high risk should receive a total minimum
dose of 50 Gy, given with the same continuous technique.

8. ADJUVANT THERAPY

The dual problems of local-regional failure following high-dose radiation
therapy and distant metastatic failure have been addressed by various
attempts to combine radiation therapy with chemotherapy. Theoretically, the
addition of chemotherapy enhances the sensitivity of local tumor in the chest,
thus making it more likely that the radiation will sterilize the tumor. Also in
theory, the addition of chemotherapy when systemic metastases are still small
microscopic deposits creates a greater likelihood of sterilizing these microde-
posits. Most combination studies have been analyzed on the basis of response
rates and median survival, usually measured in days or weeks. A complete
response (CR) is usually defined as the disappearance of all clinical evidence
of tumor and no new lesions for a minimum of four weeks. Most studies do
not require histological documentation of complete response. A partial
response (PR) is usually defined as a 50% decrease in the product of perpendicular diameters of a measurable lesion.

Carr and associates studied radiation alone versus radiation plus 5-fluorou-
racil in 188 patients. Of those with non-small cell carcinoma of the lung, 66
were treated with radiation alone, and 64 with radiation therapy plus 5-
fluorouracil [85]. 6% of 31 squamous cell carcinoma patients in each group
survived for 3 years. In adenocarcinoma patients, there were no survivors at 3
years among 19 patients treated with radiation as compared to 13% surviving
3 years among 15 patients treated with the combination therapy. For large cell
undifferentiated carcinoma, the survival at 3 years was 6% of 16 patients
treated with radiation alone, versus no survivors in 18 patients treated with
combination therapy [85].

Bergsagel and associates reported a randomized study of patients treated
with radiation alone versus radiation plus cytoxan [32]. In a group of 74
patients, 56 of whom had squamous cell or large cell undifferentiated carcinoma, and 18 of whom had their diagnosis established by cytology only, the
3–6 months' survival was significantly longer with combination treatment.
After six months, however, there was no significant difference. The authors

indicated that the time of appearance of metastatic disease seemed to be delayed by chemotherapy, but not prevented by it. For purposes of this latter analysis, oat-cell carcinoma patients were not separated from the remainder of the patients reviewed.

Berry and associates[86] reported the results of a three-arm randomized trial comparing radiation therapy alone versus procarbazine alone versus a four-drug combination of nitrogen mustard, procarbazine, velban and prednisone. There were 5 oat-cell patients and 143 non-oat cell patients in the study. No further breakdown was given of the distribution by cell type among the three treatment categories. Staging information by category was also not given; however, it appears from some of the clinical information that at least 25% of the patients had metastatic disease. The authors indicated that patients receiving the combination chemotherapy had an improved quality and duration of survival over those receiving radiation alone or single-agent chemotherapy. The radiation delivered was, however, clearly insufficient by current standards.

In a randomized study Landgren and associates compared split-course irradiation (30 Gy in 10 fractions over two weeks, 4-week rest, then repeat) to the same radiation plus hydroxyurea[54]. They noted absolutely no difference in survival.

Palmer and Kroening reported a comparison of radiation therapy alone to radiation therapy plus procarbazine[87]. This was a non-randomized study of 66 patients, all of whom had a performance status of 80% or better. The over-all response rate (CR + PR) for both groups of patients was 66%. When the patients were subclassified according to the extent of primary tumor and extent of lymph node metastases, it was noted that for each group, radiation therapy was generally, though not statistically, slightly better than the radiation therapy-chemotherapy combination.

Byar and associates[88] reported results of a European Organization for Research and Treatment of Cancer (E.O.R.T.C.) randomized trial of radiation therapy alone versus radiation therapy and cytoxan in 187 patients. The over-all response rate was 66%, with no difference between the treatment arms.

Petrovich and associates analyzed the results of the Veterans Administration Lung Cancer Group (VALG) Protocol 13-L in a number of publications[89–91]. They compared radiation therapy alone, given in various time-dose schedules, to radiation therapy plus CCNU (Lomustine) plus hydroxyurea. Sixty-nine of the 345 patients (20%) had oat cell carcinoma. They were not classified separately in the data analysis, so that this data does not represent pure non-small cell carcinoma of the lung. The authors noted a statistically significant difference in median survival (20.4 weeks versus 73.1 weeks) in favor of patients receiving the higher radiation doses[89]. Because

Table 8. Treatment schema-Southwest Oncology Group Protocol #7635.

Week	0	1	2	3	4	5	6	7	8	9	10	11	12	13	14	15
Regimen A																
Radiation therapy	×	×														
Levamisole 100 mg/M²/day; PO			×	×	×	×	×	×	×	×	×	×	×	×	×	×, etc. to 2 years
Regimen B																
Radiation therapy	×	×														
Adriamycin 50 mg/M²; IV					×			×	×				×		×, etc. to 450 mg/M²	
Regimen C																
Radiation therapy	×	×														
Adriamycin 50 mg/M²; IV							×	×				×		×, etc. to 450 mg/M²		
Levamisole 100 mg/M²/day ×2; PO			×	×	×	×	×	×	×	×	×	×	×	×	×	
Regimen D																
Radiation therapy	×	×					×	×								

In Regimen A, levamisole is given on any two consecutive days of each week starting on the last day of the first radiotherapy session. It is omitted during the second radiotherapy session and is restarted on the last day of this session and continues on any two consecutive days of each week thereafter.

In Regimen C, levamisole is given as in Regimen A but is omitted on the days that adriamycin is given.

Radiation therapy: 30 Gy in 10 fractions over two weeks followed by a 21-28 day rest period. The radiation course was then repeated with the final 12 Gy delivered through a reduced field where possible.

Source: unpublished data, Southwest Oncology Group.

of this result, the authors have adopted as the standard for all future Veterans Administration Lung Group protocols a dose of 60 Gy delivered in six weeks at the rate of 2 Gy per day, 5 days per week [91]. The median survival of 153 patients receiving radiation alone was 6.3 months, compared to 7.2 months for 164 patients receiving radiation therapy plus chemotherapy. However, 11% of patients receiving radiation alone survived 30 months, whereas only 4% of patients receiving radiation plus chemotherapy survived 30 months.

Sealy reported on two studies of combined chemotherapy and radiation therapy [92]. Nitrogen mustard and methotrexate were used for squamous cell carcinoma and large cell undifferentiated carcinoma, while cytoxan and methotrexate were used for adenocarcinoma. The response rate (CR + PR) was about 30% for all three cell types in the radiation-alone group; however, it was much lower in the radiation therapy plus chemotherapy group for squamous cell and large cell undifferentiated carcinomas. The reason for this difference in response rate is not clear. The median survival was longer for all three cell types in the radiation-alone group. In the second study, in which large cell undifferentiated carcinoma and adenocarcinoma were treated with radiation versus radiation plus cytoxan, methotrexate and CCNU, the response rates and median survival were identical for the two arms, while the toxicity was much greater in the radiation therapy plus chemotherapy group.

In 1976, the Southwest Oncology Group (SWOG) undertook a study to test the efficacy of chemotherapy with and without immunotherapy added to radiation therapy. The schema for this protocol, SWOG 7635, is presented in Table 8. Patients were stratified by Southwest Oncology Group performance status (Table 6) and by whether or not surgery had been attempted. As of August 1, 1979, 124 patients had been registered, of whom 94 were eligible for analysis of their response, toxicity, remission duration, and survival (Southwest Oncology Group Protocol 7635, preliminary analysis, August 1, 1979, unpublished data). The response rate (CR + PR) varied from 17 to 33% (Table 9). This was not statistically significant (p = .635). There was also no statistically significant difference in response rate according to performance status, surgical status, immunotherapy status or chemotherapy status (Table 10). Although not statistically significant, the best survival was seen in patients receiving radiation therapy alone (Fig. 7). Other currently active cooperative group studies are listed in Table 11.

CONCLUSION

To date there has been no demonstrated benefit from the addition of chemotherapy and/or immunotherapy to radiation therapy in the control of

Table 9. Preliminary analysis, August 1979 — Southwest Oncology Group Protocol #7635 — Limited squamous cell carcinoma of the lung-response rates by treatment arm.

Treatment arm	CR + PR Evaluated	Percentage response
Radiation + Levamisole	7/24	29
Radiation + Adriamycin	8/24	33
Radiation + Adriamycin + Levamisole	4/23	17
Radiation alone	7/23	30

$P = 0.635$.
Southwest Oncology Group Protocol 7635, preliminary analysis, August 1, 1979, unpublished data. CR = complete response, PR = partial response.

regionally inoperable non-small cell cancer of the lung. The few studies which seem to demonstrate an advantage to chemotherapy were compared to inadequate radiation therapy. However, radiation therapy alone will never ultimately benefit those patients who already have microscopic but undetected systemic disease. Furthermore, the maximum tolerable radiation dose will by itself frequently be insufficient to control many tumors locally within the chest. The rationale of adding chemotherapy in localized disease is to improve long-term survival by improving local control rate and by controlling subclinical distant metastases. But the promise of this theory will never be realized until optimal combinations of radiation and chemotherapy are developed. In the opinion of the authors, three developments are necessary before any

Table 10. Preliminary analysis, August 1979 — Southwest Oncology Group Protocol #7635 — Limited squamous cell carcinoma of the lung-response rate by treatment variable.

Variable	CR + PR Number evaluated	Percentage response	P-value
Chemotherapy			
Adriamycin	12/35	34	
No adriamycin	14/29	48	0.256
Immunotherapy			
Levamisole	11/33	33	
No levamisole	15/31	48	0.221
SWOG performance status			
1-4	0/5	0	
5-7	10/23	43	
8-10	16/39	41	0.177

Southwest Oncology Group Protocol 7635, preliminary analysis, August 1, 1979, unpublished data.

Table 11. Currently active cooperative group and major institutional studies of regional (limited) non small cell carcinoma.

Cooperative group or institution	Protocol number	Regimen
Eastern (ECOG)	3578	Radiation therapy ± Cytoxan, Adriamycin, Methotrexate and Procarbazine ± Upper half body radiation (800 rad-single dose)
Radiation Therapy (RTOG)	7811	Radiation therapy ± Levamisole (immunostimulant)
	7814 7917	Radiation therapy ±Misonidazole (radiation sensitizer)
	7807	Radiation therapy: Photons vs neutrons
	7907	Radiation therapy: Photons alone vs neutrons alone vs neutrons and photons
Southeast (SEG)	76 LUN 308	Radiation therapy ± C Parvum (immunostimulant) ± Levamisole
Veterans Administration (VALG)	15-L	Radiation therapy: Two different time dose schemes ± prophylactic cranial radiation
Mayo Clinic	782602	Radiation therapy ±Cytoxan, Adriamycin, and Cis-Platinum or Cytoxan, Adriamycin, Cis-Platinum and Triazinate
Working Party for Lung (WPL)	7812	Short course intensive radiation vs protracted radiation

Based on data compiled as of December 1, 1979.

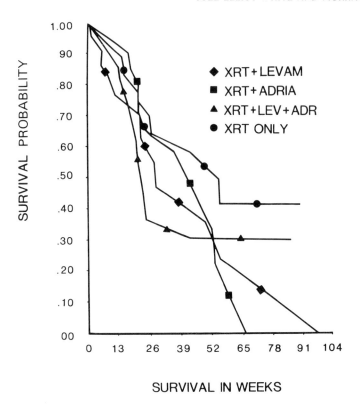

SURVIVAL IN WEEKS

Fig. 7. Southwest Oncology Group Protocol 7635, Limited Squamous Cell Carcinoma of the Lung: Survival of Eligible Patients, preliminary analysis, August, 1979, unpublished data. XRT = radiation therapy, ADR = adriamycin, LEVAM = levamisole.

Treatment Arm	Number of Failures	Total Eligible	Median Survival (weeks)
XRT Alone	9	23	55
XRT +ADR +LEVAM	14	23	22
XRT +LEVAM	12	24	29
XRT +ADR	13	24	42

improvement will appear in the results of combination therapy. 1) More effective chemotherapeutic agents, for use either singly or in combination, must be found. 2) More extensive laboratory study of cell kinetics under varying combinations of radiation therapy and chemotherapy must be carried out. 3) Because full-course radiation therapy combined with intensive chemotherapy leads to excessive toxicity, it will be necessary to develop optimal radiation time-dose schemes for use in conjunction with chemotherapy. The best time-dose scheme for radiation therapy alone may not necessarily be the best time-dose scheme for radiation therapy used in combination with chemotherapy, and the best choice may also vary according to the chemotherapy agents employed. Future protocols should consider these facts.

9. PROPHYLACTIC RADIATION

With the high incidence of undetected distant dissemination at the time of presentation, the question has been raised whether treatment results can be improved by prophylactically irradiating sites at high risk.

The rationale for such prophylactic radiation is exemplified by the work of Shipley and associates [93], who studied Lewis lung carcinoma. This tumor is a poorly differentiated squamous cell carcinoma that arose spontaneously in the lung of a C57BL mouse in 1951, and has been maintained in that strain ever since. Shipley and his associates compared the radiosensitivity of small tumors to that of large tumors. They found approximately a threefold difference, with the small tumors much more radiosensitive than the larger ones. These authors felt that the difference in sensitivity was primarily due to hypoxia in about 36% of the cells of the larger tumors. Hypoxia was essentially non-existent ($<0.5\%$) in the smaller tumors.

If this animal model holds true, prophylactic radiation for microscopic undetected metastasis should be effective. Such efficacy has been demonstrated in oat cell carcinoma of the lung [94, 95]. Brain metastasis occurs less frequently in non-small cell carcinomas than in small cell carcinomas [24, 29, 30]. However, in non-small cell carcinomas, it is not infrequent for the brain to be the only metastatic site [24, 96].

Hilaris and associates reported the brain as the site of failure in 30% of 49 patients undergoing interstitial implantation for unresectable tumors [97]. Newman and Hansen reported a higher incidence (Table 12) of brain meta-

Table 12. Incidence of brain metastasis in non-small cell carcinoma of the lung.

Histopathology	Number of patients	Percentage with brain metastasis
Squamous cell	95	13.7
Adenocarcinoma	55	25.4
Large cell undifferentiated carcinoma	51	29.4

Modified from Newman and Hansen, 1974 (29).

Table 13. Influence of site of origin of lung carcinomas on the incidence of brain metastasis at presentation.

Site	Number metastasis / Number patients (Percentage)
Apical	11/12 (92)
Peripheral	5/9 (56)
Intermediate	3/6 (50)
Central	20/62 (32)

6 of the apical tumors had single metastasis, 2 asymptomatic; 4 central tumors had single metastasis, and 5 had asymptomatic metastasis. From Tomlinson and associates, 1979 (98).

stasis with adenocarcinoma and large cell undifferentiated carcinoma than with squamous cell carcinoma [29]. Tomlinson and associates found the location of the primary tumor (Table 13) a significant factor in the incidence of neurologic presentation [98]. The lower incidence with central tumors may be a result of the fact that more of them are squamous cell type. These authors also noted that a high percentage of the apical tumors had single metastasis, and that over-all 9% of the patients with metastasis were asymptomatic.

Regardless of cell type, the neurologic effects of brain metastasis are devastating. Rosenmann and Choi compared prophylactic cranial radiation (PCR) in 24 patients to therapeutic radiation in 31 patients, all of whom had oat cell carcinoma [95]. Those who required therapeutic radiation had a significant decrease in their functional status and quality of life as measured by the Karnofsky performance scale, and one half of this group relapsed within a few months. Only one of the prophylactically irradiated patients developed metastasis. Most of the PCR group maintained their initial high Karnofsky score until shortly before death. Deeley and Edwards noted that 'significant' palliation was obtained in 47% of patients completing treatment for brain metastasis [96]. However, 30% of their 87 patients with clinical metastasis were too ill to receive or complete therapy. The mean survival was about 4.5 months. Newman and Hansen noted only 30% 'good' response in 41 patients therapeutically irradiated, with the remainder remaining debilitated [29].

Cox and associates reported a Veterans Administration Lung Group (VALG) study (Table 14) in which patients with all cell types were randomized to treatment with or without prophylactic cranial radiation [99]. The decrease in clinical metastasis was all the more remarkable considering the low dose employed – 20 Gy in 10 fractions over two weeks. Further study of prophylactic cranial radiation is required.

Because of the high incidence of other systemic metastatic sites (Table 1), similar prophylactic irradiation to other high-risk areas such as the liver, upper abdomen, and lungs should be given consideration. This possibility has

Table 14. Frequency of brain metastasis-VALG prophylactic cranial radiation (PCR) study.

No PCR	PCR
11/98 (11%)	4/101 (4%)

P = 0.054
Data from Cox and associates, 1978 (99).

already been suggested by others [34, 100–102]. Because of low tolerance and large volume, however, the bone marrow could not presently be encompassed at one time. Alternative methods of managing undetected bone marrow metastases are discussed elsewhere in this volume.

10. INTERSTITIAL IRRADIATION

A further attempt to improve local control of regional lung cancer has involved the implantation of various types of radioactive sources directly into the tumor itself (Table 15). The advantage of this procedure is that it delivers a very high dose of radiation to the tumor, while sparing much of the surrounding normal tissue.

Hilaris and associates evaluated 105 patients with unresectable non-apical lung cancer. Approximately half of these patients were implanted with radon-222 and the other half with iodine-125. Local control was found to be dependent on stage: 80% of the 10 patients with stage I and II obtained local control, while only 46% of 95 patients with stage III disease obtained local control. The two-year survival was 50% for stages I and II, and 9% for stage III. In contrast to the non-apical lung cancers, Hilaris and associates reported disease-free 5-year survivals for 9 of 15 apical lung cancer patients who were implanted with iodine-125 [103]. One patient, who died at 11 1/2 years after implantation, was found at autopsy to have remained free of disease. Among another similar group of patients who were implanted after failure of external radiation therapy there were no 5-year survivors. George [104] reported 70% local control in over 100 patients treated with implantation of iridium-192 following failure of full-course external radiation. The duration of local control was not given. Gibbons [105] reported a 5-year survival of 5% for a group of 200 patients implanted with gold-198.

CONCLUSIONS

Implantation techniques have the advantage of delivering a relatively high dose to a small volume while sparing normal tissues. The rapid fall-off of

Table 15. Interstitial radiation of inoperable lung cancer.

Author	Type of tumor implanted	Agent implanted	Number of patients	Local control	Survival
Hilaris et al. (97)	Unresectable, non-apical lung cancer	Radon 222 or Iodine 125	53 52	8/10 stage I & II 44/95 (46%) stage III	50% 2 year stage I & II 9% 2 year stage III
Hilaris et al. (103)	Partially resected or unresected apical lung cancer	Iodine 125	15	. . .	9/15 disease free ⩾ 5 years
Gibbons (105)	Inoperable, unspecified location	Gold 198	200	. . .	20% 2 years 5% 5 years
George (104)	Residual or recurrent after full course external radiation	Afterloading Iridium 192	Over 100	70%	. . .

Not all authors reported both local control and survival.

dose at the periphery of the implanted volume, however, can also be a disadvantage, because microextensions of tumor at the edges of the volume will receive an insufficient dose of radiation. It is the opinion of the authors that the best local control would be obtained by some combination of interstitial and external radiation therapy. Interstitial and intracavitary therapy were very popular in the early history of radiation treatment of cancer. However, with the advent of megavoltage radiation therapy and its marked superiority to kilovoltage therapy in ability to deliver high-dose external radiation, utilization of interstitial techniques rapidly fell into disrepute. In recent years, however, the failure of megavoltage radiation to produce all the hoped-for improvements in cure rates has led to a renaissance in interstitial radiation therapy at some centers. It is likely that interstitial radiation in various forms will be utilized with increasing frequency in the coming decade in selected groups of patients for whom the technique is appropriate.

11. PALLIATIVE RADIATION THERAPY

The major proportion of patients with inoperable lung cancer seen in the radiation therapy department will have symptoms which require palliation [16, 106, 107]. Many of these symptoms are anticipatory of a shortened survival span [16, 18]. However, their relief for the duration of a patient's survival can improve the quality of remaining life significantly.

Pooled data from a number of authors (Table 16) indicates that relief of symptoms will occur in approximately 70% of patients [15, 46, 47, 75, 86,

Table 16. Palliation of symptomatic loco-regional lung cancer-pooled data.

Symptom	Number relieved Number of patients*	Percentage relieved
Hemoptysis	202/271	75
Cough	274/406	67
Pain	117/201	58
Superior vena cava syndrome	137/159	86
Dyspnea	269/353	76
Atelectasis	28/75	37
Arthralgia/pain due to hypertrophic osteoarthropathy	10/11	91
Vocal cord paralysis	2/76	3
General overall symptomatic relief	1221/1779	69

* The number of patients in each category varies according to subject(s) discussed by included authors (15, 46, 47, 75, 86, 106, 108, 109, 110, 111, 112, 113, 114, 115, 116, 117, 118, 119, 120).

106, 108–120]. Barton and associates reported complete symptom relief in 20% of patients, and moderate symptom relief in 50% of patients [108]. Berry and associates [86] indicated that 52% of lung cancer patients who received no initial treatment had uncontrolled symptoms until their death [86]. The frequency of relief of individual symptoms has varied somewhat from series to series and is partially dependent on radiation dose and treatment volume [15, 46, 75, 86, 108, 110, 111, 113, 114, 120]. The highest incidence of symptomatic relief was found in pain and arthralgia due to hypertrophic pulmonary osteoarthropathy [116–118]. The symptom least frequently relieved was vocal cord paralysis, with improvement shown in only 2 patients out of 76 treated in two different series [15, 116].

However, the apparent difference between authors in the frequency of response of certain symptoms is also in part a function of the method of reporting. Slawson and Scott [116] reported improvement of atelectasis in only 3 out of 44 patients. On the other hand, Hackenthal [119] reported improvement in 25 out of 51 patients. Hackenthal's data, however, does not completely separate objective improvement of atelectasis from decrease in the size of the primary tumor mass. Therefore, accurate assessment of the number of patients in whom atelectasis actually improved is not possible from his data. Furthermore, variation between series in the reported ability to relieve specific symptoms may be a function of the length of time the symptoms have been present [121].

Dysphagia as a specific symptom is usually due to mediastinal invasion or mediastinal lymph node metastasis. While Schulz [107] reported that this symptom was usually relieved, it was not reported as a specific symptom in most of the series reviewed, possibly because it is not a frequent early symptom. Green and Kern reported dysphagia to have occurred in 2 out of 46 patients with post-resection recurrence of tumor, with no relief obtained by radiation therapy in either patient [111].

Although early in the century, superior vena cava syndrome appeared to be due most often to benign disease, approximately 85% of current cases are found to be caused by bronchogenic carcinoma [75]. While it presents distressing physical signs and symptoms, superior vena cava syndrome is not necessarily fatal. Deeley found that patients with superior vena cava syndrome who received radical radiation therapy in the absence of distant metastases had the same survival as a similar group of patients without superior vena cava syndrome [67]. Rubin and Ciccio reported more rapid improvement in symptoms when comparing a group of patients treated with an initial high daily dose to a similar group treated by routine fractionation [115]. By the end of treatment, however, relief of symptoms occurred in 79% of patients in each group. Perez and associates indicated that the response rate increased as the radiation dose was raised [75]. Four patients received 6000 rad and all

Table 17. Site of obstruction in patients with superior vena cava syndrome.

Site	Percentage
Superior Vena Cava (SVC)	36
Innominate Veins (INV)	27
Subclavian Veins (SUB)	18
SVC + INV	6
INV + SUB	9
SVC + INV + SUB	4

Based on 45 patients undergoing phlebography. Modified from Howard, N., 1971 (122).

achieved a complete response, with total disappearance of both the syndrome and the tumor. Two of these patients eventually relapsed in the primary tumor site, but the other two did not. Variation in the response rate of superior vena cava syndrome can also be attributed to the occurrence of thrombosis of the vena cava in some patients [109]. Another reason for failure to respond may be inadequate treatment volume [122]. Howard pointed out that the treatment volume may be inadequate in approximately 60% of superior vena cava patients (Table 17), because the site of obstruction may not necessarily be in the superior vena cava, and so would not be included in the ordinary treatment volume.

The response rate of pain also varies considerably, ranging from 24% [86] to 72% [111, 113]. Morris and Abadir pointed out that with Pancoast type tumors in particular, high-dose radiation therapy is required to obtain adequate pain relief [113].

Although some authors suggest that inoperable asymptomatic bronchogenic carcinoma patients should receive no treatment [86, 123], it is the clinical impression of the authors that symptoms due to obstructive processes, such as atelectasis or obstructive pneumonitis, are generally relieved if treated in a relatively early phase of the obstruction, whereas they are seldom relieved if the process has been long-standing [121].

CONCLUSIONS

It is the opinion of the authors that patients with regionally inoperable or unresectable non-small cell carcinoma of the lung should receive radiation therapy not only for relief of symptoms, but to avoid impending symptoms. Cases in which superior vena cava syndrome, obstructive pneumonitis, atelectasis, dysphagia, and vocal cord·paralysis are not relieved by radiation therapy represent cases in which the pathophysiological process has permanently disrupted or destroyed the normal anatomy. In these instances, even though radiation therapy may achieve tumor regression, this is insufficient to reverse the symptoms because the normal anatomy can no longer be restored. Therefore, patients who do not display indications of short life expectancy, such as marked weight loss and low performance status, should be given the benefit of attempted definitive therapy.

12. COMPLICATIONS

Gross[57] discussed the effects of radiation on lung tissue and divided them into two phases: 1) an acute phase, which he designates as radiation pneumonitis, and 2) a late phase, which he calls radiation fibrosis.

The clinical symptoms associated with radiation pneumonitis are cough and occasionally hemoptysis, but in almost all cases the cardinal symptom is dyspnea. Fever and chest pain may also be associated. The onset of acute cor pulmonale indicates a fatal outcome.

The acute stage may persist for as little as a week, and then subside without sequelae, or it may last for a month and subside gradually. In severe cases, dyspnea may progress to respiratory failure and death in a matter of days.

Radiation fibrosis occurs in almost all patients who receive radiation to the lung, and it manifests itself as X-ray changes. These changes may not be associated with symptoms. All patients with radiation pneumonitis progress to radiation fibrosis, but X-ray changes of radiation fibrosis can be present in a patient who did not manifest any symptoms of radiation pneumonitis.

Symptoms of radiation fibrosis include dyspnea on exertion, reduced exercise tolerance orthopnea, cyanosis, and sometimes chronic cor pulmonale and finger clubbing.

Spread of tumor must be differentiated from radiation pneumonitis. The differential diagnosis is sometimes difficult, because it is dependent on correlating the knowledge of the effects of all the variables in a particular case: field size, field shape and dose rate and timing of radiation.

Other pulmonary complications of radiation to the lung are pleural effusion, pneumonitis outside the radiation field and spontaneous pneumothorax.

Treatment of acute radiation pneumonitis consists of the administration of corticosteroids and antibiotics.

Bennett and associates[124] reported cases of acute radiation pneumonitis, and summarized the factors associated with this complication. They reiterated that the incidence of this complication was dose-related, and that although 2/3 of patients had X-ray changes of fibrosis, the symptoms of acute pneumonitis were in the range of 3–15%. They pointed out that radiation pneumonitis does not always follow the portal size, and that diffuse extensive radiation pneumonitis can occur. The authors discussed the relationship of lymphatic blockage associated with pneumonitis or mediastinal malignancy as being a factor in diffuse radiation pneumonitis, but their review does not demonstrate any good evidence to support this theory. They also discussed the possibility that some patients may demonstrate hypersensitivity to radiation, and that this can manifest itself as diffuse bilateral pneumonitis even with low doses.

Brady and associates [125] reported a study of pulmonary functions in relationship to radiation pneumonitis and could not find any correlation. Green and associates [68] studied patients with carcinoma of the lung and chronic pulmonary disease treated by radiotherapy. Of 303 patients receiving radiotherapy to the primary malignancy in the lung, 41 had chronic pulmonary disease. Seven out of 31 patients who received 30 Gy or more and who survived three months or longer had radiation pneumonitis. Two had peripheral lesions, and five had central lesions. One patient died of radiation pneumonitis, and one patient died of cardiorespiratory shock near the end of treatment. The authors were unable to correlate field size with the occurrence of radiation pneumonitis.

Hellman and associates [126] reported on complications in a series of 132 patients with inoperable carcinoma of the lung. They received 40 Gy to the primary lesion and mediastinum and a boost dose of 15–20 Gy to the primary and adjacent hilum. In addition 50 Gy was given to the supraclavicular nodes. There were no deaths due to radiation fibrosis at the doses given, although five patients had cough and dyspnea, which abated with time.

These authors also reported the incidence of esophagitis associated with dysphagia during treatment. The incidence was 12% when doses less than 40 Gy were given, 28% with doses of 40–50 Gy, 41% with doses of 50–55 Gy and 46% in those patients receiving doses greater than 55 Gy to the esophagus. There were no late esophageal strictures.

Radiation myelitis is a serious complication of radiation for carcinoma of the lung. Locksmith and Powers [127] reported 178 patients who received 40 Gy in 3 weeks. Six cases of transverse myelitis were observed. All patients who had this complication were treated with a field which was greater than 10 cm in length. The complication rate was 12.5% in this series.

Scruggs and associates [56] reported a series of cases in which a group of 48 patients were treated with a split-course technique consisting of 20 Gy in 5 days, followed after two weeks' rest by a second course of 20 Gy in 8 days. They reported two patients with myelitis, at 9 and 30 months, and two patients with congestive cardiac failure secondary to lung fibrosis, both of whom required large fields for large tumors.

Abramson and Cavanaugh [48] reported a series of 271 patients with carcinoma of the lung who were treated by a split-course technique of 20 Gy in five days, repeated after three weeks' rest. They stated that a spinal cord block was used. Four patients developed myelitis in 8–24 months post-irradiation. In this series, the supraclavicular area received a similar course of radiation in some cases. The authors attributed the four cases to overlap of mediastinal and supraclavicular fields.

CONCLUSIONS

It is the opinion of the authors that serious complications are usually avoidable if special care is taken with technique, such as avoiding overlapping fields, and if special attention is paid to time-dose-volume relationships.

13. SUMMARY AND CONCLUSIONS

This chapter summarizes the past experience and present state of the art of the management of non-oat cell carcinoma of the lung. In the opinion of the authors, at the present time, all patients who are in good physical condition and who have regionally inoperable non-metastatic disease, should be given the benefit of a protracted, continuous high-dose (60 Gy in 6 weeks or equivalent) course of radiation. To date randomized studies of such patients have not proven any benefit from chemotherapy. Therefore, the authors feel such treatment should be confined to research protocols.

More investigation must be carried out in the area of optimal radiation dose and time-dose schemes. Further advances in radiotherapy may be dependent on advances in chemotherapeutic agents and in the use of other modalities such as radioprotectors, radiosensitizers, more densely ionizing radiation (i.e., heavy particles), and non-ionizing radiations (i.e., hyperthermia and red light).

ACKNOWLEDGEMENT

The authors wish to express their gratitude to Charlotte E. Egerer for her editorial and secretarial assistance in the preparation of the manuscript.

REFERENCES

1. Hall LA: Case of tumor in the chest. Boston Med and Surg J 13:295-297, 1835.
2. Salter H: Diseases of the chest. Lancet 2:1-4, 1869.
3. Cleaves MA: Radium: with a preliminary note on radium rays in the treatment of cancer. J Adv Therapy 21:667-682, 1903.

4. Edwards AT: The surgical treatment of intrathoracic new growths. Br Med J 1:827-830, 1932.
5. Ormerod FC: Malignant disease of the bronchus. J Laryngol Otol 48(2):733-743, 1933.
6. Ormerod FC: The pathology and treatment of carcinoma of the bronchus. J Laryngol Otol 52:733-745, 1937.
7. Leddy ET, Moersch HJ: Roentgen therapy for bronchogenic carcinoma. JAMA 115(26):2239-2242, 1940.
8. Hocker AF, Guttmann RJ: Three and one-half years' experience with the 1,000 kilovolt roentgen therapy unit at Memorial Hospital. Am J Roentgenol 51:83-94, 1944.
9. Blomfield GW: Experience with two million volt x-ray therapy and a preliminary assessment of clinical results. Proc R Soc Med 46:219-224, 1953.
10. Bromley LL, Szur L: Combined radiotherapy and resection for carcinoma of the bronchus. Lancet 2:937-941, 1955.
11. Bloedorn FG, Cowely RA, Cuccia CA, Mercado R, Wizenberg MJ, Linberg EJ: Preoperative irradiation in bronchogenic carcinoma. Am J Roentgenol 92:77-87, 1964.
12. Bloedorn FG: Rationale and benefit of preoperative irradiation in lung cancer. JAMA 196(4):340-341, 1966.
13. Smart J, Hilton G: Radiotherapy of cancer of the lung: results in a selected group of cases. Lancet 1:880-881, 1956.
14. Roswit B, Patno ME, Rapp R, Veinbergs A, Feder B, Stuhlbarg J, Reid CB: The survival of patients with inoperable lung cancer: a large-scale randomized study of radiation therapy versus placebo. Radiology 90:688-697, 1968.
15. Rubin P, Ciccio S, Setisarn B: The controversial status of radiation therapy in lung cancer. Proc Nat Cancer Conf 6:855-865, 1970.
16. Caldwell WL, Bagshaw MA: Indications for and results of irradiation of carcinoma of the lung. Cancer 22(5):999-1004, 1968.
17. Eisert DR, Cox JD, Komaki R: Irradiation for bronchial carcinoma: reasons for failure. I. Analysis of local control as a function of dose, time, and fractionation. Cancer 37:2665-2670, 1976.
18. Lanzotti VJ, Thomas DR, Boyle LE, Smith TL, Gehan EA, Samuels ML: Survival with inoperable lung cancer: an integration of prognostic variables based on simple clinical criteria. Cancer 39:303-313, 1977.
19. Perez CA, Stanley K, Mietlowski W, Rubin P, Kramer S, Brady L, Perez-Tamayo R, Brown S, Concannon J, Seydel HG, Rotman M, Hanson W: Prognostic factors influencing the effect of irradiation in non-oat cell unresectable carcinoma of the lung. A randomized study by the Radiation Therapy Oncology Group. Presented at the 21st annual meeting of the American Society of Therapeutic Radiologists, October 24, 1979, New Orleans, Louisiana. Abstract #4.
20. Abadir R, Muggia FM: Irradiated lung cancer: an autopsy analysis of spread pattern. Radiology 114:427-430, 1975.
21. Budinger JM: Untreated bronchogenic carcinoma. Cancer 11:106-116, 1958.
22. Knights EM: Metastatic tumors of the brain and their relation to primary and secondary pulmonary cancer. Cancer 7:259-265, 1954.
23. Line DH, Deeley TJ: The necropsy findings in carcinoma of the bronchus. Br J Dis of Chest 65:238-242, 1971.
24. Loumanen RKJ, Watson WL: Autopsy findings lung cancer – a study of 5000 Memorial Hospital cases. Saint Louis, C V Mosby, 1968, p 504-513.
25. Matthews MJ, Kanhouwa S, Pickren J, Robinette D: Frequency of residual and metastatic tumor in patients undergoing curative surgical resection for lung cancer. Cancer Chemother Rep 4(2): 63-67, 1973.

26. Ochsner A, Debakey M: Significance of metastasis in primary carcinoma of the lungs. J Thoracic Surg 11(4):357-387, 1942.
27. Rissanen PM, Tikka U, Holsti LR: Autopsy findings in lung cancer treated with megavoltage radiotherapy. Acta Radiol Ther 7:433-442, 1968.
28. Warren S, Gates O: Lung cancer and metastasis. Arch Pathol 78:467-473, 1964.
29. Newman SJ, Hansen HH: Frequency, diagnosis, and treatment of brain metastases in 247 consecutive patients with bronchogenic carcinoma. Cancer 33(2):492-496, 1974.
30. Muggia FM, Chervu LR: Lung cancer: diagnosis in metastatic sites. Semin Oncol 1(3):217-228, 1974.
31. Matthews MJ, Pickren J, Kanhouwa S: Who has occult metastases? Residual tumor in patients undergoing surgical resections for lung cancer. In: Perspectives in lung cancer. Frederick E. Jones Memorial Symposium in Thoracic Surgery, Yohn DS (ed), Basel, Karger, 1977, p 9-17.
32. Bergsagel DE, Jenkin RDT, Pringle JF, White DM, Fetterly JCM, Klaassen DJ, McDermot RSR: Lung cancer: clinical trial of radiotherapy alone vs. radiotherapy plus cyclophosphamide. Cancer 30:621-627, 1972.
33. Cox JD, Yesner R, Mietlowski W, Petrovich Z: Influence of cell type on failure pattern after irradiation for locally advanced carcinoma of the lung. Cancer 44:94-98, 1979.
34. Komaki R, Cox J, Eisert DR: Irradiation of bronchial carcinoma. II. Pattern of spread and potential for prophylactic radiation. Int J Radiat Oncol Biol Phys 2:441-446, 1977.
35. Ghilezan N, Milea N, Tamburlini S: Telecobalt therapy for malignant lung tumours. Acta Radiol (Ther) 15(5):394-400, 1976.
36. Abe M, Yabumoto E, Nishidai T, Takahashi M: Trials of new forms of radiotherapy for locally advanced bronchogenic carcinoma. Strahlentherapie 153(3):149-158, 1977.
37. Brady LW, Cander L, Evans GC, Faust DS: Carcinoma of the lung: results of supervoltage radiation therapy. Arch Surg 90:90-94, 1965.
38. Stanford W, Spivey CG, Larsen GL, Alexander JA, Besich WJ: Results of treatment of primary carcinoma of the lung: analysis of 3,000 cases. J Thorac Cardiovasc Surg 72(3):441-449, 1976.
39. Johnson RRJ: Radiotherapy—primary and/or adjuvant modality. In: Perspectives in lung cancer. Frederick E. Jones Memorial Symposium in Thoracic Surgery, Yohn DS (ed), Basel, Karger, 1977, p 74-81.
40. Guttmann R: Radical supervoltage therapy in inoperable carcinoma of the lung. In: Modern radiotherapy: carcinoma of the bronchus, Deeley TJ (ed), New York, Appleton-Century-Crofts, 1971, p 181-195.
41. Emami B, Munzenrider JE, Lee DJ, Rene JB: Radical radiation therapy of advanced lung cancer: evaluation of prognostic factors and results of continuous and split course treatment. Cancer 44:446-456, 1979.
42. Salazar OM, Rubin P, Brown JC, Feldstein ML, Keller BE: Predictors of radiation response in lung cancer. Cancer 37:2636-2650, 1976.
43. Deeley TJ: Clinical trial to compare two different tumour dose levels in the treatment of advanced carcinoma of the bronchus. Clin Radiol 17:299-301, 1966.
44. Deeley TJ: Controlled clinical trials in the treatment of carcinoma of the bronchus. In: Proceedings of the Second Congress of the European Association of Radiology, Amsterdam, June 14-18, 1971, p 314-318.
45. Ruderman AI: Prerequisites for effective radiotherapy for lung cancer. Cancer Treat Rep 60(10):1475-1477, 1976.
46. Fingerhut AG, Chin FK, Shultz EH: Radical radiation therapy for cancer of the lung. Chest 60(3):244-245, 1971.
47. Garland LH: Radiation therapy of cancer: current results with megavoltage and orthovoltage. Am J Roentgenol 86(4):621-639, 1961.

48. Abramson N, Cavanaugh PJ: Short-course radiation therapy in carcinoma of the lung: a second look. Radiology 108:685-687, 1973.
49. Abramson N, Cavanaugh PJ: Short-course radiation therapy in carcinoma of the lung. Radiology 96:627-630, 1970.
50. Aristizabal SA, Caldwell WL: Radical irradiation with the split-course technique in carcinoma of the lung. Cancer 37:2630-2635, 1976.
51. Guthrie RT, Ptacek JJ, Hass AC: Comparative analysis of two regimens of split course radiation in carcinoma of the lung. Am J Roentgenol 117(3):605-608, 1973.
52. Hazra TA, Chandrasekaran MS, Colman M, Prempree T, Inalsingh A: Survival in carcinoma of the lung after a split course of radiotherapy. Br J Radiol 47:464-466, 1974.
53. Holsti LR: Clinical experience with split-course radiotherapy: a randomized clinical trial. Radiology 92:591-596, 1969.
54. Landgren RC, Hussey DH, Barkley HT, Samuels ML: Split-course irradiation compared to split-course irradiation plus hydroxyurea in inoperable bronchogenic carcinoma – a randomized study of 53 patients. Cancer 34:1598-1601, 1974.
55. Lee RE, Carr DT, Childs DS: Comparison of split-course radiation therapy and continuous radiation therapy for unresectable bronchogenic carcinoma: 5 year results. Am J Roentgenol 126(1):116-122, 1976.
56. Scruggs H, El-Mahdi A, Marks RD, Constable WG: The results of split-course radiation therapy in cancer of the lung. Am J Roentgenol 121(4):754-760, 1974.
57. Gross NJ: Pulmonary effects of radiation therapy. Ann Intern Med 86(1):81-92, 1977.
58. Rey G, Haase W: Ueber den einfluss der strahlenqualitaet auf die ueberlebenschance bei inoperablem bronchial-carcinom. Roentgenblaetter 30:202-210, 1977.
59. White JE, Livingston R, Reed RC: Combined modality treatment for limited squamous carcinoma of the lung: phase III. Southwest Oncology Group Protocol 7635, activated March 7, 1977.
60. White JE, McCracken JD, Reed R: Combined chemotherapy/radiation therapy immunotherapy for small cell (oat cell) carcinoma of the lung: phase III. Southwest Oncology Group Protocol 7628, activated October 28, 1976.
61. Perez CA, Seydel HG, Concannon J: Phase III randomized adjuvant immunotherapy with levamisole (NSC#177023) and radiation therapy, vs. radiation therapy plus placebo in unresectable epidermoid, adenocarcinoma and large cell undifferentiated carcinoma. Radiation Therapy Oncology Group Protocol 78-11, activated October 5, 1978, unpublished data.
62. Perez CA, Simpson J, Phillips T: Phase III study to compare misonidazole combined with irradiation or radiation therapy alone in the treatment of locally advanced (stage III) non-oat cell lung cancer. Radiation Therapy Oncology Group Protocol 79-17, activated September 4, 1979, unpublished data.
63. Perez C, Phillips T: Phase I/II protocol to study the value of misonidazole combined with radiation in the treatment of locally advanced lung cancer. Radiation Therapy Oncology Group Protocol 78-14, activated August 15, 1978, unpublished data.
64. Cooley WE, Silverman S: Radiation therapy in bronchiolar alveolar cell carcinoma: a case report. Cancer 34:1077-1079, 1974.
65. Emami B, Melo A, Carter BL, Munzenrider JE, Piro AJ: Value of computed tomography in radiotherapy of lung cancer. Am J Roentgenol 131:63-67, 1978.
66. Deeley TJ: The treatment of carcinoma of the bronchus. Br J Radiol 40(479):801-822, 1967.
67. Deeley TJ: The treatment of carcinoma of the lung by radiotherapy. Postgrad Med J 49:717-722, 1973.
68. Green N, Iba G, Shirey JK: The clinical experience of patients with carcinoma of the lung and chronic pulmonary disease treated by radiotherapy. Radiology 111:189-192, 1974.

69. Bowen TE, Zajtchuk R, Green DC, Brott WH: Value of anterior mediastinotomy in bronchogenic carcinoma of the left upper lobe. J Thorac Cardiovasc Surg 76(2):269-271, 1978.

70. Goldberg EM, Shapiro CM, Glicksman AS: Mediastinoscopy for assessing mediastinal spread in clinical staging of lung carcinoma. Semin Oncol 1(3):205-215, 1974.

71. Hutchinson CM, Mills NL: The selection of patients with bronchogenic carcinoma for mediastinoscopy. J Thorac Cardiovasc Surg 71(5):768-773, 1976.

72. Whitcomb ME, Barham E, Goldman AL, Green DC: Indications for mediastinoscopy in bronchogenic carcinoma. Am Rev Respir Dis 113:189-195, 1976.

73. Brantigan OC: Pretreatment clinical staging of carcinoma of the lung. Am Surg 42(1):66-70, 1976.

74. Huber CM, DeGiorgi LS, Levitt SH, King ER: Carcinoma of the lung: an evaluation of the scalene node biopsy in relation to radiation therapy of the supraclavicular region. Cancer 29(1):84-89, 1972.

75. Perez CA, Presant CA, Van Amburg AL: Management of superior vena cava syndrome. Semin Oncol 5(2):123-134, 1978.

76. Perez CA: Radiation therapy in the management of carcinoma of the lung. Cancer 39:901-916, 1977.

77. Logie MB, Kinzie JJ: Carcinoma of the lung: management by irradiation. Radiol Clin North Am 11(1):243-255, 1973.

78. Ellis F: Dose, time and fractionation: a clinical hypothesis. Clin Radiol 20:1-7, 1969.

79. Scanlon PW: The effect of mitotic suppression and recovery after irradiation on time-dose relationships and the application of this effect to clinical radiation therapy. Am J Roentgenol 81:433-455, 1959.

80. Scanlon PW: Initial experience with split-dose periodic radiation therapy. Am J Roentgenol 84:632-644, 1960.

81. Scanlon PW: Split-dose radiotherapy. Prog Clin Cancer 2:143-163, 1966.

82. Levitt SH, Bogardus CR, Ladd G: Split-dose intensive radiation therapy in the treatment of advanced lung cancer: a randomized study. Radiology 88:1159-1161, 1967.

83. Salazar OM, Rubin P, Brown JC, Feldstein ML, Keller BE: The assessment of tumor response to irradiation of lung cancer: continuous versus split-course regimes. Int J Radiat Oncol Biol Phys 1:1107-1118, 1976.

84. Thomlinson RH, Gray LH: The histological structure of some human lung cancers and the possible implications for radiotherapy. Br J Cancer 9:539-549, 1955.

85. Carr DT, Childs DS, Lee RE: Radiotherapy plus 5-FU compared to radiotherapy alone for inoperable and unresectable bronchogenic carcinoma. Cancer 29:375-380, 1972.

86. Berry RJ, Laing AH, Newman CR, Peto J: The role of radiotherapy in treatment of inoperable lung cancer. Int J Radiat Oncol Biol Phys 2:433-439, 1977.

87. Palmer RL, Kroening PM: Comparison of low dose radiation therapy alone or combined with procarbazine (NSC-77213) for unresectable epidermoid carcinoma of the lung, stage T3, N1, N2, or M1. Cancer 42:424-428, 1978.

88. Byar D, Kenis Y, Van Andel JG, de Jong M, Laval P, Marion L, Couette JE, Longueville J: Results of a E.O.R.T.C. randomized trial of cyclophosphamide and radiotherapy in inoperable lung cancer: prognostic factors and treatment results. Eur J Cancer 14:919-930, 1978.

89. Petrovich Z, Mietlowski W, Ohanian M, Cox J: Clinical report on the treatment of locally advanced lung cancer. Cancer 40:72-77, 1977.

90. Petrovich Z, Ohanian M, Cox J: Clinical research on the treatment of locally advanced lung cancer: final report of VALG protocol 13 limited. Cancer 42: 1129-1134, 1978.

91. Cox JD, Eisert DR, Komaki R, Mietlowski W, Petrovich Z: Patterns of failure following

treatment of apparently localized carcinoma of the lung. In: Lung cancer: progress in therapeutic research, Muggia F, Rozencweig M (eds), New York, Raven Press, 1979, p 279-288.

92. Sealy R: Combined radiotherapy and chemotherapy in non-small cell carcinoma of the lung. In: Lung cancer: progress in therapeutic research, Muggia F, Rozencweig M (eds), New York, Raven Press, 1979, p 315-323.

93. Shipley WU, Stanley JA, Steel GG: Tumor size dependency in the radiation response of the Lewis lung carcinoma. Cancer Res 35: 2488-2493, 1975.

94. Moore TN, Livingston R, Heilbrun L, Eltringham J, Skinner O, White J, Tesh D: The effectiveness of prophylactic brain irradiation in small cell carcinoma of the lung: a Southwest Oncology Group study. Cancer 41:2149-2153, 1978.

95. Rosenmann J, Choi NC: The quality of life following therapeutic versus elective brain irradiation in small cell undifferentiated carcinoma of lung. Presented at American Society of Therapeutic Radiologists 21st annual meeting, October 24, 1979.

96. Deeley TJ, Edwards JMR: Radiotherapy in the mangement of cerebral secondaries from bronchial carcinoma. Lancet 1:1209-1213, 1968.

97. Hilaris BS, Martini N, Batata M, Beattie EJ: Interstitial irradiation for unresectable carcinoma of the lung. Ann Thorac Surg 20(5):491-500, 1975.

98. Tomlinson BE, Perry RH, Stewart-Wynne EG: Influence of site of origin of lung carcinomas on clinical presentation and central nervous system metastases. J Neurol Neurosurg Psychiatry 42(1):82-88, 1979.

99. Cox JD, Petrovich Z, Paig C, Stanley K: Prophylactic cranial irradiation in patients with inoperable carcinoma of the lung: preliminary report of a cooperative trial. Cancer 42:1135-1140, 1978.

100. Salazar OM, Rubin P, Keller B, Scarantino C: Systemic (half-body) radiation therapy: response and toxicity. Int J Radiat Oncol Biol Phys 4:937-950, 1978.

101. Rubin P: The radiotherapeutic approach: reappraisal and prospects. In: Lung cancer: progress in therapeutic research, Muggia F, Rosencweig M (eds), New York, Raven Press, 1979, p. 333-340.

102. Fitzpatrick PJ, Rider WD: Half body radiotherapy. Int J Radiat Oncol Biol Phys 1:197-208, 1976.

103. Hilaris BS, Luomanen RK, Mahan GD, Henschke UK: Interstitial irradiation of apical lung cancer. Radiology 99:655-660, 1971.

104. George FW: Current status and recent advances in the radiotherapy of lung cancer. Chest 71(5):635-637, 1977.

105. Gibbons JRP: Interstitial irradiation in carcinoma of the lung. Panminerva Med 18:62-63, 1976.

106. Line D, Deeley TJ: Palliative Therapy. In: Modern radiotherapy: carcinoma of the bronchus, Deeley TJ (ed), New York, Appleton-Century-Crofts, 1971, p 298-306.

107. Schulz MD: Palliation by radiotherapy. JAMA 196(10):850-851, 1966.

108. Barton HL, McGranahan GM, Jordan GL: The evaluation of roentgen therapy in the management of non-resectable carcinoma of the lung. Dis Chest 37:170-175, 1960.

109. Davenport D, Ferree C, Blake D, Raben M: Response of superior vena cava syndrome to radiation therapy. Cancer 38:1577-1580, 1976.

110. Green N, Melbye RW, Kern W: Radiotherapy for suspected lung cancer not proved by tissue diagnosis. Chest 64(4):476-479, 1973.

111. Green N, Kern W: The clinical course and treatment results of patients with post resection locally recurrent lung cancer. Cancer 42:2478-2482, 1978.

112. Mincer F, Botstein C, Schwarz G, Zacharopoulos G, McDougall R: Moving strip irradiation in the treatment of extensive neoplastic disease in the chest. Am J Roentgenol 108(2):278-283, 1970.

113. Morris RW, Abadir R: Pancoast tumor: the value of high dose radiation therapy. Radiology 132:717-719, 1979.

114. Rubenfeld S, Kaplan G: Treatment of bronchogenic cancer with conventional x-rays according to a specific time-dose pattern. Radiology 73(5):671-678, 1959.

115. Rubin P, Ciccio S: High daily dose for rapid decompression. In: Modern radiotherapy: carcinoma of the bronchus, Deeley TJ (ed), New York, Appleton-Century-Crofts, 1971, p 276-297.

116. Slawson RG, Scott RM: Radiation therapy in bronchogenic carcinoma. Radiology 132:175-176, 1979.

117. Steinfeld AD, Munzenrider JE: The response of hypertrophic pulmonary osteoarthropathy to radiotherapy. Radiology 113:709-711, 1974.

118. Semple T, McCloskie RA: Generalized hypertrophic osteoarthropathy in association with bronchial carcinoma. Br Med J 1:754-759, 1955.

119. Hackenthal P: Zur Palliativbestrahlung des bronchialkarzinoms. Strahlentherapie 3:190-196, 1960.

120. Guttmann RJ: Two million volt irradiation therapy for inoperable carcinoma of the lung. Cancer 8:1254-1260, 1955.

121. White JE, Boles M, Gibbs ML: Emergencies in radiation therapy – the first 24 hours. Exhibit presented at the American Medical Association meeting, December 10-13, 1977.

122. Howard N: Superior mediastinal obstruction: value of phlebography. In: Modern radiotherapy: carcinoma of the bronchus, Deeley TJ (ed), New York, Appleton-Century-Crofts, 1971, p 266-275.

123. Brashear RE: Should asymptomatic patients with inoperable bronchogenic carcinoma receive immediate radiotherapy? No. Am Rev Respir Dis 117:411-414, 1978.

124. Bennett DE, Million RR, Ackerman LV: Bilateral radiation pneumonitis, a complication of the radiotherapy of bronchogenic carcinoma (report and analysis of seven cases with autopsy). Cancer 23:1001-1018, 1969.

125. Brady LW, Germon PA, Cander L: The effects of radiation therapy on pulmonary function in carcinoma of the lung. Radiology 85:130-134, 1965.

126. Hellman S, Kligerman MM, von Essen CF, Scibetta MP: Sequelae of radical radiotherapy of carcinoma of the lung. Radiology 82:1055-1061, 1964.

127. Locksmith JP, Powers WE: Permanent radiation myelopathy. Am J Roentgenol 102:916-926, 1968.

7. Small Cell Anaplastic Carcinoma of the Lung: Staging

HEINE H. HANSEN and PER DOMBERNOWSKY

INTRODUCTION

The presence and the type of metastases in patients with cancer are important predictable parameters for the clinical course of a malignancy, and in addition they have major indications for planning of the therapeutic strategy. Since surgery is the main curative treatment for lung cancer, much attention has been focused on the pattern of the local regional involvement. In particular, the size of the primary tumor as well as the status of regional lymph nodes as expressed in the TNM system according to the classification of the WHO and the American Joint Committee on Cancer Staging and End Results Reporting have been the subject for detailed analysis [1, 2].

The data collected by the Joint Committee include at present information from more than 2000 patients with lung cancer, from six medical centers. In the latter study it was demonstrated that in contrast to epidermoid carcinoma, adenocarcinoma and large-cell anaplastic carcinoma, the prognosis for small cell carcinoma was independent of whether the patient presented with stage I, II or III disease with a median survival for all stages being less than 6 months. Furthermore 84% of 360 patients with small cell anaplastic carcinoma presented with stage III disease defined as a primary tumor more extensive than T_2 or any tumor with metastases to the lymph nodes in the mediastinum or with distant metastases. Similar information has also been gathered from other surgical centers applying the TNM classification for small cell anaplastic carcinoma [3]. Because of the lack of applicability of the TNM-system to small cell carcinoma other types of staging systems have been applied. The most widely used system was proposed first by the VA-Lung Cancer Study Group [4]. In this classification patients with inoperable lesions

Supported by grants from the Boel Foundation

R.B. Livingston (ed.), Lung cancer 1, 157–168. All rights reserved.

were categorized as having either 'limited disease' i.e., disease confined to
one hemithorax including ipsilateral positive scalene lymph nodes or 'extensive disease' consisting of the remaining patients with non-resectable disease.
This staging system was introduced primarily due to its suitability to radiotherapy, the main modality of non-surgical therapy at the introduction of this
staging system. It is of special interest that by using this system the VA-Lung
Cancer Study Group demonstrated, that the median survival time from diagnosis in 118 untreated patients with 'limited' and 'extensive' small cell
carcinoma was 3,1 and 1,4 months, respectively [4, 5]. Also in patients receiving intensive therapy with combination chemotherapy with or without radiotherapy the survival is significantly better for patients classified as having
'limited disease' compared to patients with 'extensive' disease [6–8].

The classification system of the VA-Lung Cancer Study Group or a slight
modification of it i.e., including also patients with bilateral positive scalene or
supraclavicular lymph nodes into the 'limited disease' category but excluding
patients with pleural involvement has later been used also by others [9, 10].
Also in the latter studies, where rigorous staging procedures were utilized, a
significant difference in survival was noted comparing the two stages of the
disease.

The classification is still highly important for prognostification. However, it
has lost some of its significance in the overall planning of therapy for patients
with small cell anaplastic carcinoma in recent years, compared to when it was
initially introduced, because systemic therapy with combination chemotherapy
has emerged as the main modality of treatment for this type of lung cancer.
However, with the improved therapeutic results obtained within the last 10
years resulting in 4–5 times prolongation of median survival time including
long-term survival in a small group of patients the importance of staging
patients with small cell carcinoma might be of increasing value again. This is
based on the fact, that staging procedures are important not only in order to
determine the presence of a complete remission, but also in determining the
necessary duration of treatment for achieving a remission of years' duration,
if not 'a cure' [11].

For small cell carcinoma, the staging procedures have naturally focused on
the most common anatomic location for extrathoracic metastatic spread.
Based on autopsy data from the literature for small cell anaplastic carcinoma,
the location for metastatic spread includes abdominal lymph nodes (57%), liver
(62%), bone (38%), adrenals (39%), kidneys (22%), brain (37%), and pancreas
(31%) [12]. In addition to the pancreas, small cell carcinoma also has a great
tendency to metastasize to other endocrine organs. In one autopsy series
including 102 patients with small cell anaplastic carcinoma, Matthews found,
that 18 had metastases to the thyroid, 15 to the pituitary, 7 to the testis and 1
to the parathyroid glands [13]. Thus the metastatic spread is wide, and it is

also well established that it occurs early. In another autopsy study also by Matthews *et al.*, it was observed, that among 19 patients with small cell anaplastic carcinoma who died within 1 month of so-called curative surgery, 63% had dissemination outside one lung with a similar organ distribution as mentioned above[14].

The methods used to detect metastatic spread may vary among different investigators according to the availability of techniques, the expenses of the procedures and the therapeutic implications attached to the staging. It is obvious that when performing comparative clinical trials, the demand for vigorous staging procedures is much more imperative, than when one is treating patients outside clinical trials. In the following some of the most frequently used staging procedures by organ system will be discussed.

BONE METASTASES

In addition to hematologic and biochemical examination the following methods are available for screening of bone metastases: bone marrow aspiration or biopsy, radio-isotopic bone scan and radiographic bone survey.

Of the hematologic elements neither levels of hemoglobin nor white blood cell counts are indicative for bone marrow involvement, whereas the presence of thrombocytopenia heralds bone marrow metastases. In one study 6 of 35 patients with bone marrow involvement had thrombocytopenia in contrast to none of a comparable control group without bone marrow involvement[15]. In another study by Ihde *et al.* [16], the platelet counts were found to be markedly lower in marrow-positive patients than in marrow-negative patients with both groups having extensive disease. Blood cell indices, serum folate and vitamin B-12 levels determined before therapy did not vary significantly among bone marrow positive and bone marrow negative patients, while alkaline phosphatase values were significantly elevated in marrow positive patients compared to marrow-negative patients.

In a number of studies of patients with solid tumors, the presence of a leucoerythroblastic blood picture consisting of myeloblasts, neutrophilic myelocytes or erythroblasts in the circulating blood has been indicative of malignant infiltration of the bone marrow, which is also the case for small cell carcinoma[15–17].

The high propensity of small cell anaplastic carcinoma to metastasize to the bone marrow was first demonstrated by bone marrow examination in 1971 by Hansen and Muggia[17], and subsequently in a number of other studies[18–23]. The bone marrow examination was initially performed from the posterior iliac crest with a modified Silverman needle using the technique of McFarland and Damashek, but also aspiration from the sternum has been used [24]. More recently other techniques using the Jamshidi or the Radner needle have been employed. These techniques permit larger biopsy specimens and/or are less traumatic. When performing the bone marrow examination, it is recommended to obtain biopsy specimens, touch imprint of the biopsy, bone marrow aspiration with smears from the aspirate and clot specimens. With these techniques a great deal of material is available for histopathologic examination. The touch preparations are of special value by providing a rapid method for diagnosis particularly when aspiration is unobtainable because of 'dry-tap.'

In one study, detection of tumor cells in aspirates alone was noted in 1/3 of all bone marrow positive patients compared with less than 10% by biopsy only, thus indicating that bone marrow aspiration and biopsy are complementary in the detection of bone marrow metastases in this disease [15]. Similar observations have also been made by Lymann et al. [25].

At histopathologic evaluation a remarkable feature of small cell anaplastic carcinoma compared to other cell types of lung cancer, is the osteoblastic and myelofibrotic process associated with the bone marrow metastases. These changes resemble those associated with prostatic cancer and breast malignancies, and they are not observed nearly as frequently in other cell types of lung cancer[12]. The new bone formation and fibrotic changes are even observed in untreated patients with bone marrow metastases and they remain in the marrow in spite of eradication of tumor cells by combination chemotherapy [12, 16]. The pathological bone abnormalities are also reflected on X-rays of the bones in patients with small cell anaplastic carcinoma, where osteoblastic changes are much more frequent than in the other types of lung cancer [12].

The question of performing more than one bone marrow examination has also been the subject of investigations in small cell anaplastic carcinoma as in studies of malignant lymphomas. In one study including 89 patients an approximately 30% increase was noticed in bone marrow involvement when bilateral bone marrow examination was performed as compared with the unilateral procedure [26].

In addition to bone marrow examination, bone scanning has emerged as a very valuable diagnostic method for osseous metastases. A number of radioactive compounds have been used as bone seekers and today it is well recognized that bone scan in general is much more sensitive than X-ray for the early detection of metastatic osseous disease. The most frequently used radioisotopes are 90^m Technetium polyphosphate and diphosphonate complexes giving a minimal radiation dose.

Comparing bone marrow examination, radioisotope bone scans and radiographic bone survey for detection of spread to the osseous system in patients with lung cancer, it is evident from a comparative study that the value of

Table 1. Comparisons between bone scans, bone surveys, and bone marrow examinations at time of diagnosis in 22 patients with small cell carcinoma.
Reproduced with permission from Hansen [12].

	Bone survey all negative		
	Scan positive	Scan negative	Total
Bone marrow positive	6	5[3]	11[4]
Bone marrow negative	3[1]	8	11
Total	9[2]	13	22

[1] Two patients became positive later.
[2] Six patients developed signs of bone involvement on x-ray 1-6 months later.
[3] Bone scan became positive later in 3 patients.
[4] X-ray showed later evidence of osteoblastic or osteolytic lesions in 8 patients.

bone survey as a routine investigation is much overrated [12]. For patients having recently diagnosed small cell anaplastic carcinoma it is an almost useless screening procedure as compared with bone marrow examination in particularly if the latter is combined with bone scans. The results of such a comparative study of the 3 methods in 22 consecutive patients with small cell anaplastic carcinoma clearly demonstrate the superiority of bone scan and bone marrow examination as compared with the radiographic bone survey. In the latter study none of the patients with small cell anaplastic carcinoma had positive radiographic bone survey at the time of diagnosis, in spite of the findings of bone marrow metastases in 11 of 22 patients. Later the bone survey become positive with the occurrence of osteoblastic changes in 6 of the 22 patients (Table 1) [12].

CNS-METASTASES

Metastases to the CNS-system occur more frequently in patients having small cell anaplastic carcinoma than in patients with other cell types of lung cancer. At the time of diagnosis, the frequency of CNS-metastases is approximately 10% in large non-selected series, while the incidence at autopsy varies between 28–55% [27]. In autopsy studies both intracranial and extracranial metastases are present. Table 2 summarizes the location of intracranial metastases at autopsy in two studies including information concerning the focality of the metastases [28, 29]. The most frequent locations of intracranial CNS-metastases include the cerebellum, cerebrum and pituitary glands.

The occurrence of extracranial metastases is dominated by leptomeningeal

Table 2. ₁Location of intracranial metastases at autopsy in small cell anaplastic carcinoma.

	Hirsch *et al.* [28] (N = 33)	Nugent *et al.* [29] (N = 55)	Total (N = 88)(%)
Location of metastases			
Cerebrum alone	7	9	16 (18)
Cerebellum alone	4	0	4 (5)
Brainstem	3	–	3 (3)
Pituitary glands alone	4	6	10 (11)
Multiple intracranial metastases	15	40	65 (24)

carcinomatosis, extradural or intradural locations or both [29]. The frequency in a recent autopsy study is reported to be 28% [29]. Autopsy data have also revealed that leptomeningeal metastases usually are associated with the presence of either intracranial or intraspinal disease [29].

The incidence of CNS-metastases might be influenced by age, as observed by Burgess *et al.* [30], who in an autopsy study of 177 patients with small cell anaplastic carcinoma including 70 patients with a positive brain autopsy found that among patients 70 years or more, the frequency of brain metastases was 3% as compared to 42% in patients less than 70 years (p < 0.001).

Within recent years screening and early detection of CNS-metastases in small cell carcinoma have become of increasing interest. This is based on the observation that the improved treatment results with longer survival of patients with small cell carcinoma has increased the frequency of CNS-metastases [29]. The increasing frequency has subsequently resulted in a number of studies investigating the use of prophylactic methods such as brain irradiation.

A number of screening procedures have been used in these studies for detection of CNS-metastases, but unfortunately, most of them have been found to be of minimal or no value as screening procedures in asymptomatic patients with normal neurological evaluation. The procedures examined include electroenchephalograms, lumbar puncture with the determination of protein and cells for cytologic examination and brain scans with 99^m-Tc-pertechnetate or other radioisotopes. Most of these studies include patients with various histologic cell types of lung cancer [31–33]. More recently the same techniques have been tested specifically in patients with small cell anaplastic carcinoma, again with disappointing results. In two studies including 51 and 35 patients with small cell carcinoma, brain scan was found to be of no value in patients having normal neurological examination [25, 34]. Furthermore, in 120 patients with small cell anaplastic carcinoma, who underwent 310 routine brain scans at weeks 0, 6, 12, 24 and 48 after start of treatment, only 6 of 310 scans were found positive in asymptomatic patients. In the same study routine pretreatment lumbar puncture was performed in 56 consecutive asymptomatic patients, all being normal [29].

Recently computerized tomography has been introduced, often replacing brain scan with 99^m-Tc-pertechnetate. Computerized tomography permits detection of minor differences in absorption in various tissues and the success of this technique has been impressive in neuro oncology. Preliminary data using computerized tomography which compare it with other procedures in patients with small cell anaplastic carcinoma are now emerging. In one study the CT-scan was evaluated as a preoperative procedure in a series of 50 patients with bronchogenic carcinoma including 16 patients with small cell anaplastic carcinoma. All patients were neurologically asymptomatic and they had all normal skull roentgenograms and radionuclide brain scans. Three of the 50 patients (6%) were discovered on CT-scan to have metastases located to the cerebellum, occipital lobe and corpus callosum, respectively [35]. Further studies to elucidate the usefulness of CT-scan for CNS-metastases in small cell carcinoma are in progress and awaited with great interest. Another option for improvement of the CNS-diagnostic procedures includes the determination of 'ectopic markers' in the cerebrospinal fluid. In an exploratory study ACTH and calcitonin were measured in the cerebrospinal fluid in 22 patients with small cell carcinoma, including 14 patients with CNS-metastases. The concentrations of ACTH were found to be significantly elevated in patients with CNS-metastases compared to patients without, while no difference was observed for calcitonin [36].

LIVER METASTASES

In the detection of liver metastases the clinical examination and the biochemical variables such as serum glutamicoxaloacetic transaminase (S-GOT), serum bilirubin, serum alkaline phosphatase, prothrombine time and serum lactic dehydroxygenase (S-LDH) are the most important non-invasive methods in the routine clinic.

For the biochemical tests it is obviously that the positive findings, may be caused by the presence of non-malignant hepatic disorders, such as cirrhosis or fatty degeneration of the liver, which occur with a high incidence in patients with lung cancer [37]. In a study including 190 patients with small cell anaplastic carcinoma, who as a part of different staging procedures underwent peritoneoscopy with liver biopsy, it was demonstrated, that in patients with histologic verified liver metastases, alkaline phosphatase was increased in 71%, S-GOT in 56% and S-LDH in 79% compared with elevated values in 14, 0 and 16% of patients without demonstrable liver metastases [38]. The findings of abnormal values in 2 of the following three liver function tests: Alkaline phosphatase, S-GOT and S-LDH were indicative of the presence of liver metastases in 16% of patients with histologic verified metastases and in 3% of patients without liver metastases. All three of the above biochemical tests were positive in 52% of patients with liver metastases and in 0% in patients without liver metastases.

Concerning liver scans, 99^m Tc-sulfur colloid has been the most commonly used among the isotopes in the scintigraphic evaluation of the liver. After the initial optimism concerning this method in the early diagnosis of hepatic metastases, it is now evident that there are several limitations in the use and evaluation of liver scans: 1) the lesion must be larger than 1-2 centimeters in diameter to be visualized on the scintigram; 2) the procedure is non-specific with benign conditions resulting in abnormal scan; and 3) subjective interpretation can influence its reliability.

Comparing liver function tests with liver scans, it was observed by Wittes *et al.* in a series of 23 patients with small cell carcinoma that no patient with normal liver function tests had a focally abnormal liver scan[34].

It is thus not surprising that most investigators, who have been using liver scans as a routine procedure for staging of patients with lung cancer including larger series of patients with small cell carcinoma conclude that this method should not be considered as a routine screening procedure for patients, who present with clinically normal liver function tests[34, 37, 38].

Furthermore, comparing liver scintigraphy and peritoneoscopy with liver biopsy, Van Houtte and De Jager observed in a study including 59 patients with small cell carcinoma, that 13 cases with positive scintigram had a negative peritoneoscopy and moreover, in 6 patients with negative liver scan, peritoneoscopy showed liver metastases[39].

How then to document the presence of hepatic metastases in small cell carcinoma? It is possible that ultrasonography with fine-needle aspirations might be useful and also important in small cel anaplastic carcinoma, but no data are yet available. At present, the use of more invasive procedures such as peritoneoscopy with liver biopsy still remains the most reliable method short of laparotomy in the detection of liver metastases; even this procedure also is hampered by certain limitations.

For instance only lesions on the surface of the liver can be inspected, and the posterior surface is excluded from visualization. In addition, the presence of diffuse peritoneal adhesions may limit the use of the procedure.

Even with the above mentioned limitations in mind, peritoneoscopy has been shown to be of definite value in the detection of liver metastases in patients with small cell anaplastic carcinoma. In the first study hepatic metastases were observed in 8 of 19 untreated patients (45%)[37]. In a subsequent and larger study that included 190 previously untreated patients hepatic metastatic disease was detected in 21% with adequate liver biopsy and an additional 9% of all patients had macroscopic signs of liver metastases. Biopsy could not be performed in the latter group for technical reasons either because of thrombocytopenia or because of the anatomic locations of the lesions. Usually the liver metastases were visualized on the surface of the liver, but in 10% of the patients with positive liver biopsy the metastases were not macroscopically visible under the exposed surface of the liver[38].

DETECTION OF METASTASES AT OTHER SITES

Other sites with frequent metastases at autopsy include, within the thorax, the mediastinal lymph nodes, and extrathoracic sites such as the upper retroperitoneal lymph nodes, adrenals, pancreas and the kidneys.

In the evaluation of mediastinal lymph nodes chest tomography and/or mediastinoscopy has been used and appreciated for decades, while the other organs are not easily assessable for specific diagnostic procedures. The methods used in the evaluation of these regions include procedures such as ultrasound guided biopsy of the pancreas, lymphangiography of retroperitoneal lymph nodes etc., but these methods have not yet been tested in small cell anaplastic carcinoma.

Recently it has been observed that ^{67}Gallium accumulates with a high incidence in tumors including the primary tumor and mediastinal metastases from lung cancer. The procedure has also been evaluated in the detection of extrathoracic malignant spread in patients with small cell anaplastic carcinoma with somewhat conflicting results. In a study by Brereton et al.[40] 47 patients with untreated small cell anaplastic carcinoma had a ^{67}Gallium scan performed. The result of this procedure was compared with other radioisotope-scans of the liver, brain and bone, and in addition bilateral posterior iliac crest bone marrow examination with aspiration and biopsy was performed. Twenty-seven separate sites of extrathoracic metastases were identified in 16 patients by means other than gallium scan. Of these 27 extrathoracic sites, however, only 2 demonstrated an abnormal gallium accumulation, both present in the same patient, and both more evident on bone scan. Accordingly, the authors conclude that whole-body scan with ^{67}Gallium was inferior to the other methods used to detect extrathoracic tumor deposits. On the contrary Bitran et al.[41], indicate that a ^{67}Gallium scan had an overall sensitivity of 59% with a specificity of 100% in extrathoracic sites. The discrepancies comparing the two studies may be explained by differences in techniques, but it has also to be emphasized that in none of the studies invasive procedures were performed in order to verify the malignant nature of abnormalities observed at the scintigrams.

To which degree of introduction of whole body CT-scan might influence the staging of patients with small cell anaplastic carcinoma is still uncertain and the results of ongoing studies are not available yet in details. Noteworthy, however, is that for demonstration of mediastinal involvement one study with 18 patients having various types of lung cancer found a false negative rate of 80%, when CT-scan was correlated with mediastinoscopy [42].

The future role and need for the different staging procedures in general in small cell anaplastic carcinomas might be difficult to assess at the time being because of major changes in treatment strategy with more and more emphasis on the systemic treatment. However, in order to proceed with the goal of achieving an improved treatment, staging will remain important for assessment of complete remission, the relapse pattern, and for determination of the duration of treatment necessary to induce a possible 'cure.'

REFERENCES

 1. TNM classification of malignant tumors. Geneva, International Union against Cancer, 1968.
 2. Mountain CF, Carr DT, Anderson WAD: A system for the clinical staging of lung cancer. Amer J Roentgenol 120:130-139, 1974.
 3. Larsson S: Pretreatment classification and staging of bronchogenic carcinoma. Scand J Thorac and Cardiovasc Surg Suppl 10, 1973.
 4. Roswitt B, Patno ME, Rapp R: The survival of patients with inoperable lung cancer: A large-scale randomized study of radiation therapy versus placebo. Radiology 90:688-697, 1968.
 5. Green RA, Humphrey E, Close H et al.: Alkylating agents in bronchogenic carcinoma. Amer J Med 46:516-524, 1969.
 6. Livingston RB, Moore TN, Heilbrun L et al.: Small-cell carcinoma of the lung: Combined chemotherapy and radiation. Ann Intern Med 88:: 194-199, 1978.
 7. Cohen MH, Ihde DC, Bunn PA, Jr: Cyclic alternating combination chemotherapy for small cell bronchogenic cercinoma. Cancer Treat Rep 63:163-170, 1979.
 8. Cooksey JA, Bitran JD, Desser RK: Small-cell carcinoma of the lung: the prognostic significance of stage on survival. Europ J Cancer 15:859-865, 1979.
 9. Hansen HH, Dombernowsky P, Hansen M et al.: Chemotherapy of advanced small cell anaplastic carcinoma. Superiority of a four-drug combination to a three-drug combination. Ann of Intern Med 89:: 177-181, 1978.
10. Hansen HH, Dombernowsky P, Hirsch   et al.: Prophylactic irradiation in bronchogenic small-cell anaplastic carcinoma. A comparative trial of localized versus extensive radiotherapy including prophylactic brain irradiation in patients receiving combination chemotherapy. Cancer 1980. In press.
11. Hansen M, Hansen HH, Dombernowsky P: Long-term survival in small cell carcinoma of the lung. JAMA 1980. In press.
12. Hansen HH: Bone metastases in lung cancer. Copenhagen, Munksgaard, 1974.
13. Matthews MJ: Problems in morphology and behaviour of bronchopulmonary malignant disease, in Israel L, Chahanian P (eds): Lung Cancer. Facts, Problems and Prospects. New York, Academic Press, 1976, PP. 23-62.

14. Matthews MJ, Kanhouwa S, Pickren J et al.: Frequency of residual and metastatic tumor in patients undergoing curative surgical resection for lung cancer. Cancer Chemother Rep 4:63-67, 1973.

15. Hirsch F, Hansen HH, Dombernowsky P et al.: Bone-marrow examination in the staging of small-cell anaplastic carcinoma of the lung with special reference to subtyping. Cancer 39:2563-2567, 1977.

16. Ihde DC, Simms EB, Matthews MJ et al.: 'Bone marrow metastases in small cell carcinoma of the lung: Frequency, description, and influence on chemotherapeutic toxicity and prognosis.' Blood 53:677-686, 1979.

17. Hansen HH, Muggia FM: Early detection of bone-marrow invasion in oat-cell carcinoma of the lung. N Engl J Med 284:: 962-963, 1971.

18. Eagan RT, Maurer LH, Forcier RJ et al.: Small cell carcinoma of the lung: Staging, paraneoplastic syndromes, treatment, and survival. Cancer 33:527-532, 1974.

19. Präuer HW, Rastettet J, Sauer E et al.: Ergebnisse der ungezielten Beckenkamm-Biopsie bei Patienten mit Bronchus-Karzinom. Munch Med Wochenschr 117:1821-1824, 1975.

20. Bagley CM, Roth GJ: Dubious value of marrow biopsy in small cell carcinoma. Proc AACR 17:198, 1976.

21. Abeloff MD, Ettinger DS, Baylin SB et al.: Management of small cell carcinoma of the lung. Therapy, staging and biochemical markers. Cancer 38:1394-1401, 1976.

22. Choi CH, Carey RW: Small cell anaplastic carcinoma of the lung. Cancer 37:2651-2657, 1976.

23. Anner RM, Drewinko B: Frequency and significance of bone marrow involvement by metastatic solid tumors. Cancer 39:1337-1344, 1977.

24. Gutierrez AC, Vincent RG, Sandberg AA et al.: Evaluation of sternal bone marrow aspiration for detection of tumor cells in patients with bronchogenic carcinoma. J Thorac and Cardiovasc Surg 77:392-395, 1979.

25. Lyman GH, Williams CC: Evaluation of the extent of disease in undifferentiated small cell bronchogenic carcinoma (USCBC). Amer Fed Clin Res p 389, 1979 (Abstract).

26. Hirsch FR, Hansen HH, Hainau B: Bilateral bone-marrow examination in small cell anaplastic carcinoma of the lung. Acta Path Microbiol Scand Sect A 87:59-62, 1979.

27. Bunn PA Jr, Nugent JL, Matthews MJ: Central nervous system metastases in small cell bronchogenic carcinoma. Sem Oncol 5:314-322, 1978.

28. F Hirsch et al.: unpublished data.

29. Nugent JL, Bunn PA, Matthews MJ et al.: CNS-metastases in small cell bronchogenic carcinoma. Increasing frequency and changing pattern with lengthening survival. Cancer 44:0333-0341, 1979.

30. Burgess RE, Burgess VF, Dibella NJ: Brain metastases in small cell carcinoma of the lung. JAMA 242:2084-2086, 1979.

31. Hayes TP, Davis LW, Raventos A: Brain and liver-scans in the evaluation of lung cancer patients. Cancer 27:362-363, 1971.

32. Pedersen HE, Hjelms E, Struve-Christensen E et al.: Intracranial metastasis from cancer of the lung. J. Thorac Cardiovasc. Surg. 65:159-164, 1973.

33. Kies MS, Baker AW, Kennedy PS: Radionuclide scans in staging of carcinoma of the lung. Surg Gynec Obstet 147:175-176, 1978.

34. Wittes RE, Yeh SDJ: Indications for liver and brain scans. Screening tests for patients with oat cell carcinoma of the lung. JAMA 238:: 506-507, 1977.

35. Jacobs L, Kinkel WR, Vincent RG: 'Silent' brain metastases from lung carcinoma determined by computerized tomography. Arch Neurol 34:690-693, 1977.

36. Hansen M, Hansen HH, Almqvist S et al.: Cerebrospinal fluid in patients with CNS-metastases from small cell bronchogenic carcinoma. Europ J Cancer. In press.

37. Margolis R, Hansen HH, Muggia FM *et al.*: Diagnosis of liver metastases in bronchogenic carcinoma. Cancer 34:1825-1829, 1974.
38. Dombernowsky P, Hirsch FR, Hansen HH *et al.*: Peritoneoscopy in the staging of 190 patients with small-cell anaplastic carcinoma of the lung with special reference to subtyping. Cancer 41:2008-2012, 1978.
39. Van Houtte P, De Jager R: Correlation between liver scintigraphy and peritoneoscopy in small cell carcinoma of the lung. Unpublished data.
40. Brereton HD, Line BR, Londer HN: Gallium scans for staging of small cell lung cancer. JAMA 240:666-667, 1978.
41. Bitran JD, Bekerman C, Pinsky S, *et al.*: Gallium 67 scans in small cell carcinoma. JAMA 241:1106, 1979.
42. Underwood GH, Hooper RG, Axelbaum SP *et al.*: Computed tomographic scanning of the thorax in the staging of bronchogenic carcinoma. N Engl J Med 300:777-778, 1979.

8. Small Cell Bronchogenic Carcinoma: A Review of Therapeutic Results

PAUL A. BUNN, Jr. and DANIEL C. IHDE

INTRODUCTION

Small cell bronchogenic carcinoma (SCBC) accounts for 20–25% of all lung cancers in the United States. It is estimated that there are 20,000–25,000 cases per year. Recent studies have shown that SCBC is biologically different from the other lung cancer cell types [1, 2]. The natural history and response to therapy are also markedly different from the non-small cell histologic groups [1, 3]. Untreated patients have median survivals of only 6–17 weeks and less than 1% of patients are alive 5 years following surgical treatments [4–6]. Radiotherapy alone has been shown to be superior to surgery alone for patients with limited disease stages; however, mean survival for these early stage patients treated with radiotherapy alone is short (43 weeks), and less than 1–5% of patients are alive at 5 years [1, 6]. Systemic chemotherapy has made a dramatic impact on survival. Several useful reviews of single agent and combination chemotherapy have recently been published [1, 7–10].*

In this manuscript, we will review reports of chemotherapy given alone or in combination with surgery or radiotherapy. Emphasis will be placed on randomized trials. Articles with predominantly previously treated patients or with less than 10 patients given a particular therapy will not be included. We will also not include data reported only in abstract form except for randomized trials of particular importance.

The stage of disease (limited versus extensive), the performance status, and prior therapy are the well established prognostic factors in SCBC. For the purpose of this manuscript, we will rely on definitions of limited and exten-

---

* Abbreviations of chemotherapeutic and biologic agents discussed in this manuscript are provided in Table 1.

R.B. Livingston (ed.), Lung cancer 1, 169–208. All rights reserved.
Copyright © 1981 Martinus Nijhoff Publishers bv, The Hague/Boston/London.

Table 1. Abbreviations used for chemotherapeutic and biologic agents.

Abbreviation	Agent
ADR	doxorubicin (Adriamycin®)
BCG	Bacille Calmette Guerin vaccine
BCNU	bis-chloroethyl-nitrosourea
BLEO	bleomycin
BUS	busulfan
CCNU	cyclohexyl-chloroethyl-nitrosourea
CDDP	cis-diamminedichloro-platinum
Cparv	Corynebacterium parvum
CTX	cyclophosphamide (Cytoxan®)
DBD	dibromodulcitol
DTIC	dimethyl-triazeno-imidazole-carboxamide
EMET	dehydroemetine
5FU	5-fluorouracil
HDCTX	high dose cyclophosphamide (60 mg/kg × 2)
HDMTX	high dose methotrexate (with citrovorum factor rescue)
HMM	hexamethylmelamine
HN2	mechlorethamine (nitrogen mustard)
HU	hydroxyurea
IFOS	ifosfamide
MeCCNU	methylcyclohexyl-chloroethyl-nitrosourea
MER	methanol extractable residue (of BCG)
MTX	methotrexate
PCZ	procarbazine
PRED	prednisone (or prednisolone)
STZ	streptozotocin
THY	thymosin Fraction V
VCR	vincristine
VLB	vinblastine (Velban®)
VM-26	demethyl-thenylidene-glucopyranosyl-epipodophyllotoxin
VP-16	demethyl-ethylidene-glucopyranosyl-epipodophyllotoxin

sive disease used by the authors. In general, limited disease is defined as disease confined to one hemithorax which can be encompassed in a single radiation port. Different authors include or exclude supraclavicular nodes and pleural effusions. Any spread beyond these limits is defined as extensive disease. We will provide results by stage, limited versus extensive, except in a few instances where the majority of patients had limited or extensive disease and results by stage were not provided. Unfortunately, most articles do not provide response and survival data by performance status so this data cannot be included. Future articles clearly should provide response and survival data both by stage and by performance status. In early studies when median survivals were less than 6 months and few, if any, patients lived beyond

2 years, survival data was usually given in days or weeks and 2-year disease-free survival data were not included. Current active combination chemotherapy regimens consistently provide median survials of 8–18 months and some 2-year disease-free survivors. Thus, we will list median survival data in months and will provide the number of 2-year disease-free survivors when available. Since a minority of SCBC patients are cured, the median survival figures might not be influenced by better therapy which is curative in only a few patients. The 2-year disease-free survival will clearly demonstrate such differences. For this reason, future reports should provide long-term follow-up and 2-year disease-free survival information.

CHEMOTHERAPY AS SURGICAL ADJUVANT TREATMENT

The autopsy demonstration of distant metastases in 70% of patients dying within 30 days of 'curative' surgical resection for SCBC [11] supports attempts to eradicate metastatic disease with chemotherapy following operative removal of the primary tumor. Early randomized trials of surgical adjuvant chemotherapy, however, were conducted with single drugs in relatively low doses, treatment that is clearly not optimal for SCBC. In addition, since the marked chemotherapeutic responsiveness of small cell cancer was not appreciated at the time many of the trials were begun, results were sometimes specifically analyzed for this cell type only in retrospect [12].

By the time substantial evidence was accrued that aggressive combination chemotherapy was the mainstay of drug treatment of this tumor, surgical resection of small cell pulmonary cancer had largely been supplanted by primary therapy with radiation, drugs, or both. Thus, trials utilizing what would now be considered optimum adjuvant chemotherapy were never performed. Nonetheless, the clinical studies which have been completed are suggestive of drug benefit [12–15].

In three of the four prospective randomized trials of surgical adjuvant chemotherapy for SCBC published in the 1970's (Table 2), survival of treated patients was superior to the survival of randomized controls managed solely by surgery. In the trials which suggested benefits from chemotherapy, statistical analysis of survival differences between treated and control groups was not provided [12, 14] or yielded insignificant results [15], perhaps due to the small numbers of patients studied. Despite these facts, the data are intriguing.

Patients entered in the trial reported by Higgins had tumors that could not be diagnosed at preoperative bronchoscopy and perhaps were less massive [12]. Beneficial effects were probable from chemotherapy that consisted of only two courses of intravenous CTX administered over 5 weeks. More

Table 2. Randomized trials of surgical adjuvant chemotherapy in small cell carcinoma of the lung.

Reference	Treatment	Duration	No. patients	% survival			
				2yr	3yr	4yr	5yr
MRC[13]	BUS	2 years	14	21			
	CTX		9	0			
	Placebo		16	12			
Higgins[12]	CTX	5 weeks	32	28	22	16	
	Control		26	11	8	4	
Shields[14]	CTX/MTX	18 months	9		33		
	CTX	18 months	6		17		
	Control		3		0		
Karrer[15]	CTX + 5FU + VLB + MTX	3 years	22	25*			37
	Control		16	0			0

* Actuarial projection.

prolonged chemotherapy was administered in the trials reported by Shields *et al.* [14] and Karrer *et al.* [15]. However, leukopenia was induced in only 10% of treated patients[15] or after 10–24% of courses of chemotherapy[14]. Despite this relatively modest chemotherapeutic toxicity, the results of both studies suggest benefit from drug treatment. In the only trial which fails to support the efficacy of adjuvant chemotherapy[13], the therapeutic programs consisted of daily oral alkylating agents, almost surely an inferior mode of administration.

For reasons already discussed, it is extremely improbable that a prospective randomized trial comparing immediate post-resection aggressive combination chemotherapy with a policy of waiting until recurrence to begin such treatment will ever be initiated in patients with SCBC. Recently, two groups of authors[16, 17] have presented several patients who received combination chemotherapy following surgical resection of apparently limited stage tumor with intrathoracic regional lymph node involvement. Long-term disease-free survival was reported in 4 patients. In addition, a large randomized chemotherapy trial in SCBC found superior survival in patients who had previously undergone pulmonary surgery[18]. Since many patients with limited disease presently fail initially in the primary tumor site, whether treated with chemotherapy alone or chemotherapy plus chest irradiation, the role of surgical resection as adjunctive treatment to chemotherapy, rather than the opposite traditional conception, probably deserves prospective evaluation.

RANDOMIZED TRIALS OF RADIATION ALONE VERSUS CHEMOTHERAPY ALONE

When it became apparent that both chemotherapy and radiotherapy were active modalities, three randomized trials comparing radiotherapy alone with chemotherapy alone were performed [19–21]. These trials are of interest but are outdated since the chemotherapy employed was greatly inferior to current chemotherapy regimens which produce far better survivals whether combined with irradiation or not (vide infra). Two trials were confined to patients with limited disease and employed single agent chemotherapy (CTX or BCNU) [19, 20]. In both trials, survival was superior in patients receiving chemotherapy (median survival = 26–29 weeks) versus radiotherapy (median survival = 10–22 weeks). In the third trial, patients were not adequately staged although the majority were limited [21]. Combination chemotherapy $(HN_2 + VLB + PCZ + PRED)$ was used and survival was significantly shorter in patients receiving the combination chemotherapy (median 14 weeks versus 31 weeks for radiotherapy alone).

RADIOTHERAPY ALONE VERSUS RADIOTHERAPY PLUS CHEMOTHERAPY (Table 3)

By the early 1970's it was appreciated that metastatic dissemination was the most frequent cause for failure of radiation therapy even in patients with limited disease. It was thus logical to compare radiation therapy alone with radiation plus systemic chemotherapy. The results of 6 such randomized trials of radiation therapy alone versus radiation therapy plus chemotherapy are shown in Table 3 [22–28]. Each of these trials included only patients with limited disease, although most did not employ extensive staging procedures and the Medical Research Council trial included a few patients with bone marrow involvement [27]. The earliest trial reported by Carr et al. employed 5FU, an agent without documented activity in SCBC, and only one or two courses were used. Not surprisingly, no differences in one or two year survival were noted [22]. The trials of Bergsagel et al. [23] and Host et al. [24] found the addition of cyclophosphamide to radiation improved early survival with statistically improved median survival, but did not infuence late survival. Similarly, Petrovich et al. found that CCNU and hydroxyurea improved early and median survival, but had no effect on 1 or 2 year survival [25, 26]. More recent trials have added more effective drug combinations $(CTX + MTX + CCNU$ and $CTX + MTX + ADR)$ to radiation. In these trials, the combined modality therapy also improved median survival [27, 28]. In addition, the one and two year survivals and the number of patients without distant metastases were improved in the combined modality arms. The results of radiation therapy alone were quite similar in these trials with median

Table 3. Randomized trials of radiation therapy alone versus radiation therapy plus chemotherapy.

Radiation[1]		Chemotherapy	Reference	No. Patients	Median survival (mos.)	% 1 year survival	% 2 year survival	% distant mets, 1 year
4,500-5,000, 1, 2, B		None	Carr [22]	27	NR	19	11	NR
		5FU		31	NR	23	6	NR
4,000-5,000, 1 C		None	Bergsagel [23]	14	5.0	NR	NR	NR
		CTX[2]		27	10.0	NR	NR	NR
4,000, 1 B		None	Host [24]	36	5.5	20	10[3]	NR
		CTX		39	8.5	30	10[3]	NR
5,000-6,000, 1 B		None	Petrovich [25, 26]	34	5.0	28	10	NR
		CCNU+HU		35	9.0	28	7	NR
3,000, 1 A		None	MRC [27]	121	6.0	18	8[4]	79
		CTX+MTX+CCNU		115	10.0	34	26[4]	57
5,500, 1 B		None	Matthiessen [28]	14	NR	NR	NR	65
		CTX+MTX+ADR		11	NR	NR	NR	25

[1] Dose in rads; 1 = continuous, 2 = split course, A = prior to chemotherapy, B = concurrent with chemotherapy, C = between chemotherapy courses.

[2] Total of 2 groups given either 4 or 8 doses.

[3] % 1.5 year survival.

[4] 1 year disease free survival.

NR = not reported.

survivals of 5–6 months, 1 year survivals of 18–28% and 2 year survivals of 8–11%. These randomized trials document the superiority of combined radiation therapy-chemotherapy over radiation alone when effective chemotherapy is used. Even the most recent of these combined modality trials used doses of chemotherapy which have been shown to be inferior to larger doses in randomized studies employing chemotherapy alone (vide infra).

SINGLE AGENT CHEMOTHERAPY

The failure of surgery or radiation therapy to cure more than 1–2% of patients with apparently localized SCBC [1, 5, 6] can be ascribed in the majority of instances to the presence of distant metastatic disease at the time of diagnosis. Hence, systemic chemotherapy is the logical cornerstone of treatment.

The major impetus for aggressive investigation of the value of chemotherapy in SCBC was provided by the Veterans Administration Lung Cancer Study Group in 1969. Green *et al.* [29] demonstrated that three courses of intravenous CTX given over a period of 9 weeks significantly prolonged the median survival of patients with extensive stage disease, when compared to a similar group of patients receiving a placebo. Although the survival prolongation was short, from a median of 1.5 to 4 months, it represented a doubling of lifespan for the entire treated population, results that cannot even begin to be approached in other cell types of lung cancer with the much more complex and intensive chemotherapeutic regimens in use today.

One characteristic of tumors which are highly responsive to drug therapy is that a large number of agents will produce objective tumor regressions. Documentation of the activity of a variety of single agents in small cell carcinoma was well reviewed by Broder *et al.* [7] in 1977, and will only briefly be considered here. At the time of that review, 11 drugs were considered to be active in small cell carcinoma. Only seven, however, fulfilled the criteria of evaluation in 40 or more patients with an overall response rate of 15% or more, including at least 2 studies with 10 or more patients which demonstrated at least 20% objective responses. These agents include CTX, HN2, ADR, MTX, HMM, VP-16, and VCR. Only two of them, VCR and to a lesser extent HMM, do not have myelosuppression as their major acute dose-limiting side effect, hampering efforts to construct drug combination regimens with non-overlapping toxicities. Another limitation of single agent chemotherapy in SCBC is illustrated by the fact that despite high overall response rates to these drugs, especially in previously untreated patients, only 19 of 753 patients (2.5%) treated with one of these seven single agents experienced complete tumor regressions [7, 30].

As of late 1977, four other agents were presumed to be active in this tumor on the basis of two or more trials, although they fail to fulfill the more demanding criteria outlined in the previous paragraph. They include PCZ and three nitrosoureas, CCNU, BCNU, and MeCCNU. Although the total response rate to CCNU as a single agent as tabulated by Broder et al. [7] was only 14%, CCNU plus CTX have produced improved response rates and survival when compared in a randomized fashion to CTX alone [18], and CCNU was the only one of the three nitrosoureas which significantly improved survival in extensive stage small cell cancer when compared (after correction for performance status) to placebo-treated controls of the Veterans Administration Lung Cancer Study Group [31].

The search for more and hopefully more active single agents is clearly justified in patients with small cell cancer. Thus, it is surprising how little additional information on the activity of other agents has been published since the review of Broder et al. [7].

DBD, which may act as a bifunctional alkylating agent, was reported to produce a 24% objective response rate and yield similar survival results to HMM in a randomized trial conducted in poorly characterized patients [32]. Although results were available for only one trial conducted with the alkylating agent IFOS in Broder's review [7], no further confirmatory small cell-specific studies have been published.

STZ is a nitrosourea which could be a valuable addition to SCBC treatment regimens, since it lacks myelosuppressive properties. Unfortunately, it failed to demonstrate activity in two Phase II trials in patients who had progressed on combination chemotherapy [33, 34]. VM-26, an epipodophyllotoxin like VP-16, the most recently introduced active agent, was inactive in one Phase II trial [35].

The only other new agent for which recent results have been published other than in abstract form is CDDP, and data on its activity in small cell cancer are conflicting. Cavalli et al. [36] reported a 36% response rate in 11 patients who had failed combination chemotherapy, while Dombernowsky et al. [37] observed only 3/28 partial responses (median duration 2 months) in a similar patient population. Over one-third of the patients in the latter study received CDDP in less than standard doses. Despite this lack of clear documentation of single agent activity, CDDP is already being used in combination regimens in previously untreated patients [38].

HDMTX is similarly being added to first-line combination chemotherapy programs with little more than anecdotal evidence of single agent activity [39], much less any demonstration of superiority to usual doses of MTX and some suggestion that administration of MTX in this fashion as part of a drug combination is no better than standard doses of the agent [40]. HDMTX is of potential interest in prevention of central nervous system metastases since high but not standard doses of the drug yield cytotoxic concentrations in the cerebrospinal fluid.

Phase II disease-specific trials of newer and previously untested drugs that are active in other tumors are definitely needed in SCBC. Agents which produce minimal or no myelosuppression would be especially good candidates for study.

COMBINATION CHEMOTHERAPY

Superiority to Single Agent Treatment

Complete tumor responses are a prerequisite to prolonged disease-free survival in SCBC and any other human cancer. In small cell cancer, treatment with single chemotherapeutic agents very infrequently produces complete responses [7, 39], as previously discussed. In contrast, combination chemotherapy yields 25–50% complete responses in previously untreated patients (see Tables 4, 5). Thus, one would expect not only more frequent tumor responses but also superior survival in patients given combination chemotherapy as opposed to single agents, and in collected results from the literature this is indeed the case. A limited number of prospective randomized trials have directly addressed the question of the superiority of combination treatment.

Edmonson *et al.* [18] observed a statistically significant improvement in overall (complete plus partial) and complete response rate when CCNU was added to CTX; median survival was very modestly prolonged as well, an improvement of borderline significance. Lowenbraun *et al.* [41] compared the combination of CTX + ADR + DTIC to CTX alone and found a highly significant improvement in overall response rate from 12% to 59% when the combination was compared to the single agent; the combination significantly prolonged median survial by almost 3 months, although additional patients given CTX + ADR + DTIC without randomization were included when the survival curves were analyzed.

In the two studies just mentioned, radiotherapy was not part of the treatment program. Two other randomized trials have evaluated combination vs. single agent treatment when some [42] or all [40] patients received chest irradiation in addition to drugs. Eagan *et al.* [42] failed to note differences in either response rate or survival when VP-16 alone was compared to two 3-drug combinations. However, 5/5 patients failing VP-16 had later responses to one of the combination regimens, essentially rendering this trial a comparison between initial versus delayed combination chemotherapy. Perhaps because of small patient numbers randomized to CTX alone, the trial of Maurer *et al.* [40] did not demonstrate that response rates or survival were improved when CTX was compared to CTX + VCR + MTX. Further treat-

Table 4. Combination chemotherapy in limited disease: Randomized and non-randomized trials.

Chemotherapy	Reference	No. patients	No. CR+PR	No. CR	MED SURV (mos)	No. 2-yr DFS
3 drugs:						
CTX+ADR+VP-16(±MER)	Aisner[46]	9	7	4	5.0+	TE
CTX+ADR+VCR	Stevens[47]	18	12	8	11.5	1*
CTX+ADR+DTIC/ ±HU+MTX+VCR	Lowenbraun[41]	61	38	NR	9.5	TE
Totals		88	57/88 (65%)	12/27 (44%)	5.0 − 11.5	1/18 (6%)
4 or more drugs:						
CTX+MTX+CCNU/VCR+ADR+ PCZ/±VP-16+IFOS (±THY)	Cohen[48]	19	19	14	14.0	1
CTX+MTX+CCNU+VCR	Hansen[49]	69	63	NR	14.0	TE
CDDP+VP-16/CTX+ADR+VCR	Sierocki[38]	21	21	11	10.0+	TE
CTX+ADR+MTX+CCNU/VCR+ BLEO+EMET (+Cparv)	Israel[50]	34 (16 E)	28	19	10.5+	4*
HDCTX/CTX+VCR+MTX+BCNU	Ettinger[51]	15	12	4	6.5	0
Totals		158 (16 E)	143/158 (91%)	48/89 (54%)	6.5 − 14.0	5/68 (7%)
	Grand totals (all L patients)	246 (16 E) (7% E)	200/246 (81%)	60/116 (52%)	5.0 − 14.0	6/86 (7%)

Abbreviations: CR = complete response, PR = partial response, MED SURV = median survival, DFS = disease-free survival, NR = not reported, TE = too early, E = extensive, * = more patients too early, + = MED SURV not yet reached, L = limited.

ment was not standardized after patients failed CTX. Later during this study, the 3 drugs were randomly compared to a 2-drug combination, with VCR eliminated. When all patients are combined and those receiving 3 drugs are compared to those given 1 or 2 drugs, higher overall response rates for 3 drugs were noted in limited disease and higher overall responses plus minor responses in extensive disease. These trends were of borderline or actual statistical significance, respectively. When difficulties in interpretation of the results of all four randomized trials are taken into account, the superiority of combination chemotherapy seems evident. Nonetheless, the results of combination treatment in the larger studies are less striking than those observed in many trials from single institutions (see Tables 4, 5), presumably because some of the randomized studies include many patients previously failing radiotherapy [18, 41].

One randomized study has addressed the question of whether the individual components of a drug combination are better given simultaneously or sequentially. Alberto *et al.* [43] found that overall response rates increased from 36% to 62% (borderline significance) when the combination of CTX + MTX + VCR + PCZ was administered simultaneously. Virtually all investigators currently employ simultaneous administration.

Optimum Number of Drugs in the Combination

Two randomized studies in patients with extensive disease have sought to determine the optimum numbers of drugs which should be administered simultaneously. Both were conducted by Hansen *et al.* [44, 45]. The first trial compared CTX + MTX + CCNU to a combination consisting of only the first 2 agents. Although the 3-drug regimen had a higher overall response rate (52% vs. 31% of all entered patients responded) and was associated with 2 months prolongation of median survival, neither difference was statistically significant [44]. A more recent study [45] tested whether the addition of VCR improved the results which could be achieved with CTX + MTX + CCNU. Although overall response rates to the 2 combinations were quite similar, patients receiving 4 drugs experienced a 1.5 month increase in median survival (7.5 vs. 6 months) which was statistically significant; long-term disease-free survival was seen only with the VCR-containing combination. The probable superiority of the combination of CTX + MTX + VCR to CTX + MTX, at least in terms of response rate, has already been mentioned [40]. Although the results of randomized trials utilizing chemotherapy alone discussed up to this point [18, 44, 45] are consistent with the derivation of successive benefit from adding one, two, and then three additional drugs to therapy with CTX alone, this advantage could be present only when new drugs are added to relatively less myelosuppressive treatment regimens. Approximaely 30–50% of the patients of Hansen *et al.* [44, 45] never experienced leukopenia below the level

Table 5. Combination chemotherapy in extensive disease: Randomized and non-randomized trials.

Chemotherapy	Reference	No. patients	No. CR + PR	No. CR	MED SURV (mos)	No. 2-yr DFS
2 drugs:						
CTX + CCNU	Edmonson[18]	106 (18 L)	46	13	4.5	TE
CTX + MTX	Hansen[44]	29	9	NR	5.5	0
CTX + MTX	Straus[52]	19 (4 L)	17	10	14.5	NR
CCNU + ADR	Trowbridge[53]	16 (5 L)	10	6	7.5 +	TE
CTX + VCR	Holoye[54]	23	14	6	6.0	0**
Totals		193 (27 L)	96/193 (50%)	35/164 (21%)	4.5-14.5	0/52 (0%)
3 drugs:						
CTX + ADM + DTIC/ ±HU + MTX + VCR	Lowenbraun[41]	146	81	NR	6.5	TE
CTX + MTX + CCNU	Hansen[45]	52	36	NR	6.0	0
CTX + MTX + CCNU (high dose)	Cohen[55]	23 (4 L)	22	7	10.5	2
CTX + MTX + CCNU (standard dose)	Cohen[55]	9 (1 L)	4	0	5.0	0
CTX + MTX + CCNU	Hansen[44]	33	17	NR	7.5	0**
VCR + CTX + MTX	Eagan[42]	9	5	NR	7.0	0
VCR + ADR + BLEO	Eagan[42]	13	5	3	8.5	TE
CTX + ADR + DTIC	Saiontz[56]	18	12		4.5	0
CTX + ADR + VP-16 (±MER)	Aisner[46]	21	14	7	5.0 +	TE
CTX + ADR + VCR	Holoye[57]	25	15	7	6.5	TE
CTX + ADR + VCR (+BCG)	Holoye[73]	15	13	6	9.5	TE
Totals		364 (5 L)	224/364 (62%)	30/111 (27%)	4.5-10.5	2/144 (1%)

Table 5 (continued)

Chemotherapy	Reference	No. patients	No. CR+PR	No. CR	MED SURV (mos)	No. 2-yr DFS
4 or more drugs :						
CTX+MTX+CCNU+VCR CTX+MTX+CCNU/ VCR+ADR+PCZ/±VP-16+IFOS (±THY)	Hansen [45]	53	39	NR	7.5	1
CTX+ADR+VCR+BLEO	Cohen [48]	42	38	15	9.5	3
CTX+MTX+VCR+PCZ/CTX± MTX+VCR+PCZ	Einhorn [58]	29 (4 L)	22	6	8.0	TE
CTX+MTX+CCNU+VCR	Alberto [43, 59]	53 (26 L)	33	NR	7.0	0**
CTX+MTX+CCNU+VCR/ADR+VP-16	Dombernowsky [60]	73	59	NR	9.0	TE
CDDP+VP-16/CTX+ADR+VCR	Dombernowsky [60]	73	66	NR	9.0	TE
PCZ+VCR+CTX+CCNU	Sierocki [38]	17	15	7	9.0	TE
HDCTX/CTX+VCR+MTX+BCNU	Williams [61]	12	11	5	11.0	1*
CTX+ADR+VP-16/BCNU+ VCR+MTX+PCZ	Ettinger [51]	9	4	0	4.0+	0
MTX+ADR+CTX+CCNU	Abeloff [62]	15	13	3	7.5+	TE
MTX+VCR+CTX+ADR (±BCG or Cparv)	Chahinian [63]	15 (4 L)	13	5	10.0	TE
CTX+VCR+PCZ+PRED	Sarna [64]	29 (7 L)	20	8	10.0	0**
	Nixon [65]	13 (4 L)	11	5	9.5	TE
	Totals	433 (45 L)	344/433 (79%)	54/181 (30%)	4.0+ – 11.0	5/198 (3%)
	Grand totals (all E patients)	990 (77 L) (8% L)	664/990 (67%)	119/456 (26%)	4.0+ – 14.5	7/394 (2%)

Abbreviations as in Table 4; in addition, ** = actuarial projection.

of 2–3000/μl, and in fully half platelet counts below 100,000/μl w
recorded. Since many current combination regimens produce great
of myelosuppression, it is conceivable that increasing drug doses co
efficacious as adding additional agents to a 2- or 3-drug combinati

Tabular Results from the Literature

The results of combination chemotherapy in SCBC reported thro
are listed in Tables 4 and 5. A total of 1,236 patients (246 limited
extensive stage) given drug combinations without chest irradiation a
able for analysis [18, 38, 41–65, 73].

The overall objective response rate (complete plus partial responses)
these tabulated reports is 81% in limited disease and 67% in extensive
disease. More importantly, twice as many complete responses (52% vs. 26%)
are induced by chemotherapy in limited as opposed to extensive disease.
Median survival of patients with limited disease is almost always superior to
the life span of extensive disease patients, as has been shown in many
individual reports [18, 41], and exceeds 12 months in some recent
trials [48, 49]. Disease-free survival 2 years from the beginning of therapy, a
reasonable measure of intermediate- to long-term efficacy, can clearly be
achieved in a small minority of patients given combination chemotherapy
alone. The fraction of patients with sufficient observation time who remain in
complete remission at 2 years is 7% in limited disease and 2% in extensive
disease, indicating that the prospects for prologed survival with chemotherapy
are not hopeless even in the latter group of patients. Because so many reports
are published with short follow-up periods, these tabulated estimates of 2-year
disease-free survival are clearly imprecise.

The combination regimens are segregated in the Tables by the number of
drugs which they contain. Reports of 2-drug combinations in limited disease
have not appeared. Both overall and complete response rates appear to
increase in both limited and extensive disease as the number of drugs in the
combination is increased from 2 to 3 to 4 or more. There is no readily
apparent improvement in results with 5 or more drugs. Lengthening of
median survival with increasing numbers of drugs is not so obvious as the
increase in response rates. In view of the obvious limitations of collected data,
it would be hazardous to suggest that the administration of more than 3 or 4
drugs simultaneously is beneficial.

Similarly, whether any specific drugs need be included in a combination
regimen for optimal results is uncertain. Virtually every published regimen
contains CTX. It is clearly impossible to conclude that any single combination
is superior, and it is possible that the addition of any two or three other active
agents to CTX will produce fairly equivalent therapeutic effects with equivalent degrees of myelosuppression.

Effect of Response on Survival

A powerful predictor of survival on combination chemotherapy is the response to treatment. A virtually universal finding in reported studies in SCBC is that patients with complete or partial response live significantly longer than those with stable disease or disease progression [18, 41, 44, 45, 48, 50, 55]. Furthermore, in contrast to other cell types of lung cancer in which patients with disease stability often have similar or even superior survival to patients with objective tumor response, SCBC patients with stable disease have only minimal survival advantage over those with disease progression [18, 43]. More recent intensive regimens induce such a high frequency of objective responses that distinctions between disease stability and progression are not usually made, but in most reports it is clear that the major survival advantage is derived from complete rather than partial responses [48, 50, 55].

Time Course of Objective Response

The poor survival of patients with disease stability on combination chemotherapy compared with the life span of objective responders is consistent with the relatively rapid growth rate of SCBC compared to other types of lung cancer. As might be predicted from knowledge of the latter fact, tumor regressions on chemotherapy occur quickly. When high doses of CTX + MTX + CCNU were employed, maximum response to treatment occurred within 3 weeks (after 1 cycle of drugs) in 8 of the 18 patients who eventually responded to chemotherapy; after another 3 weeks, the remaining 10 patients had achieved their maximum tumor regression [55]. Numerous other authors [18, 38, 51, 57, 62] who analyzed their data in this fashion have observed that maximum response to chemotherapy occurs in virtually all patients within 5 to 8 weeks. In fact, some groups have been unable to increase the objective response rate by introducing a new, presumably non-cross resistant drug regimen within the first 2 to 3 months of therapy [38, 51, 62].

Intensity of Chemotherapy

Most combination regimens in current use produce substantial myelosuppression, and present therapeutic results seem clearly superior to those attained with less aggressive single agent and combination regimens in common use 5 to 10 years ago. Only one prospective randomized trial, however, has directly addressed the question of the value of increasing drug dosages. Cohen *et al.* [55] compared the results of CTX + MTX + CCNU in standard outpatient doses with those achieved by doubling the doses of these agents and administering them in an inpatient setting. Overall response rate and median survival were significantly superior in the high-dose chemotherapy group, and, more importantly, complete responses and 2-year disease-free survival were noted only with the more intensive regimen. Whether greater escalations in the intensity of chemotherapy will produce further improvement in results, however, is uncertain. Many groups now employ drug doses that produce myelosuppression of a degree that at least approaches that reported by Cohen et al. [55], and this can often be accomplished in an outpatient setting. Ettinger et al. [51] and Abeloff et al. [62] have escalated the doses of CTX, with or without ADR + VP-16, to levels 1 1/2 to 2 times that employed by Cohen et al. [55] without observing any striking benefits in terms of an increase in complete responses. The regimen of CTX + ADR + VP-16 has been administered with less than half the amount of CTX used by Abeloff et al. [62], with what appear to be quite similar results [46].

Alternating Non-Cross Resistant Regimens

One likely mechanism for relapse from response to chemotherapy in small cell carcinoma is the development of drug resistance by the tumor. Several investigators, therefore, have attempted to prolong remission duration and hopefully survival by introduction of a new, non-cross resistant drug regimen after initial tumor response but prior to disease progression. The usual strategy has been to alternately administer the two combination regimens. Cohen et al. [48] in a one-armed study found that the administration of VCR + ADR + PCZ at Week 7 after initial treatment with CTX + MTX + CCNU increased the complete response rate from 42 to 74% in limited disease and from 24 to 36% in extensive disease. Introduction of a third regimen of VP-16 + IFOS in a randomized fashion at Week 13 produced no further complete responses and had no effect on survival compared with further therapy with only the first two combinations. However, despite the increased complete response rate, overall survival with this program was not different from the group's previous study, which employed CTX + MTX + CCNU until tumor progression, followed by VCR + ADR + PCZ [55]. This was explained by the short survival of patients who attained a late complete response to the second drug regimen, compared with those who achieved complete tumor regression in the first 6 weeks [48].

Two prospective randomized studies have tried to assess the value of alternating 2 drug combinations as opposed to giving only a single combination until disease progression. Although duration of response [60] and time to disease progression [41] were significantly prolonged by early introduction of an additional regimen, median survival was not affected. The results of all these studies are consistent with the concept that only complete responses which are achieved early in the course of treatment have major clinical impact.

Maintenance Chemotherapy

Most investigators have continued to administer chemotherapy in SCBC until disease progression or, in complete responders, for 12 to 24 months. Whether such protracted treatment is necessary is unknown, but the probability is that it is not, at least for some patients. Johnson et al. [66] employed an intensive combined modality program of CTX + ADR + VCR and simultaneous chest and prophylactic cranial irradiation, with continuation of chemotherapy in complete responders for only 2–4 months. Actuarial disease-free survival at 2 years in limited disease was 30%, as good or better than other studies of CTX + ADR + VCR and chest/prophylactic cranial irradiation in which chemotherapy was continued for 14 [67] or 24 [68] months. Only one randomized study has evaluated the necessity of maintenance chemotherapy. Maurer et al. [40] randomized complete responders at 6 months to continued versus no additional chemotherapy until relapse. Although survival was significantly improved in limited disease patients receiving maintenance chemotherapy, the results are difficult to interpret since duration of remission was not. It seems likely that much shorter durations of maintenance treatment than those customarily employed may be sufficient; this point could profitably be addressed in further prospective studies.

Treatment of Superior Vena Cava Obstruction

Superior vena cava syndrome, of which lung cancer is presently the most common cause, is customarily considered a radiotherapeutic emergency. Two recent reports [69, 70] make clear that combination chemotherapy alone is excellent treatment in patients with SCBC who have not previously been exposed to drug treatment. Dombernowsky et al. [70], who noted that the syndrome was present at diagnosis in 11.5% of 225 consecutive patients, treated 22 patients with combination chemotherapy alone; complete response of the syndrome occurred in 95% in a median of 14 days. The results of Kane et al. [69] in fewer patients are similar. It is appropriate to treat SCBC patients presenting with superior vena cava syndrome with chemotherapy alone, reserving irradiation for failures of chemotherapy, if the treatment policy of an individual institution would not otherwise mandate chest irradiation.

Sites of Relapse

Determination of sites of relapse from a chemotherapy program, particularly relapses from a complete remission, may be of value in identifying areas of disease for which other measures to improve local control (such as irradiation) might be considered. Many reports of sites of relapse combine results in patients with disease progression after complete and partial response, or in patients with limited and extensive disease. Distinctions are not always made between initial and subsequent sites of relapse. The chest is certainly the most common site of disease progression, but it is relatively easy to monitor and simultaneous relapse in extrathoracic sites can be overlooked unless specifically investigated. Cohen et al. [55] reported that 42% of relapses in a population predominantly composed of patients with extensive disease occurred solely in the chest. In a later study of relapses from complete response only [48], 71% of relapses in limited and 56% of relapses in extensive disease were diagnosed solely in the chest. However, 6/10 patients with solely local relapse developed extrathoracic disease progression within 4–10 weeks. Tumor progression sites in 6/9 patients of Williams et al. [61] treated only with chemotherapy were solely in the chest, but a similar proportion (5/9) of relapses confined to the thorax was evident in patients who were randomized to receive additional chest irradiation. Central nervous system metastases, particularly in the brain, often develop in patients who do not receive prophylactic cranial irradiation, but the great majority of disease progression in the brain is accompanied by growth of extracranial tumor [71, 72]. Central nervous system relapses are frequent even with drug treatment including lipophilic agents such as CCNU [71] which penetrate the blood-brain barrier (vide infra).

Toxicity

Myelosuppression from effective combination chemotherapy is virtually universal, in large part because hematologic toxicity is induced by all but one of the active agents in this disease. Toxic deaths from present relatively intensive combination chemotherapy programs range from 0 to 6% [45, 48, 50, 51, 58, 62]. Early diagnosis and treatment of leukopenia-associated infection should be the major focus of a program to reduce toxicity of chemotherapy. Severe thrombocytopenia with agents currently employed is less common. Non-hematologic toxicities of drug combinations are usually not different from the specific toxicities of the single agents. This is not true when chemotherapy is combined with irradiation.

Immunotherapy as an Adjunct to Chemotherapy

Most forms of immunotherapy in animal tumor systems are of major efficacy only when the total body tumor burden is small. Thus, small cell carcinoma, a neoplasm in which complete responses to chemotherapy are achieved relatively frequently, might be an ideal candidate for immunotherapeutic approaches. Uncontrolled studies by Israel et al. [50], Einhorn et al. [68], and Holoye et al. [73] utilized Cparv or BCG in conjunction with combination chemotherapy with or without chest irradiation, but the contribution of the microbiologic agent to the results obtained could not be evaluated. In most of the few prospective randomized studies which have been performed, a therapeutic role for the immunologic agent has not been demonstrated. MER [46] and BCG or Cparv [64] failed to improve response rate or survival when added to combination chemotherapy regimens in a randomized fashion. In another study employing combination chemotherapy and chest irradiation, addition of BCG did not increase the response rate [74]. One positive prospective trial evaluating a putative immunotherapeutic agent has been reported. Cohen *et al.* [75], in a small number of patients, found that administration of THY twice weekly for 6 weeks in a dose of 60 mg/m² led to improved survival (not due to a higher complete response rate) in small cell carcinoma patients receiving combination chemotherapy. Further studies are indicated, particularly those which attempt to evaluate some immunologic parameters in treated and untreated patients, but for the moment any role of immunotherapy in this disease remains speculative.

COMBINED MODALITY THERAPY: CHEMOTHERAPY PLUS RADIATION THERAPY

Nonrandomized Trials of Combined Modality Therapy in Limited Disease

Combined modality studies were based on the premise that SCBC is usually systemic in nature, making systemic chemotherapy necessary, and that the chemotherapy often fails in sites of bulk disease. Thus radiation therapy was given to the primary site in the chest. The results of nonrandomized trials employing radiation therapy and chemotherapy in limited disease are shown in Table 6, which is divided into studies with 1, 2, 3, and 4 or more drugs. In both studies with a single drug (CTX) and radiation therapy, median survivals (11–12 months) are superior to the results in randomized trials with radiation therapy alone, but there were no 2 year disease-free survivors [40, 76]. Trials employing 2 drugs plus radiation have produced complete responses in 42% of patients and median survivals of 9.5 to 18 months [40, 54, 77–79]. These results are consistently superior to trials using radiation with a single drug, and 2 year disease-free survivals of approximately 20% were found.

Trials of radiation with 3 drug combinations of CTX and VCR with either ADR, MTX, or CCNU have produced slightly higher complete response rates (58% versus 42%) with median survivals more consistently in excess of 13 months when compared to 2 drug regimens [40, 66–68, 73, 80–84]. However, the fraction of patients with 2 year disease-free survival is similar in the 2 and 3 drug groups (≈ 20%).

Using the 3 drug combination of CTX + VCR + ADR, with and without BCG, Holoye *et al.* found median survivals of 9–12 months; these survival differences were not significant [57, 73]. The 3 drug combination employing CCNU rather than ADR produced results similar to trials with ADR [80, 81]. The largest of the 3 drug trials, reported by Livingston *et al.* for the South-

Table 6. Non-randomized trials with combined modality therapy in limited disease[1].

Therapy Radiation[2]	Chemotherapy	Reference	No. patients	No. CR+PR	No. CR	MED SURV (mos)	No. 2-yr DFS
1 drug:							
3,200, 1C	CTX	Maurer[40]	15	8	4	11	NR
NR, 1C	CTX	Hattori[76]	11	5	3	12	0
		Totals	26	13/26 (50%)	7/26 (27%)	11.0-12.0	0/11 (0%)
2 drugs:							
3,200, 1C	CTX+MTX	Maurer[40]	41	21	14	9.5	NR
6,000, 2C	CTX+VCR	Holoye[54]	16	15	8	12.0	3
4,000, 2C	CTX+VP-16	Eagan[79, 42]	12	11	4	13.0	4
4,000, 2C	ADR+VP-16	Eagan[79, 42]	10	9	3	12.0	1
3,000-4,500, 1,2C	CTX+ADR	Herman[77, 78]	10	10	8	18.0	1
		Totals	89	66/89 (74%)	37/89 (42%)	9.5-18.0	9/48 (19%)
3 drugs:							
3,200, 1C	CTX+VCR+MTX	Maurer[40]	12	7	6	9.0	NR
3,200, IC	CTX+VCR+HDMTX	Maurer[40]	47	29	22	9.0	NR
2,400, 1C	CTX+VCR+CCNU	King[80, 81]	18	17	14	13.5	3[3]

Table 6. (Continued)

Therapy		Reference	No. patients	No. CR+PR	No. CR	MED SURV (mos)	No. 2-yr DFS
Radiation²	Chemotherapy						
4,000, 2C	CTX+VCR+ADR	Holoye [57]	17	14	11	9.0	3
4,500, 2C	CTX+VCR+ADR	Livingston [82]	108	81	44	12.0	NR
3,600, 2C	CTX+VCR+ADR (+BCG)	Einhorn [17, 68, 83]	19	NR	17	17.0	5
3,000, 1B	CTX+VCR+ADR	Greco [67]	32	32	29	14.0+	3*
3,000-4,500, 1A, B, C	CTX+VCR+ADR	Johnson [66, 84]	36	28	27	18.5	10
4,500, 2C	CTX+VCR+ADR (+BCG)	Holoye [73]	15	11	5	12.0	TE
		Totals	304	219/285 (77%)	175/304 (58%)	9.0-18.5	24/122 (20%)
4 or more drugs:							
2,800-3,200, 1A	CTX+VCR+PCZ+PRED	Nixon [65]	11	11	8	6.0	0
3,000, 1A, C	CTX+VCR+ADR+MTX	Wittes [85]	33 (14 E)	24	5	10.0	NR
3,000, 1B	CTX+VCR+ADR/ CCNU+MTX	Jackson [72]	17	NR	6	10.0	2
4,500, 2C	CTX+VCR+CCNU/ ADR+VCR	Ginsberg [81]	12	12	6	NR	2³
		Totals	73 (14 E)	47/56 (84%)	25/73 (34%)	6.0+ -12.0	4/40 (10%)
		Grand totals (all L patients)	492 (14 E) (3% E)	345/456 (76%)	244/492 (50%)	6.0+ -18.5	37/221 (17%)

¹ Abbreviations as in Tables 4 and 5.
² Total dose in rads; 1 = continuous; 2 = split course; A = prior to chemotherapy, B = concurrent with chemotherapy; C = between chemotherapy courses.
³ 18 months.

west Oncology Group, had lower complete response rates and shorter median survivals than single institution studies employing similar regimens [82]. The relative contribution of poor risk factors, different radiotherapy techniques, and different amounts of chemotherapy to these inferior results cannot be determined. This study employed a lower dose of VCR and/or CTX than each of the other trials except the Einhorn trial [68].

In two sequential randomized trials by Maurer *et al.*, patients received identical radiotherapy with a single drug (CTX), 2 drugs (CTX+MTX), or 3 drugs (CTX+VCR+MTX or HDMTX) [40]. There were no statistically significant differences in response rates or survivals. However, all patients alive at 2 years received 2 or 3 drugs; and when the 3-drug regimens are combined and compared to the one- and two-drug regimens combined, there is a trend toward superior complete response rate, 48% versus 32% (P = 0.09).

The combined modality treatments employing combinations of 4 or more drugs are more difficult to interpret because there were few patients, results were often not divided by stage, and follow-up was short [65, 81, 85]. Response rates and fractions of patients with 2 year disease-free survival are similar to 3 drug trials. Median survivals are in the 12 month range.

In summary, while the majority of recent trials have used 3-drug combinations, there are no striking differences between trials using 2, 3 or 4 drugs. Overall, 50% of the patients achieved a complete response, and 76% an objective response; median survivals in general range from 9–18 months and almost 20% of patients have 2 year disease-free survival. These results are clearly superior to results from trials using radiation alone or radiation with less intensive chemotherapy. However, the results are similar to those achieved in some recent trials with combination chemotherapy alone in patients with limited disease (Table 4).

Nonrandomized Trials of Combined Modality Therapy in Extensive Disease

The results of combined modality therapy in extensive disease are summarized in Table 7, and are clearly inferior to the results in limited disease. Overall, only 21% of patients had a complete remission (versus 50% in limited patients) and median survivals were in the 6–10.5 month range. Only 5 patients are reported to have 2 year disease-free survival although the majority of reports do not provide this information.

In the randomized studies of the Cancer and Leukemia Group B reported by Maurer *et al.*, there were no statistical differences in response rates or survival in groups receiving 1, 2, or 3 drugs, but there was a trend toward higher response rates in multiple drug regimens compared to a single drug (P = 0.04) [40]. In the randomized trial reported by Alexander *et al.* comparing a 3-drug regimen (CTX+VCR+MTX), with a 4-drug regimen (CTX+VCR+CCNU+PCZ), there was no difference in response rates but

Table 7. Non-randomized trials of combined modality therapy in patients with extensive disease[1].

Therapy		Reference	No. patients	No. CR + PR	No. CR	MED SURV (mos)	No. 2-yr DFS
Radiation	Chemotherapy						
1 drug							
3,200, 1C	CTX	Maurer[40]	12	1	1	4.0	NR
NR, 1C	CTX	Hattori[76]	12	5	1	7.5	0
		Totals	24	6/24 (25%)	2/24 (8%)	4.0-7.5	0/12 (0%)
2 drugs							
3,200, 1C	CTX+MTX	Maurer[40]	40	9	4	4.5	NR
3,000-4,500, 1,2C	CTX+ADR	Herman[77, 78]	17	10	3	3.0	0
		Totals	57	19/57 (33%)	7/57 (12%)	3.0-4.5	0/17 (0%)
3 drugs							
3,200, 1C	CTX+VCR+MTX	Maurer[40]	25	6	3	5.5	NR
3,200, 1C	CTX+VCR+HDMTX	Maurer[40]	33	12	3	5.5	NR
3,200-5,000 1A, B, C	CTX+VCR+MTX	Eagan[87]	26 (4 L)	22	14	9.5	0
3,000-3,500, 1A, C	CTX+VCR+MTX	Bitran[88]	18 (1 L)	13	3	9.5	TE
3,000, 1C	CTX+VCR+MTX	Alexander[86]	11 (1 L)	7	2	10.0	NR
2,400, 1C	CTX+VCR+CCNU	King[80, 81]	19	11	4	10.5	1
3,000, 1C	CTX+VCR+ADR	Livingston[82]	250	140	35	6.0	0**
3,600, 2C	CTX+VCR+ADR (+BCG)	Einhorn[17, 68, 83]	39	NR	9	9.0	1

Table 7 (continued)

Therapy		Reference	No. patients	No. CR + PR	No. CR	MED SURV (mos)	No. 2-yr DFS
Radiation	Chemotherapy						
3,000, 1B	CTX+VCR+ADR	Greco [89]	20	NR	11	10.0	0**
3,000-4,500, 1A, B, C	CTX+VCR+ADR	Johnson [66, 84]	35	21	14	10.5	0
3,000-4,500, 1, 2, A, B, C	CTX+VCR+ADR	Cox [90, 91]	22	22	NR	10.0	1
		Total	498 (6 L)	254/439 (50%)	98/476 (21%)	5.5-10.5	3/411 (1%)
4 or more drugs							
3,000, 1A	CTX+VCR+PCZ+BCNU	Abeloff [92]	24 (7 L)	15	8	6.0+(10.5 L)	0**
3,000, 1C	CTX+VCR+PCZ+CCNU	Alexander [86]	12 (1 L)	9	5	14.0	0
NR, 1C	CTX+VCR+MeCCNU+BLEO	Osieka [94]	26 (? L)	24	12	10.0	NR
NR	CTX+VCR+ADR+HDMTX	Burdon [95, 96]	46 (10 L)	28	8	8.5	NR
4,000-5,000 1A, C	CTX+VCR+ADR+MTX+ PRED	Gilby [93]	35	20	NR	7.5	NR
3,000, 1B	CTX+VCR+ADR/CCNU +MTX	Jackson [72]	12	NR	4	5.5	2
		Totals	155 (18 L)	96/143 (67%)	37/120 (31%)	5.5-14.0	2/48 (4%)
		Grand totals (all E patients)	734 (24 L) (3% L)	375/663 (57%)	144/667 (21%)	3.0-14.0	5/488 (1%)

1 Abbreviations as in Tables 4, 5, and 6.

patients treated with the 4-drug regimen had a median survival of 11 months vs. 10 months for those treated with 3 drugs (P = 0.055)[86].

In nonrandomized trials, the results from the 3 and 4 drug trials appear superior to results of 1 and 2 drug trials though few patients received 1 or 2 drugs [76–78, 80–96]. As in limited disease, there are no striking differences between trials with 3 or 4 drugs. The results in terms of response, survival, and disease-free survival are similar or slightly inferior to those reported in patients with extensive disease treated with chemotherapy alone (Table 5). In summary, the value of adding radiation therapy to combination chemotherapy in either limited or extensive disease cannot be determined from the non-randomized studies.

Randomized Trials of Combined Radiation Therapy
Plus Chemotherapy versus Chemotherapy Alone

To determine whether the addition of radiation therapy to chemotherapy is beneficial, randomized trials of combined modality treatment versus chemotherapy alone have been initiated. Unfortunately, the results of only one trial have been published, although preliminary results of 3 trials currently in progress or recently completed have been presented (Table 8). Three trials were restricted to patients with limited stage disease [47, 49, 97]. In the Einhorn trial which employed CTX + VCR + ADR with or without split course sandwich radiotherapy (total dose 3600 rads), the response rates were higher in the combined modality group but there was no advantage in median or long-term survival [47]. In the Hansen trial with CTX + VCR + CCNU + MTX with or without 4000 rads in a split course sandwich technique, there were no differences in response rates but patients receiving chemotherapy alone had a significantly superior survival (14 months median versus 11 months, P < 0.01)[49]. The National Cancer Institute trial reported by Cohen *et al.* employing CTX + MTX + CCNU, alternating with VCR + ADR + PCZ with or without 4000 rads to the chest given concurrently in a continuous course beginning on day 1 reached the opposite conclusion [97]. The complete response rate was 77% in the combined treatment group and 46% in the chemotherapy alone group. Disease free survival at 18 months was 4/8 in the combined group and 1/9 in the chemotherapy group. There was a trend in overall survival favoring the combined group (P = .15). In patients with extensive disease, randomized trials have found no benefit to the addition of radiation. In the Stanford experience reported by Williams *et al.*, response, survival, and the pattern of sites of initial relapse were not different in groups receiving CTX + VCR + CCNU + PCZ alone or the same drugs plus 3000 rads given in 2 weeks after 2 or 3 cycles of chemotherapy [61]. Actual two year survival was limited to the chemotherapy alone arm in this study. Einhorn has stated that results of a randomized study failed to demonstrate survival

Table 8. Randomized trials of chemotherapy alone versus chemotherapy plus radiation therapy.

Chemotherapy	Radiation[1]	Reference	No. patients[2]	No. CR+PR	No. CR	MEDIAN SURVIVAL (mos)	No disease free, 2 years
CTX+VCR+MTX+CCNU	4,000, 2C	Hansen[49]	65	57	NR	11	NR
	None		69	63	NR	14	NR
CTX+VCR+ADR	3,500, 2C	Stevens[47]	14	14	10	13	2
	None		16	12	8	12	1
CTX+MTX+CCNU/VCR+ADR+PCZ	4,000, 1B	Cohen[97]	14	NR	11	NR	4/8[3]
	None		14	NR	6	NR	1/9
CTX+VCR+PCZ+CCNU	3,000, 1C[4]	Williams[61]	13	9	5	9	NR
	None		12	11	5	11	1

[1] Dose in rads; 1 = continuous, 2 = split course, B = concurrent with chemotherapy, C = between chemotherapy cycles.
[2] All limited stage in first 3 trials, all extensive in last trial.
[3] No. disease free at 18 mo/No. 18 mo after onset of therapy.
[4] Radiation also given to sites of metastatic disease.

advantage for chest radiotherapy in patients with extensive disease, given CTX + VCR + ADR alone or with irradiation, but details of the results of this trial have not been published [68].

Dose, Schedule, and Timing of Radiotherapy

The most appropriate dose, schedule and timing of radiotherapy with chemotherapy are unknown. Cox and coworkers at Wisconsin have shown that the total dose of radiotherapy (when given in a continuous technique) needed for local control is less when radiotherapy is combined with combination chemotherapy than when radiation is used alone [90, 91]. They recommend 3750 rads (1750 rets) as sufficient for local control. McMahon et al., using split course irradiation in a randomized study, found that total doses of 4000-4500 rads produced longer survival and relapse-free survival than total doses of 3000 rads [78]. If one compares the nonrandomized studies shown in Table 6, there is no difference in complete response rate, median survival or 2 year disease-free survival for patients receiving <3200 rads, 3200 rads, 3500-3600 rads, or >4000 rads.

In the early randomized study of radiation therapy versus 5-FU plus radiation therapy, there was no difference in survival for combined modality patients receiving radiation therapy in a continuous or split course [22]. In the nonrandomized trials listed in Tables 6 and 7, there are no striking differences between those receiving continuous and those receiving split course radiotherapy.

In a nonrandomized study with radiation therapy (4000–5000 rads) and a 5-drug combination, survival was identical whether radiotherapy was given first or between the second and third courses of chemotherapy [93]. Similarly, Wittes et al. found no survival differences whether a 4-drug regimen was given prior to, after, or simultaneously with radiation therapy [85]. The best approach for combining chemo- and radiotherapy cannot be determined by reviewing the nonrandomized trials in Tables 6 and 7. For example, the Greco trial [67, 89] used continuous radiation (3000 rads/ 10 fractions/2 weeks) given concurrently with the 3-drug combination of CTX + VCR + ADR, while the Einhorn trial [68, 83] used split course irradiation (total dose 3600 rads in 12 fractions over 7 weeks) sandwiched between cycles of the same drugs. Response, survival and toxicity results were very similar in the 2 trials. The nonrandomized trial of Johnson et al. was designed to determine the best approach for the delivery of combined modality radiotherapy [66, 84]. The results were not conclusive, but there was a suggestion that patients receiving concurrent irradiation and chemotherapy had better local control than patients receiving radiation after 4–5 cycles of chemotherapy or sandwiched between chemotherapy cycles. These patients also had more toxicity (vide infra). Patients receiving 3000 rads over 3 weeks concurrently with chemotherapy (both starting day 1) seemed to have the best survival with acceptable toxicity. One could argue that the randomized trials also suggest concurrent combined modality therapy is most appropriate since the concurrent study showed benefit from combined modalities while the 2 studies with 'sandwich' therapy showed no benefit. Clearly the most appropriate techniques for combining chemotherapy and radiotherapy are unknown, and randomized trials are sorely needed. This is particularly apparent in reviewing the toxicity data.

Toxicity

There is no question that toxicities encountered in combined modality approaches are greater than when either modality is used alone. In certain circumstances, the toxicities may be particularly enhanced by the concurrent administration of both modalities. Both modalities may cause nausea and vomiting, malaise, lethargy and alopecia. The reader is referred to reviews of toxicities of each modality alone, and these will not be discussed in detail in this text. Particular toxicities encountered in combined modality trials will be considered.

Dysphagia and esophagitis have been reported in many patients in all combined modality trials. In most trials employing radiotherapy prior to chemotherapy or in between chemotherapy cycles, esophagitis, although frequent, has been mild. For example, Livingston *et al.* [82, 98] reported mild esophageal toxicity in 5%, and Einhorn *et al.* [68, 83] in 50%. Trials with concurrent chemotherapy have had considerably more toxicity. In the trial of Johnson *et al.*, esophagitis of moderate to severe degree developed in 46/71 patients [66]. Esophageal strictures developed in 3 patients, all of whom had concurrent chemotherapy. In the Memorial Hospital experience reported by Chabora *et al.* severe esophagitis developed in 6/8 patients receiving concurrent therapy, 2/5 receiving chemotherapy within 1 week of radiotherapy, and 0/9 receiving chemotherapy more than 2 weeks after radiotherapy [99]. Greco *et al.* reported mild to moderate esophagitis in 20/26 patients receiving concurrent therapy although none was severe [67]. In the current NCI trial with concurrent combined modality therapy, severe esophagitis developed in 2 of the first 7 patients. Subsequently, an esophageal block was used after 2000 rads and there has been no severe toxicity in the next 7 patients [97].

In their initial report, Johnson *et al.* also reported that skin toxicity was enhanced in patients receiving concurrent therapy; 17 of 21 patients had enhanced radiation skin reactions [84]. Others have found skin toxicity to be less of a problem, even with concurrent therapy. For example, the Greco (2/26 with moist desquamation) and current NCI trials have had no severe skin reactions after concurrent therapy [67, 89, 97]. With sandwich therapy,

Moore *et al.* [98] reported mild skin toxicity in less than 1% and Einhorn *et al.* [68] found no severe toxicity.

Pulmonary toxicity, fibrosis and/or pneumonitis is reported in nearly all combined modality trials and has frequently been severe. Pulmonary fibrosis developed in 5 of 13 patients receiving combined modality therapy with BLEO + CTX + VCR + ADR and was fatal in 3 [100]. In contrast, none of 29 patients receiving the same drugs without radiation developed this complication. Pulmonary toxicity was noted in 26/71 patients in another trial using these same drugs without bleomycin and was fatal in 12 of these 26 patients [66]. For reasons which are not entirely clear, others have noted less toxicity even when the same drugs were used. Moore *et al.* found significant pulmonary complications in 3% of patients, half of which were fatal [98].

It has been suggested that patients receiving ADR and radiation to the mediastinum are at increased risk for cardiac toxicity. In a recent retrospective review, Von Hoff *et al.* noted no significant increase in dose adjusted cardiac toxicity in this group [101]. Cardiac toxicity has been reported in most trials employing ADR but does not appear to be more of a problem than in trials using ADR without radiation. Moore *et al.* found cardiac symptoms in only 7/383 patients and only one patient died from cardiac failure [98].

All combined modality trials report significant hematopoietic toxicity with suppression of all marrow elements. Most trials were designed to produce hematopoietic toxicity. However, in most trials, the degree of toxicity and the frequency of subsequent infection have been acceptable. The most significant toxicity was reported by Johnson *et al.* who repeated chemotherapy cycles as soon as the WBC recovered to 3500 cells/μl rather than at set intervals [66, 84]. In this trial, 85% of patients had severe neutropenia ($<1000/\mu$l), 39% severe thrombocytopenia ($<50,000/\mu$l), and 80% required packed red cell transfusions. While 51/71 patients had at least one febrile episode with leukopenia, documented sepsis was found in only 5 and pneumonias in 6. At the other extreme, Moore *et al.*, with slightly lower drug doses given less often, found only 27% of patients had a WBC $<1000/\mu$l and only 9/383 had sepsis [98]. In other trials, the degree of hematopoietic suppression and frequency of infection were intermediate between these studies.

While much of the hematopoietic toxicity is related to the chemotherapy, the radiation plays a significant role. Irradiation of the intrathoracic region and skull affects 20–25% of the functioning bone marrow [102]. Abrams has reported that the addition of radiotherapy to a 3 drug chemotherapy combination produces significantly more myelosuppression and also a significant reduction in the level of circulating hematopoietic colonies formed on soft agar [103].

A 'CNS syndrome' consisting of memory loss for recent events (100%), tremor (97%), somnolence (73%), slurred speech (54%), and myoclonus

(41%) in various combinations was observed in 35 of 71 patients by Johnson *et al.* [66, 84]. These patients were treated with concurrent chemotherapy, chest irradiation, and cranial irradiation, and the syndrome was most severe in patients given a midline cranial dose of 3000 rads. This syndrome has not been reported by others, although most have given cranial irradiation later in the clinical course.

All trials report some cases of fatal treatment related complications. These vary in frequency from 3–4% [67, 82, 89, 98] to as high as 24% in the studies of Johnson *et al.* [66]. In most series, less than 10% of patients die from treatment-related toxicity. Criticisms of these toxicities must be tempered by the fact that nearly all patients have objective responses, and that these patients generally have symptomatic improvement, improvement in performance status and can usually return to work on a part-time or full-time basis. Development of strategies to minimize combined modality toxicities remains a major goal of future studies.

Sites of Relapse

In addition to the problems of treatment-related toxicity, the relapse patterns must be considered when evaluating combined modality treatments. In these series, the primary thoracic site remains the most common site of relapse. In the randomized trials from Stanford, the chest irradiation did not alter the pattern of sites of initial relapse [61]. In the nonrandomized trials, chest relapses are common, although they seem to be less frequent than chest relapses in patients receiving chemotherapy alone. In a recent literature review, Cohen *et al.* found no differences in the fraction of patients relapsing in nodes, liver, bone, or bone marrow, but slightly few chest relapses (33% versus 46%) in patients receiving combined modality therapy [9]. Consequently, sterilization of the primary tumor is still frequently not achieved, even with the most intensive combined modality approaches.

Combined Modality Therapy with Irradiation to Extrathoracic Sites

Relapse is common in sites in the upper abdomen, particularly the liver, adrenals, and upper abdominal lymph nodes. The randomized trial of CTX + MTX + CCNU alone versus the same 3 drugs with irradiation to the upper abdomen at weeks 6–8 and 10–12 in patients with limited disease has been reported by Hirsch *et al.* [104]. There was no difference in survival in the 2 groups (10 versus 9.5 months median survival). In the Stanford study of CTX + VCR + CCNU + PCZ alone versus the same drugs plus radiation therapy for patients with extensive disease, patients randomized to combined modality received radiotherapy (1,500–2,500 rads) to involved sites outside the chest in addition to standard chest irradiation [61]. There was no difference in sites of relapse or survival in this study between irradiated and non-irradiated patients.

Prophylactic Cranial Irradiation (PCI)

As early as 1973, Hansen and coworkers at the National Cancer Institute recognized that central nervous system (CNS) metastases were more frequent in SCBC than the other histologic groups of lung cancer and suggested that trials with prophylactic or elective cranial irradiation (PCI) be instituted [105, 106]. Four randomized trials with or without cranial irradiation have since been completed and the results are summarized in Table 9 [40, 72, 104, 107]. In addition, a number of nonrandomized trials have used elective cranial irradiation and the results of these trials are contrasted with nonrandomized trials not utilizing cranial irradiation [27, 78, 84, 85, 89, 104, 108]. Many of these latter trials included drugs that crossed the blood brain barrier and it was felt these drugs might reduce the frequency of CNS metastases. Results from the first two randomized trials in this table were published first, and supported the view that cranial irradiation significantly reduced the frequency of CNS relapse but did not influence survival [40, 72]. Since that time, results of two additional randomized trials have shown no benefit for PCI in either CNS relapse rate or in survival [104, 107]. The dose and timing of PCI does not seem to explain the differences; one positive and one negative trial used radiotherapy at the onset of therapy [72, 107], while in one positive and one negative trial it was given at week 8 or 12 [40, 104]. The dose of radiation therapy was 3000 rads in the 2 positive studies and 4000 and 2000 rads in the negative studies. One of the negative studies was confined to patients with limited disease [104]. In one positive trial, there was a definite delay in the time of onset of CNS relapse while in one of the negative trials the median time of onset of CNS relapse was identical in patients with or without PCI.

In nonrandomized trials, the frequency of brain metastases appears to be lower in patients given PCI. Comparison of these results is treacherous because there was a higher frequency of patients with limited disease in the PCI trials and because the length of follow-up was different in many trials. The frequency of CNS relapse is clearly related to time post diagnosis as the studies of Nugent and Maurer have demonstrated [40, 71]. Thus, trials with short follow-up could report a falsely low frequency of CNS relapse.

CNS relapses are frequent in all areas of the neuraxis including the spinal cord and leptomeninges as well as the brain as shown by Nugent et al. [71]. PCI does not influence relapse in these sites, and relapses have been reported in as many as 10% of patients in these sites whether or not PCI was given [71, 109–111].

Ultimately, prophylactic CNS therapy is most important for patients with

Table 9. Frequency of CNS metastases in trials with and without elective cranial irradiation.

Randomized trials (4)

References	Dose (rads)	Cranial irradiation			No cranial irradiation			Relapse significance	Survival significance
		No. PTS	No. CNS Relapse	Median survival (mos)	No. PTS	No. CNS relapse	Median survival (mos)		
Jackson [72]	3000A*	14	0	9.8	15	4	7.2	P < 0.05	NS
Maurer [40]	3000B+	79	3	8.4	84	15	8.8	P < 0.009	NS
Hirsch [104]	4000B	55	5	9.5	7	56	10	NS	NS
Cox [107]	2000A	24	4	NR	21	4	NR	NS	NR
		172	12 (6.9%)		176	31 (17.6%)			

Non-randomized trials (33)

References	Cranial irradiation			No cranial irradiation		
	No. PTS	No. CNS relapse	%	No. PTS	No. CNS relapse	%
17, 78, 108	422	33	8	956	214	22
27, 85, 89, 104, 108						

+ Includes only patients with limited disease

NR = not reported
NS = not significant
PTS = patients
*A = cranial irradiation beginning at start of therapy.
B = cranial irradiation beginning week 8 or 12.

long disease-free intervals and possible cure. There are too few patients with long complete remissions in any of these studies to determine whether PCI has had an impact on these groups. In fact, in the randomized trial reported by Maurer *et al.* the benefit from PCI was primarily in extensive stage patients during the first year [40]. Further studies on the most effective dose and timing of cranial irradiation, and methods for prophylaxis of the entire neuraxis are needed.

Perspective on combined modality therapy. It is clear that combined modality treatment employing effective drug combinations is superior to irradiation alone and to combined modality treatments employing single drugs. The toxicities from combined modality therapy are enhanced compared to the use of either modality alone. It is not clear from either random or nonrandomized trials whether combined modality therapy is superior to combination chemotherapy alone. Further studies are needed to determine the best way to deliver the radiotherapy, to combine the modalities with the most effectiveness and the least possible toxicity, and to determine whether combined treatment is superior to chemotherapy alone.

FUTURE PROSPECTS

Chemotherapy: 1. New drugs. It is clear that there are limitations to all the currently available drugs, and it is unlikely that the majority of patients would be cured by even the best schedule of these drugs. Thus, drug development and the search for new active drugs are imperative. Evaluation of new and untested drugs in relapsing patients must be continued.

2. More intensive induction. It appears we may have reached a plateau in the doses of chemotherapy that can profitably be given in the first 6–8 weeks. Earlier studies established that increasing CTX dose to 1 g/m^2 or more in 3 or 4 drug combinations produced better results than were seen with lower doses. Several studies have suggested that further increases in CTX may lead to more toxicity but do not increase complete remission rate or survival. Increasing the frequency of induction doses of chemotherapy during the first 6–8 weeks may also increase toxicity without improving survival [112].

3. 'Late intensification.' Recent studies in lymphomas in dogs and in acute leukemias in humans suggest that intensive therapies with high doses of total body radiotherapy and chemotherapy can be given with acceptable toxicity and may lead to long disease-free survival ('cure') not possible without this therapy [113, 114]. Similar trials in patients with SCBC in remission after induction chemotherapy are in progress in several centers, including the National Cancer Institute and Johns Hopkins University.

4. Prevention of drug resistance. The majority of patients relapse within the first year of treatment, frequently while on therapy which initially induced remission. The mechanisms for development of resistance are unknown. Use of alternating non-cross resistant regimens may be one way to prevent resistance. There are nonrandomized trials suggesting some benefit from alternating regimens and randomized trials are in progress. Unfortunately, it appears that large differences in disease-free survival do not result from these approaches. Further studies on the mechanism of resistance and approaches to prevent it are needed.

5. New drug scheduling approaches. All studies to date have been empiric in nature. Our understanding of the cell kinetics of this tumor before and after drug perturbation is extremely limited. More information about drug scheduling in relation to tumor cell versus normal cell kinetics is needed to improve the therapeutic index.

6. Growth factors. Establishment of SCBC cells in tissue culture and after heterotransplantation allows study of hormone and protein growth factors. Knowledge of these growth factors would allow manipulation for cytotoxic purposes alone or in conjunction with chemotherapy.

Radiation Therapy: Radiation therapy should not be used as a single modality. In combined modality trials, the best timing for radiation therapy is unknown, and there are no randomized trials asking this question (e.g., concurrent day 1 versus concurrent at 6 weeks versus sandwich at 6 weeks). We do not know the best total dose, whether radiation should be split course or continuous, nor the best number of fractions for a given total dose. These questions need to be addressed in future trials.

Surgery: Earlier studies established that radiation therapy, chemotherapy or radiation and chemotherapy were superior to surgery alone. It is now clear that the primary thoracic disease is the primary relapse site, in limited disease, even in combined modality chemotherapy plus radiation therapy studies. The role of surgery in reducing bulk disease in the chest before or after chemotherapy needs to be re-addressed.

Sanctuary Sites and Sites of Bulk Disease: CNS relapse and relapse in non-thoracic sites of bulk disease are also frequent. New approaches for reduction of the tumor in these areas are needed. New approaches for prevention of spinal cord and leptomeningeal metastases are also needed.

New Modalities and Immunotherapy: There is no established benefit for current non-specific immunotherapeutic approaches. A positive effect on survival was noted in a small randomized study using thymosin fraction V [75].

This observation requires confirmation and more specific immunotherapeutic methods should be tested as they became available. Interferon and other new approaches can also be tested in relapsing patients.

Early Diagnosis and Prevention. Although this chapter has not been devoted to this subject, we must recognize that for the immediate future, the only way to substantially reduce mortality from this disease is to reduce cigarette consumption. Patients with limited disease are significantly more likely to have 2 year disease-free survival than patients with extensive disease. Currently the majority of patients in nearly all trials have extensive disease. Thus, early detection could have an important impact on survival. At present, there are no methods of proven efficacy for early diagnosis. Development of newer methods could allow earlier detection and therefore better survival results, even using the currently available therapies.

There is no doubt that the prognosis for SCBC patients in 1980 is improved over the prognosis a decade ago. Unfortunately it is not clear that therapeutic results reported in this manuscript for the period 1976–1980 are superior to those reported in similar reviews for the period 1972–1976 [1, 7]. In addition, there is still no standard treatment for this disease, and the vast majority of patients continue to die within 2 years of diagnosis. We must continue to enter patients on prospective therapeutic trials if progress is to continue in the next decade.

REFERENCES

1. Bunn PA, Cohen MH, Ihde DC *et al.*: Advances in small cell bronchogenic carcinoma. Cancer Treat Rep 61:333-342, 1977.
2. Tischler AS: Small cell carcinoma of the lung: Cellular origin and relationship to other neoplasms. Semin Oncol 5:244-252, 1978.
3. Cohen MH, Matthews MJ: Small cell bronchogenic carcinoma: A distinct clinicopathologic entity. Semin Oncol 5:234-243, 1978.
4. Zelen M: Keynote address on biostatistics and data retrieval. Cancer Chemother Rep (Part 3) 4 (2):31-42, 1973.
5. Mountain CF: Clinical biology of small cell bronchogenic carcinoma: Relationship to surgical therapy. Semin Oncol 5:272-279, 1978.
6. Fox W, Scadding JG: Medical Research Council comparative trial of surgery and radiotherapy for primary treatment of small-celled or oat-celled carcinoma of bronchus. Ten year follow-up. Lancet 2:63-65, 1973.
7. Broder LE, Cohen MH, Selawry OS: Treatment of bronchogenic carcinoma. II. Small cell cancer. Cancer Treat Rev 4:219-260, 1977.
8. Weiss RB: Small-cell carcinoma of the lung: Therapeutic management. Ann Intern Med 88:522-531, 1978.
9. Cohen MH, Fossieck BE, Ihde DC *et al.*: Chemotherapy of small cell carcinoma of the lung: Results and concepts. In: Lung Cancer, Muggia FM, Rozencwieg M (eds), New York, Raven Press, 1979, p 559-568.

10. Bunn PA, Cohen MH. Ihde DC *et al.*: A review of recent therapeutic trials in small cell bronchogenic carcinoma. In: Lung Cancer, Muggia FM, Rozencwieg M (eds), New York, Raven Press, 1979, p 549-557.

11. Matthews MJ, Kanhouwa S, Pickren J *et al.*: Frequency of residual and metastatic tumor in patients undergoing curative surgical resection for lung cancer. Cancer Chemo Rep (Part 3) 4(2):63-67, 1973.

12. Higgins GA: Use of chemotherapy as an adjuvant to surgery for bronchogenic carcinoma. Cancer 30:1382-1387, 1972.

13. Medical Research Council Working Party: Study of cytotoxic chemotherapy as an adjuvant to surgery in carcinoma of the bronchus. Br Med J 2:421-428, 1971.

14. Shields TW, Humphrey EW, Eastridge CE *et al.*: Adjuvant cancer chemotherapy after resection of carcinoma of the lung. Cancer 40:2057-1062, 1977.

15. Karrer K, Pridun N, Denck H: Chemotherapy as an adjuvant to surgery in lung cancer. Cancer Chemother Pharmacol 1:145-159, 1978.

16. Meyer JA, Comis RL, Ginsberg SJ *et al.*: Selective surgical resection in small cell carcinoma of the lung. J Thorac Cardiovasc Surg 77:243-248, 1979.

17. Mandelbaum I, Williams SD, Hornback NB *et al.*: Combined therapy for small cell undifferentiated carcinoma of the lung. J Thorac Cardiovasc Surg 76:292-296, 1978.

18. Edmonson JH, Lagakos SW, Selawry OS *et al.*: Cyclophosphamide and CCNU in the treatment of inoperable small cell carcinoma and adenocarcinoma of the lung. Cancer Treat Rep 60:925-932, 1976.

19. Tucker RD, Sealy R, van Wyk C *et al.*: A clinical trial of cyclophosphamide (NSC-26271) and radiation therapy for oat cell carcinoma of the lung. Cancer Chemother Rep (Part 3) 4(2):159-160, 1973.

20. Kaung DT, Wolf J, Hyde L *et al.*: Preliminary report on the treatment of nonresectable cancer of the lung. Cancer Chemother Rep 58:359-364, 1974.

21. Laing A, Berry R: Treatment of small cell carcinoma of bronchus. Lancet 1:129-132, 1975.

22. Carr DT, Childs DS, Lee RE: Radiotherapy plus 5-FU compared to radiotherapy alone for inoperable and unresectable bronchogenic carcinoma. Cancer 29:375-380, 1972.

23. Bergsagel D, Jenkin R, Pringle J *et al.*: Lung cancer: Clinical trial of radiotherapy alone vs. radiotherapy plus cyclophosphamide. Cancer 30:621-627, 1972.

24. Host H: Cyclophosphamide (NSC-26271) as adjuvant to radiotherapy in the treatment of unresectable bronchogenic carcinoma. Cancer Chemother Rep (Part 3) 4(2):161-164, 1973.

25. Petrovich Z, Mietlowski W, Ohanian M *et al.*: Clinical report on the treatment of locally advanced lung cancer. Cancer 40:72-77, 1977.

26. Petrovich Z, Ohanian M, Cox J: Clinical research on the treatment of locally advanced lung cancer. Cancer 42:1129-1134, 1978.

27. Medical Research Council Lung Cancer Working Party: Radiotherapy alone or with chemotherapy in the treatment of small-cell carcinoma of the lung. Br J Cancer 40:1-10, 1979.

28. Matthiessen W: Controlled clinical trial of radiotherapy alone, against radiotherapy plus chemotherapy in small-cell carcinoma of the lung: Comparison of radiation damage. Scand J Resp Dis Suppl 102:209-211, 1978.

29. Green RA, Humphrey E, Close H *et al.*: Alkylating agents in bronchogenic carcinoma. Am J Med 46:516-525, 1969.

30. Cavalli F, Sonntag RW, Jungi F *et al.*: VP-16-213 monotherapy for remission induction of small cell lung cancer: A randomized trial using three dosage schedules. Cancer Treat Rep 62:473-475, 1978.

31. Wolf J: Nitrosoureas as single agents in the treatment of pulmonary cancer. Cancer Treat Rep 60:753-756, 1976.

32. Wilson WL, Van Ryzin J, Weiss AJ et al.: A Phase III study in lung carcinoma comparing hexamethylmelamine to dibromodulcitol. Oncology 31:293-309, 1975.
33. Bunn PA, Ihde DC, Cohen MH et al.: Streptozotocin in advanced small cell bronchogenic carcinoma: An ineffective nonmyelosuppressive agent. Cancer Treat Rep 62:479-481, 1978.
34. Kane RC, Bernath AM, Cashdollar MR: Phase II trial of streptozotocin for small cell anaplastic carcinoma of the lung. Cancer Treat Rep 62:477-478, 1978.
35. Samson MK, Baker LH, Talley RW et al.: VM26: A clinical study in advanced cancer of the lung and ovary. Eur J Cancer 14:1395-1399, 1978.
36. Cavalli F, Jungi WF, Sonntag RW et al.: Phase II trial of cis-Dichlorodiammineplatinum (II) in advanced malignant lymphoma and small cell lung cancer: Preliminary results. Cancer Treat Rep 63:1599-1603, 1979.
37. Dombernowsky P, Sorenson S, Aisner J et al.: cis-Dichlorodiammineplatinum (II) in small cell anaplastic bronchogenic carcinoma: A Phase II study. Cancer Treat Rep 63:543-545, 1979.
38. Sierocki JS, Hilaris BS, Hopfan S et al.: cis-Dichlorodiammineplatinum (II) and VP-16-213: An active induction regimen for small cell carcinoma of the lung. Cancer Treat Rep 63:1593-1597, 1979.
39. Greco FA, Einhorn LH, Richardson RL et al.: Small cell lung cancer: Progress and perspectives. Semin Oncol 5:323-335, 1978.
40. Maurer LH, Tulloh M, Weiss RB et al.: A randomized combined modality trial in small cell carcinoma of the lung: Comparison of combination chemotherapy-radiation therapy versus cyclophosphamide-radiation therapy, effects of maintenance chemotherapy and prophylactic whole brain irradiation. Cancer 45:30-39, 1980.
41. Lowenbraun S, Bartolucci A, Smalley RV et al.: The superiority of combination chemotherapy over single agent chemotherapy in small cell lung carcinoma. Cancer 44:406-413, 1979.
42. Eagan RT, Carr DT, Frytak S et al.: VP-16-213 versus polychemotherapy in patients with advanced small cell lung cancer. Cancer Treat Rep 60:949-951, 1976.
43. Alberto P, Brunner KW, Martz G et al.: Treatment of bronchogenic carcinoma with simultaneous or sequential combination chemotherapy, including methotrexate, cyclophosphamide, procarbazine, and vincristine. Cancer 38:2208-2216, 1976.
44. Hansen HH, Selawry OS, Simon R et al.: Combination chemotherapy of advanced lung cancer: A randomized trial. Cancer 38:2201-2207, 1976.
45. Hansen HH, Dombernowsky P, Hansen M et al.: Chemotherapy of advanced small cell anaplastic carcinoma: Superiority of a four-drug combination to a three-drug combination. Ann Intern Med 89:177-181, 1978.
46. Aisner J, Wiernik PH, Esterhay RJ: Treatment of small cell carcinoma of the lung with cyclophosphamide, adriamycin, and VP16-213 with or without MER. In: Adjuvant Therapy of Cancer, Salmon SE, Jones SE (eds), Amsterdam, Elsevier/North Holland Biomedical Press, 1977, p 245-250.
47. Stevens E, Einhorn L, Rohn R: Treatment of limited small cell lung cancer. Proc AACR and ASCO 20:435, 1979.
48. Cohen MH, Ihde DC, Bunn PA et al.: Cyclic alternating chemotherapy for small cell bronchogenic carcinoma. Cancer Treat Rep 63:163-170, 1979.
49. Hansen HH, Dombernowsky P, Hansen HS et al.: Chemotherapy versus chemotherapy plus radiotherapy in regional small cell carcinoma of the lung. A randomized trial. Proc AACR and ASCO 20:277, 1979.
50. Israel L, Depierre A, Choffel C et al.: Immunochemotherapy in 34 cases of oat cell carcinoma of the lung with 19 complete remissions. Cancer Treat Rep 61:343-347, 1977.

51. Ettinger DS, Karp JE, Abeloff MD et al.: Intermittent high-dose cyclophosphamide chemotherapy for small cell carcinoma of the lung. Cancer Treat Rep 62:413-424, 1978.
52. Straus MJ: Cytokinetic chemotherapy design for the treatment of advanced lung cancer. Cancer Treat Rep 63:767-773, 1979.
53. Trowbridge RC, Kennedy BJ, Vosika GJ: CCNU-adriamycin therapy in bronchogenic carcinoma. Cancer 41:1704-1709, 1978.
54. Holoye PY, Samuels ML: Cyclophosphamide, vincristine and sequential split-course radiotherapy in the treatment of small cell lung cancer. Chest 67:675-679, 1975.
55. Cohen MH, Creaven PJ, Fossieck BE et al.: Intensive chemotherapy of small cell bronchogenic carcinoma. Cancer Treat Rep 61:349-354, 1977.
56. Saiontz HI, Dalton RJ, Eagan RT: Cyclophosphamide, adriamycin, and DTIC polychemotherapy in advanced small cell lung cancer. Cancer Treat Rep 61:481-483, 1977.
57. Holoye PY, Samuels ML, Lanzotti VJ et al.: Combination chemotherapy and radiation therapy for small cell carcinoma. JAMA 237:1221-1224, 1977.
58. Einhorn LH, Fee WH, Farber MO et al.: Improved chemotherapy for small cell undifferentiated lung cancer. JAMA 235:1225- 1229, 1976.
59. Alberto P: Remission rates, survival and prognostic factors in combination chemotherapy for bronchogenic carcinoma. Cancer Chemo Rep (Part 3) 4(2):199-206, 1973.
60. Dombernowsky P, Hansen HH, Sorenson S et al.: Sequential versus non-sequential combination chemotherapy using 6 drugs in advanced small cell carcinoma: A comparative trial including 146 patients. Proc AACR and ASCO 20:277, 1979.
61. Williams C, Alexander M, Glatstein EJ et al.: The role of radiation therapy in combination with chemotherapy in extensive oat cell cancer of the lung. A randomized study. Cancer Treat Rep 61:1427-1431, 1977.
62. Abeloff MD, Ettinger DS, Khouri NF et al.: Intensive induction therapy for small cell carcinoma of the lung. Cancer Treat Rep 63:519-524, 1979.
63. Chahinian AP, Mandel EM, Holland JF et al.: MACC (methotrexate, adriamycin, cyclophosphamide, and CCNU) in advanced lung cancer. Cancer 43:1590-1597, 1979.
64. Sarna GP, Lowitz BB, Haskell CM et al.: Chemo-immunotherapy for unresectable bronchogenic carcinoma. Cancer Treat Rep 62:681-687, 1978.
65. Nixon DW, Carey RW, Suit HD et al.: Combination chemotherapy in oat cell carcinoma of the lung. Cancer 36:867-872, 1975.
66. Johnson RE, Brereton HD, Kent CH: 'Total' therapy for small cell carcinoma of the lung. Ann Thorac Surg 25:509-515, 1978.
67. Greco FA, Richardson RL, Snell JD et al.: Small cell lung cancer: Complete remission and improved survival. Am J Med 66:625-630, 1979.
68. Einhorn LH, Bond WH, Hornback W et al.: Long term results in combined modality treatment of small cell carcinoma of the lung. Semin Oncol 5:309-313, 1978.
69. Kane RC, Cohen MH, Broder LE et al.: Superior vena caval obstruction due to small cell anaplastic lung carcinoma: Response to chemotherapy. JAMA 235:1717-1718, 1976.
70. Dombernowsky P, Hansen HH: Combination chemotherapy in the management of superior vena caval obstruction in small call anaplastic carcinoma of the lung. Acta Med Scand 204:513-516, 1978.
71. Nugent JL, Bunn PA, Matthews MJ et al.: CNS metastases in small cell bronchogenic carcinoma. Cancer 44:1885-1893, 1979.
72. Jackson DV, Richards F, Cooper MR et al.: Prophylactic cranial irradiation in small cell carcinoma of the lung. A randomized study. JAMA 237:2730-2733, 1977.
73. Holoye PY, Samuels ML, Smith T et al.: Chemoimmunotherapy of small cell bronchogenic carcinoma. Cancer 42:34-40, 1978.
74. McCracken J, White J, Reed R et al.: Combination chemotherapy, radiotherapy, and immunotherapy for oat cell carcinoma of the lung. Proc AACR and ASCO 19:395, 1978.

75. Cohen MH, Chretien PB, Ihde DC *et al.*: Thymosin Fraction V and intensive combination chemotherapy: Prolonging the survival of patients with small cell lung cancer. JAMA 241:1813-1815, 1979.

76. Hattori S, Matsuda M, Ikegami H *et al.*: Small cell carcinoma of the lung: Clinical and cytomorphological studies in relation to its response to chemotherapy. Gann 68:321-332, 1977.

77. Herman TS, Jones SE, McMahon LG *et al.*: Combination chemotherapy with adriamycin and cyclophosphamide (with or without radiation therapy) for carcinoma of the lung. Cancer Treat Rep 61:875-879, 1977.

78. McMahon LJ, Herman TS, Manning MR *et al.*: Patterns of relapse in patients with small cell carcinoma of the lung treated with adriamycin-cyclophosphamide chemotherapy and radiation therapy. Cancer Treat Rep 63:359-362, 1979.

79. Eagan RT, Carr DT, Lee RE *et al.*: Phase II studies of polychemotherapy regimens in small cell lung cancer. Cancer Treat Rep 61:93-95, 1977.

80. King GA, Comis R, Ginsberg S *et al.*: Combination chemotherapy and radiotherapy in small cell carcinoma of the lung. Radiology 125:529-530, 1977.

81. Ginsberg SJ, Comis RL, Gottlieb AJ *et al.*: Long-term survivorship in small-cell anaplastic lung carcinoma. Cancer Treat Rep 63:1347-1349, 1979.

82. Livingston RB, Moore TN, Heilbrun L *et al.*: Small cell carcinoma of the lung: Combined chemotherapy and radiation. Ann Intern Med 88:194-199, 1978.

83. Hornback NB, Einhorn L, Shidnia H *et al.*: Oat cell carcinoma of the lung. Early treatment results of combination radiation therapy and chemotherapy. Cancer 37:2658-1664, 1976.

84. Johnson RE, Brereton HD, Kent CH: Small-cell carcinoma of the lung: Attempt to remedy causes of past therapeutic failure. Lancet 2:289-291, 1976.

85. Wittes RE, Hopfan S, Hilaris B *et al.*: Oat cell carcinoma of the lung: Combination treatment with radiotherapy and cyclophosphamide, adriamycin, vincristine, and methotrexate. Cancer 40:653-659, 1977.

86. Alexander M, Glatstein EJ, Gordon DS *et al.*: Combined modality treatment for oat cell carcinoma of the lung. A randomized trial. Cancer Treat Rep 61:1-6, 1977.

87. Eagan RT, Maurer H, Forcier RJ *et al.*: Combination chemotherapy and radiation therapy in small cell carcinoma of the lung. Cancer 32:371-379, 1973.

88. Bitran J, Golomb HM, Desser RK *et al.*: Prolonged survival of patients with extensive oat cell carcinoma treated with radiotherapy and cyclophosphamide (NSC-26271), vincristine (NSC-67574), and methotrexate (NSC-740). Cancer Treatment Rep 60:221-223, 1976.

89. Greco FA, Richardson RL, Schulman SF *et al.*: Treatment of oat cell carcinoma of the lung: Complete remissions, acceptable complications, and improved survival. Br Med J 2:10-11, 1978.

90. Cox JD, Byhardt RW, Wilson JF *et al.*: Dose-time relationships and the local control of small cell carcinoma of the lung. Radiology 128:205-207, 1978.

91. Cox JD, Byhardt R, Komaki R *et al.*: Interaction of thoracic irradiation and chemotherapy on local control and survival in small cell carcinoma of the lung. Cancer Treat Rep 63:1251-1255, 1979.

92. Abeloff MD, Ettinger DS, Baylin SB *et al.*: Management of small cell carcinoma of the lung. Therapy, staging and biochemical markers. Cancer 38:1394-1401, 1976.

93. Gilby ED, Bondy PK, Morgan RL *et al.*: Combination chemotherapy for small cell carcinoma of the lung. Cancer 39:1959-1966, 1977.

94. Osieka R, Schmidt CG, Makoski HB *et al.*: The combined modality approach in the treatment of inoperable small-cell anaplastic carcinoma of the lung. Z Krebsforsch 89:9-18, 1977.

95. Burdon JGW, Henderson MM, Moan WJ *et al.*: Combined chemotherapy and radiotherapy for the treatment of small cell carcinoma of the lung. Med J Aust 1:353-355, 1978.

96. Burdon JGW, Sinclair RA, Henderson MM: Small cell carcinoma of the lung. Chest 76:302-304, 1979.

97. Cohen MH, Lichter AS, Bunn PA *et al.*: Chemotherapy-radiation therapy (CT-RT) versus chemotherapy (CT) in limited small cell lung cancer (SCCL). Proc AACR and ASCO 21:1980 (in press).

98. Moore TN, Livingston R, Heilbrun L *et al.*: An acceptable rate of complications in combined doxorubicin-irradiation for small cell carcinoma of the lung: A Southwest Oncology Group study. Int J Radiat Oncol Biol Phys 4:675-680, 1978.

99. Chabora BM, Hopfan S, Wittes R: Esophageal complications in the treatment of oat cell carcinoma with combined irradiation and chemotherapy. Radiology 123:185-187, 1977.

100. Einhorn L, Krause M, Hornback N *et al.*: Enhanced pulmonary toxicity with bleomycin and radiotherapy in oat cell lung cancer. Cancer 37:2414-2416, 1976.

101. Von Hoff DD, Layard MW, Basa P *et al.*: Risk factors for doxorubicin-induced congestive heart failure. Ann Int Med 91:710-717, 1979.

102. Seydel HG, Creech RH, Mietlowski W *et al.*: Radiation therapy in small cell lung cancer. Semin Oncol 5:288-298, 1978.

103. Abrams RA, Lichter A, Johnston-Early A *et al.*: Enhanced suppression of peripheral blood CFU_c and white blood cell and platelet counts by regional radiotherapy in adult patients with non-hematologic malignancy. Proc AACR and ASCO 20:144, 1979.

104. Hirsch FR, Hansen HH, Paulson OB *et al.*: Development of brain metastases in small cell anaplastic carcinoma of the lung. In: CNS Complications of Malignant Disease. Kay J, Whitehouse J (eds), MacMillan Press, 1979, p 175-184.

105. Newman SJ, Hansen HH: Frequency, diagnosis and treatment of brain metastases in 247 consecutive patients with bronchogenic carcinoma. Cancer 33:492-496, 1974.

106. Hansen HH: Should initial treatment of small cell carcinoma include systemic chemotherapy and brain irradiation? Cancer Chemother Rep (Part 3) 4(2):239-241, 1973.

107. Cox JD, Petrovich Z, Paig C *et al.*: Prophylactic cranial irradiation in patients with inoperable carcinoma of the lung. Cancer 42:1135-1140, 1978.

108. Bunn PA, Nugent JL, Matthews MJ: Central nervous system metastases in small cell bronchogenic carcinoma. Semin Oncol 5:314-322, 1978.

109. Brereton HD, O'Donnell JF, Kent CH *et al.*: Spinal meningeal carcinomatosis in small-cell carcinoma of the lung. Ann Intern Med 88:517-519, 1978.

110. Greco FA, Fer MF: Oat-cell carcinoma of the lung with carcinomatous meningitis. N Engl J Med 298:1146, 1978.

111. Fox RM: Spinal cord metastasis after combination chemotherapy and prophylactic whole-brain irradiation in small cell carcinoma of the lung. Lancet 2:136, 1977.

112. Minna JD, Ihde DC, Bunn PA *et al.*: Extensive stage small cell carcinoma of the lung (SCCL): Effect of increasing intensity of induction chemotherapy. Proc AACR and ASCO, 1980 (in press).

113. Weidin PL. Storb R, Seeg HJ *et al.*: Prolonged disease-free survival in dogs with lymphoma after total body irradiation and autologous marrow transplantation consolidation of combination chemotherapy induced remissions. Blood 54:1039-1049, 1979.

114. Thomas ED, Buchner CD, Fefer A *et al.*: Marrow transplantation for acute nonlymphoblastic leukemia in first remission. N Engl J Med 301:597-599, 1979.

9. Radiation Therapy – New Approaches

OMAR M. SALAZAR and GUNAR ZAGARS

1. INTRODUCTION

Lung cancer is no longer considered to represent one single disease process. It is composed of several diseases conditioned by histopathologic forms which determine behavior, treatment and prognosis [1]. Although most oncologists accept four main pathologic forms of lung cancer (small cell, epidermoid, large cell and adenocarcinoma), therapeutic goals have allowed for a simpler general classification of lung cancer into: Small Cell Bronchogenic Carcinoma (SCBC) and Non-Small Cell Bronchogenic Carcinoma (NSCBC) with a subsequent stratification by the four main histologic forms. In addition to the clinical and surgical staging systems available for lung cancer [2], many oncologists also prefer to subclassify in broader terms by disease extent, since this also carries therapeutic implications. Consequently, SCBC and NSCBC are commonly described as: Limited disease (LD), when the tumor seems to be confined to the involved lung and draining nodal areas in the hilum, mediastinum and ipsilateral supraclavicular fossa; and extensive disease (ED), when the tumor has disseminated elsewhere.

Traditionally, local therapeutic approaches such as radiation therapy (RT) and surgery (S) have been, whenever feasible, routinely employed as primary therapy for lung cancer patients with LD. Systemic therapeutic approaches such as chemotherapy (CT) have generally constituted the primary armamentarium for lung cancer patients with ED. Secondary therapeutic approaches for the palliation of symptomatic primary and metastatic lung cancer have mainly rested on localized RT. Despite multiple advances in diagnostic and therapeutic techniques, the prognosis of lung cancer patients, even when the disease appears to only be locally advanced, has remained extremely poor. Nevertheless, the therapeutic experience of recent years has given oncologists a better knowledge and understanding of the behavior and spread patterns of the main pathological forms of lung cancer. This in turn, has helped to

R.B. Livingston (ed.), Lung cancer 1, 209–281. All rights reserved.
Copyright © 1981 Martinus Nijhoff Publishers bv, The Hague/Boston/London.

uncover major limitations with nearly every therapeutic strategy employed so far for lung cancer patients. A brief overview by each histologic group stressing these limitations follows:

1.1. Small Cell Bronchogenic Carcinoma (SCBC)

In recent years, SCBC has emerged as a distinct clinico-pathologic entity of an apparent neuro-endocrine origin and is characterized by an extremely aggressive behavior[3]. From its very early clinical stages, SCBC has been recognized to involve the draining chest nodes as well as many extrathoracic sites in a high proportion of instances[1]. Modern diagnostic techniques have allowed to classify three of every four patients presenting with SCBC as having disease outside the thorax at the time of diagnosis[4]. Because of this, SCBC is now regarded as a systemic process from the time of detection and curative surgical procedures are no longer routinely practiced. However, SCBC has been recognized for many years to be a radiosensitive tumor[1]. Localized RT achieves good intrathoracic tumor control with minimal toxicity in patients with LD-SCBC[4]. Nevertheless, the high tendency of this tumor to spread early to distant sites coupled with the inability of this local therapy to affect metastatic compartments outside its treatment portals has prevented the accepted local effectiveness of RT from achieving substantial overall survival gains in these patients. Consequently, the role of RT as a primary therapy for LD-SCBC has been obscured and has diminished considerably. Fortunately, the search for a systemic therapy for SCBC has yielded several combinations of cytotoxic agents which can now be effectively given to these patients and seem capable of achieving by themselves substantial local and distant tumor responses with moderate toxicity. Unfortunately, the use of systemic CT alone for SCBC patients has also yielded a high percentage of local chest failures and recurrences in sanctuary areas despite apparent gains in tumor responses and median survival estimates[4]. The use of elective brain irradiation (EBI) in these patients has reduced significantly the incidence of metastatic brain involvement although this has not conveyed major gains in survival presumably because of a lack of effective disease control elsewhere[5]. The use of combined therapeutic approaches with local RT and CT was geared to overcome the limitations of each individual therapy and therefore, was theoretically aimed to achieve maximum local and distant tumor control. Unfortunately, combined RT and CT approaches have also led to an increase in toxicity greater than with each therapeutic modality alone. This increase in toxicity has required subsequent adjustments in the concomitant or sequential administrations of these two therapies which could be responsible for some curtailment of their ·maximum effectiveness. Intensification of induction CT and/or localized RT for SCBC patients has achieved notable improvements in tumor responses and median survival of patients[4, 5]. Nevertheless, these aggressive attempts have also conveyed considerable fatal and life-threatening toxicity which remains difficult to accept in view of the fact that complete responders have continued to relapse and there are only a few patients who luckily remain disease-free two or more years from the initiation of therapy [4].

1.2. Non-Small Cell Bronchogenic Carcinoma (NSCBC)

This represents a conglomerate of the remaining three main histologic forms of lung cancer. A careful staging to exclude mediastinal involvement and distant metastasis in patients with small primary lung lesions can lead to hopeful probabilities of cure by surgical excision [5]. Nevertheless, these early carefully-selected cases constitute the exception and not the rule; the vast majority of patients with NSCBC are found to be inoperable, unresectable, locally advanced or already metastatic at presentation [6]. The primary therapeutic approach for NSCBC has been local RT; it has also confronted major obstacles which are responsible for relatively poor overall survival probabilities for most of these patients. The efficacy of this therapeutic modality requires careful assessment of the dose-time-volume relations employed. A curative attempt should include treatment of the adjacent draining nodal areas in the mediastinum and supraclavicular fossae because of a relatively high incidence of tumor involvement of these areas at the time of diagnosis [1]. The higher the dose delivered, the higher the local control rate although higher probabilities also exist for treatment-related complications [7]. Local chest irradiation is limited by the tolerance of certain vital normal structures to RT. Nevertheless, the minimum dose that should probably be delivered in a curative attempt with conventional daily fractionated RT is 5000 rad [8]. A well-planned curative RT attempt for LD-NSCBC patients achieves local tumor control in nearly 50% of the patients [1, 8]; however, the majority of the patients will fail in sites outside the treatment protals thus making survival a poor parameter by which to judge the efficacy of this treatment modality [1, 8]. The incidence of distant metastases in NSCBC is higher than has been expected. About one third of the patients will present with distant metastases, another third of the patients will develop this complication during the first three months after the initiation of RT, and when patients with locally advanced tumors submitted to local RT are carefully assessed, almost 80% will disseminate during the first year after therapy [6]. This represents a clear indication that patients who are found free of distant metastases at diagnosis by the available detection tests are actually harboring a substantial subclinical metastatic tumor burden at the initiation of therapy [6]. Based on these observations, similarly but not as strikingly as for SCBC, it may not be unrealistic to consider most of the NSCBC as disseminated disease from diagnosis. Unfortunately, differently from SCBC, there seems to be no proven effective combination CT that could be offered to these patients [5, 6]. In this respect, oncologists are seriously limited in their attempt to achieve substantial survival gains in NSCBC patients. As was the case for SCBC, there are many patients with NSCBC who develop metastatic brain disease and who would perhaps benefit from elective brain irradiation to this sanctuary area.

As the decade of the 1980's begins, oncologists are regrouping trying to redefine the goals that need to be achieved for lung cancer patients. It becomes evident that each therapeutic modality that has been employed for these patients is limited in one or several ways to achieve a high cure rate. The experience of recent years has taught oncologists that the best probabilities for cure may well occur with ambulatory patients who can achieve a complete tumor response early in their therapy [5]. Maintenance of the ideal disease-free status has led to recent attempts to re-stage and re-biopsy these patients to document this clinical impression [4]. With the effort to achieve the maximum possible tumor cell kill with minimal normal tissue damage, the quality of the patient's life has to be given one of the highest priorities. The morbidity of any therapeutic attempt should never outweigh the intended therapy benefits. The principal and driving goal behind a carefully combined therapeutic approach for lung cancer patients includes: effective utilization of one therapeutic modality to achieve its maximum possible benefits while also facilitating the use of other therapies which would complement or consolidate what cannot be soundly achieved by the first therapy alone. In the attempt, the quality of the patient's life should not be seriously jeopardized or compromised.

In order to understand how RT can overcome some of its limitations and broaden its scope as a primary or adjuvant therapy for lung cancer patients, some basic radiobiological principles need to be explored in the next section. The unfamiliarity of most non-radiation oncologists with many of these principles and terminology requires a substantial discussion on the subject. It is hoped that familiarization with these basic concepts will lead to a better understanding and appreciation of some of the new innovative RT approaches such as hyperbaric oxygen therapy, carbogen breathing, radiosensitizers, radioprotective agents, unconventional fractionation schedules, hemibody irradiation, increasing the tumor dose, hyperthermia, high energy RT sources, and combined modality approaches with RT.

2. THE RADIOBIOLOGY OF INNOVATIVE RADIATION THERAPY IN LUNG CANCER

Clinical RT has largely evolved along empiric lines with relatively little contribution from basic sciences. However, the virtues and limitations of classic fractionated RT are now well delineated and continuing advances in

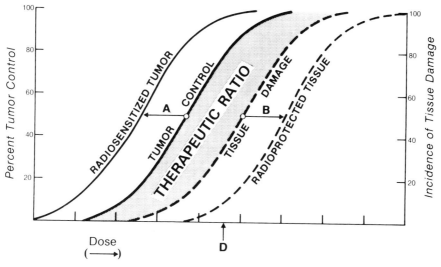

Fig. 1. Heuristic curves of tumor control and tissue damage versus radiation dose. Due to the stochastic nature of the radiation-cell interaction these curves are sigmoid. The two middle curves show tumor control and tissue damage under unmodified conditions. To achieve an 80% tumor control rate requires a dose D which produces a 40% incidence of complications. Shifting the tumor control curve to the left (A) by selective tumor radiosensitization achieved a 98% tumor control with the dose D. Shifting the tissue damage curve to the right (B) by selectively radioprotecting normal tissues leads to a 10% complication rate with a dose D.

The simultaneous achievement of A and B leads to a maximized therapeutic ratio where a dose slightly less than D achieves a 95% tumor control rate with only a 5% incidence of complications.

the art are increasingly based on concepts developed in the radiobiology laboratory. Significantly, the interaction between the radiotherapist and the radiobiologist has become a two-way interchange of problems and ideas so that neither can neglect the other's findings and pursue his field in isolation.

In clinical RT one cannot consider local tumor control and radiation-induced complications as separate and unrelated events. Tumor control can in principle always be improved by raising radiation dose and in practice this holds for bronchogenic carcinoma. However, with any increase in radiation dose, complications also increase and at sufficiently high doses any gain in tumor control is more than negated by serious radiation damage. *The central choice in radiotherapy is the choice between a high tumor control rate with attendant high complications and a lower control rate with fewer complications.* Tumor cell-kill is never the only issue. Fig. 1 is an illustration of the central goal of radiation oncology. Where tumor control and tissue damage curves are close together, as they are for bronchogenic carcinoma, there we are faced with a poor therapeutic ratio – any substantial tumor control can only be realized with significant complications. Selective tumor radiosensitization and/ or normal tissue protection will improve the therapeutic ratio. All recent radiation strategies are aimed at widening the zone between tumor control probability and complication incidence. Some approaches such as hypoxic cell sensitizers clearly aim to move the tumor control curve to the left; others such as the radioprotectors aim to move the tissue damage curve to the right and still other strategies such as densely ionizing radiation or unconventional fractionation, aim to improve the therapeutic ratio without as yet any certainty of which curve will be predominantly moved. Finally, it needs stressing that careful physical planning of tumor volume, dose distribution, and critical normal tissue exposure will of itself enhance the therapeutic ratio.

What follows is a brief overview of the major radiobiologic concepts that have impinged on new radiotherapeutic approaches to lung cancer. More comprehensive reviews are available in books by Andrews [9] and Hall [10].

2.1. Oxygen Radiobiology

Oxygen is the most potent radiosensitizing agent known – conversely, severe hypoxia is a potent radioprotective circumstance. It seems that the first demonstration of this oxygen effect was by Schwarz in 1909 [9] and though a number of sporadic observations were made in the next several decades, it was not until 1955 that, after analysis of histologic sections from human bronchogenic carcinoma, the idea that hypoxic cancer cells may be one limitation to successful RT first crystallized [11]. Since then, oxygen radiobiology has come to occupy a central role in radiation oncology.

Oxygen enhances the magnitude of the radiation effect by driving, at the time of energy exchange, radiation-produced free radicals into destructive auto-oxidative reactions. The oxygen concentration at the tumoral level at the time of radiation is a critical factor. Human tumors are composed of both oxic and hypoxic cells. Oxic cells are usually located toward the periphery of the tumor near the vascular supply (oxygen source); they are radiosensitive and are killed between fractionated radiation treatments. Hypoxic cells are not usually killed between fractionated radiation treatments. Hypoxic cells are usually located toward the center of tumors away from the capillary blood supply; they are radioresistant and although most of them are not cycling, these cells are not dead. As the oxic tumor cells are killed by fractionated radiation treatments, the distance from the oxygen supply to the hypoxic cells is shortened. The blood supply of the hypoxic cells is in fact improved and some of these tumor cells become oxic, begin to proliferate, and may give rise to tumor recurrences. Most of the RT innovations (which will be discussed in the next section of this chapter) are related to the oxygen effect and its radiobiology. Basic concepts follow:

2.1.1. Oxygen Enhancement Ratio (OER)

To achieve any given level of biologic damage, oxygenated cells require a considerably smaller radiation dose than hypoxic cells. This oxygen enhancement effect is a universal biologic phenomenon and is mediated by oxygen participating in radiochemical reactions[12]. The fundamental mechanism is uncertain; it is radiochemical and not metabolic, and is probably crucially dependent on the high electron affinity of oxygen[13, 14]. Fig. 2 illustrates typical in vitro mammalian cell survival curves under hypoxic and oxygenated conditions exposed to X or γ irradiation. The shape of both curves is identical but that under oxygen is displaced to the left by a constant factor, the oxygen enhancement ratio (OER). Thus, *OER is the ratio of radiation doses under hypoxic to oxygenated conditions to produce the same biologic effect.* OER has been determined in many biologic systems with a variety of endpoints and for sparsely ionizing (low linear energy transfer (LET)) radiation it

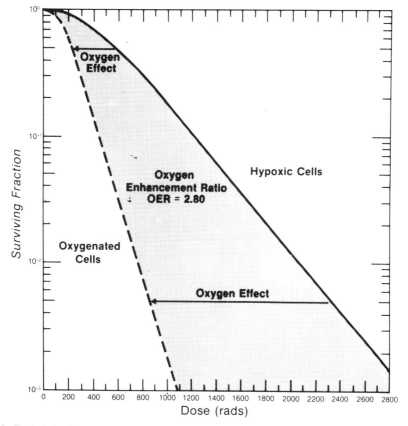

Fig. 2. Typical in vitro mammalian cell survival curves under oxygenated and hypoxic conditions. Oxygen reduces the radiation dose required to achieve any level of survival by a constant factor, the oxygen enhancement ratio (OER).

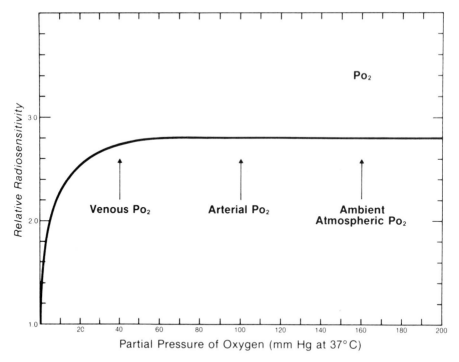

Fig. 3. Idealized diagram showing the relation between oxygen concentration and radiosensitivity. Under anoxic conditions ($Po_2 = 0$) relative radiosensitivity is assigned a value of 1.0. Full OER is taken to be 2.80. Note that full OER is virtually attained at the Po_2 of venous blood. Normal tissues are radiobiologically well-oxygenated. Pronounced hypoxic radiation resistance occurs at cellular Po_2 less than 10 mmHg.

almost always lies between 2.5 and 3.0 [9, 10]. This means that to achieve any desired level of cell survival, hypoxic cells will need a dose of 2.5 to 3.0 times greater than oxygenated cells. This oxygen effect does not occur with densely ionizing radiations (2.5 MeV alpha particles) and has only a modest role with intermediate density radiations (15 MeV neutrons) where OER is approximately 1.6 [15, 16].

OER is usually defined as the full enhancement achievable by oxygen. However, oxygenation and hypoxia are relative terms; oxygen enhancement is a function of oxygen concentration or partial pressure. Fig. 3 is a representation of the relation between oxygen pressure and radiosensitivity relative to anoxia. Virtually complete oxygen radiosensitization is achieved at $Po_2 \geq 30$ mmHg. Since normal human arterial Po_2 is 100 mmHg and normal venous Po_2 is 40 mmHg, then normal tissues are not radiobiologically hypoxic. Significant radiobiologic hypoxia implies a cellular Po_2 less than 10 mmHg.

2.1.2. The Hypoxic Fraction

Since normal tissues are radiobiologically well-oxygenated, the oxygen effect plays no part in modulating the radiation response. Tumors on the other hand do not possess an architecturally highly organized vascular stroma geared to meeting variations in oxygen demand. Indeed, many malignant growths appear to 'outgrow' their blood supply; necrosis and hemorrhage are macroscopic hallmarks of malignancy. Thomlinson and Gray [11] analyzed histologic sections of human bronchial carcinoma and drew attention to the predictable occurrence of necrosis at distances greater than 150 microns from capillaries. Calculations of the likely distance to which oxygen could diffuse through *respiring* tissue indicated that Po_2 would practically be zero at 150 to 200 microns from a capillary [17]. The implication is clear that breathing air under ambient conditions creates problems in oxygen delivery to cells no more than 150 microns from a capillary and that where intercapillary distances of more than 300 microns occur, there radiosensitivity will decrease steadily with increasing distance from the blood supply. Between the zone of well-oxygenated perivascular tumor cells and the area of frank necrosis there must occur viable (anaerobically metabolizing) and radiobiologically hypoxic cells. That such radioresistant, hypoxic but clonogenically viable, tumor cells occur has been demonstrated in almost every animal tumor system where these have been sought [9, 10]. A direct radiobiologic methodology for demonstrating hypoxic cells in human tumors is not available, however, a number of polarographic oxygen micro-electrode studies have shown critical hypoxia in many tumors [18–20].

The proportion of radiobiologically hypoxic cells in a solid tumor can be estimated from the single-dose cell survival curve when the tumor as a whole is irradiated. The hypoxic fraction, the fraction of hypoxic clonogenically viable cells expressed as a percentage of the total number of clonogenic cells, varies between 1% and 50% in various animal tumors, but the vast majority of hypoxic fractions lie between 10% and 20% [10]. The smaller the tumor is, the smaller its hypoxic fraction. As growth proceeds, the proportion of such cells rises until it achieves some value (usually between 10% and 20%) characteristic of the particular tumor and its host [21].

Figure 4 illustrates the single-dose cell survival curves obtained when whole tumors with various hypoxic fractions are irradiated with X or γ rays. The main characteristic of survival curves from such mixed cell populations is their biphasic form, with a steep initial dose-response and a shallow terminal slope at high doses. The inflection point in these curves occurs between 300 rad and 1000 rad depending on the hypoxic fraction: the larger the hypoxic component, the earlier is the break [22]. The steep initial portion is largely a manifestation of oxygenated-cell killing; the final shallow dose-response occurs when only hypoxic cells remain. Since normal tissues are well-oxygen-

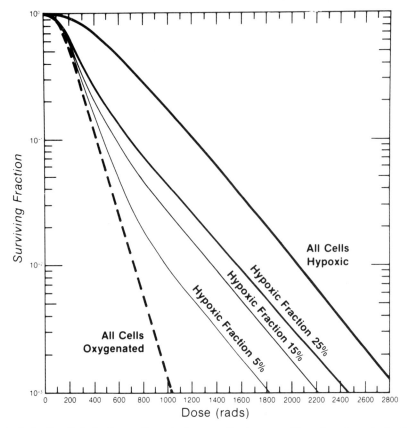

Fig. 4. A family of single dose cell survival curves for tumors with various hypoxic fractions. These are theoretic curves calculated using the multi-target single-hit model and are representative of many experimental results. The hypoxic fraction curves are biphasic with a steep dose-response initially and a terminal final slope parallel to the fully hypoxic survival curve. As hypoxic fraction rises, so the inflection region of the survival curve occurs at lower radiation doses. In theory, even at relatively low radiation doses the hypoxic fraction curves do deviate from the fully oxygenated curve.

ated, their dose-response will follow the fully oxygenated curve; tumor damage follows one of the biphasic curves. One practical implication is clear: relative to normal tissue damage, the smaller a single radiation dose is, the greater the tumor damage. For doses beyond the inflection point on the mixed oxygenated-hypoxic curve there is a pronounced therapeutically adverse divergence between tumor damage and normal tissue destruction. This is one reason why clinical radiation therapy empirically evolved small-dose fractions as the optimal mode for local control.

Good illustrations of the problems facing oxygen diffusion through respiring cells can be obtained in the laboratory with the use of microspheroids:

Small multi-cell spheroids grown *in vitro* show a fairly homogeneous cell population and their single-dose cell survival curves are typical well-oxygenated curves without any inflection; large spheroids on the other hand, have a central zone of necrosis and display biphasic survival curves indicating 15% hypoxic clonogenic cells [23].

The hypoxic fraction has one other therapeutically adverse characteristic: the vast majority of its cells are out of active mitotic cycle (variously termed as resting, G-1 block, or G-0). Thus, they are relatively inaccessible to chemotherapeutic agents, quite apart from significant problems with drug diffusion.

2.1.3. Reoxygenation

Given the nature of the single-dose cell survival curve for a mixed oxygenated-hypoxic tumor, it is clear that following any substantial dose of radiation (even as low as 200 rad), the surviving fraction will be largely hypoxic. If this state of affairs persisted then all tumors would indeed become seriously radioresistant and well beyond the reach of standard fractionated radiotherapy. However, the majority of animal tumors investigated show marked reoxygenation of hypoxic cells surviving a single radiation dose [24]. The time course of this reoxygenation is rapid and hypoxic fractions return to pretreatment values in 1 to 24 hours in most tumors [25]. This rapid reoxygenation precedes any demonstrable tumor shrinkage and its mechanism remains uncertain [25]. Reoxygenation, however, is not a universal phenomenon and, for example, did not occur in one transplantable osteosarcoma [26].

The demonstration of human tumor reoxygenation between fractions of standard radiation therapy is not amenable to direct radiobiologic study. However, a number of oxygen microelectrode studies of human cancers have shown improvement in average tumor Po_2 following small-fraction radiation doses [19]. Whether such increase in average tumor Po_2 really corresponds to the rapid reoxygenation observed in animal tumors in uncertain. Nonetheless, reoxygenation by whatever mechanism, has important therapeutic implications. By reoxygenating between radiation fractions, the hypoxic fraction will effectively remain constant until the tumor begins macroscopic regression. If regression begins early during the course of treatment, then we would expect the hypoxic fraction to fall in the later phases of treatment. Under these circumstances, the overall tumor response will be largely, but in theory not entirely, a reflection of oxygenated cell killing. The fact that many human tumors, particularly exophytic rapidly regressing lesions, are locally controlled by radiobiologically relatively low fractionated total doses (6000 to 7000 rad) suggests that under these conditions reoxygenation is efficient [27]. However, the all too frequent contrary observations that some tumors are not permanently locally controlled raises the possibility that, in these cases, reoxygenation is inadequate and persistent hypoxic cells are one limitation to successful radiotherapy.

2.2. High LET Radiobiology

All ionizing radiations deposit their energy in matter via charged particle interactions: 'collisional' interactions between high-velocity charged particles and orbital electrons of the medium. Directly ionizing radiations are beams of charged particles, e.g., electron beams, proton beams, pion beams; indirectly ionizing radiations are beams of electrically neutral particles which generate high-speed charged particles within the medium, e.g. photon beams generate electrons, neutron beams generate protons. The high-velocity charged particles deposit their energy in discrete and randomly distributed energy deposition events along their tracks. Each charged particle energy deposition event liberates an average of 60 electron volts (ev) of energy into a sphere of 30 Å diameter. As a result of the energization, this sphere contains excited and ionized molecules which rapidly transform into free radicals that may interact with biologic molecules in their vicinity – interactions with critical molecular sites (e.g. DNA) will be scored as lethal hits unless metabolic repair processes remove the damaged moiety. The initial shoulder on mammalian cell survival curves strongly suggests that for cell sterilization, more than one energy deposition event must occur within a small volume. Whether this phenomenon is to be interpreted as a single target requiring several hits or as several close targets each needing one hit or whether additive 'sublesions' are involved has not been settled [9, 28]. However, this requirement for multiplicity of interaction underlies the phenomenon of relative biologic effectiveness: radiations of different types require different absorbed doses to achieve a specified degree of effect.

2.2.1. Linear Energy Transfer (LET)

The frequency with which a charged particle interacts with electrons in a medium corresponds to the rate at which it deposits energy along its track and this is specified as linear energy transfer (LET). *LET is defined as the energy imparted to matter by one charged particle transversing some specified length.* Commonly LET is expressed in units of thousands of electron volts (KEV) per micron of particle track. LET is a complex function of velocity and charge of the ionizing particle, but simplistically it is proportional to Q^2/V where Q is the charge of the particle and V its velocity [10]. In virtually all conditions one is dealing with a spectrum of LET values even for monoenergetic radiations (noting that for any one particle LET increases as it slows down) and 'average LET' does not fully define a beam. Nevertheless, this concept permits qualitative understanding of the importance of ionization density. Fig. 5 is a schematic representation of the average spacings between

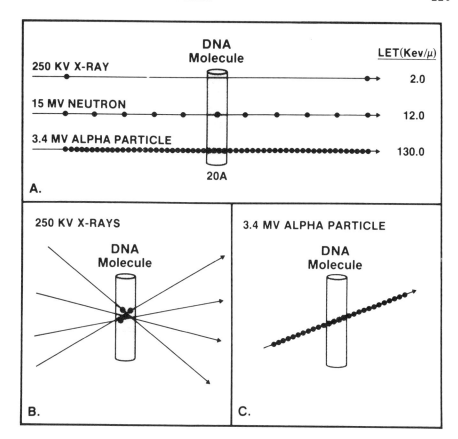

Fig. 5. A. A heuristic diagram of the frequency of ionizing events along the paths of ionizing particles of different LET.

B. If inactivation of a DNA molecule requires four ionizations in a small volume then four independent low LET tracks will have to deposit energy in a specified portion of its track.

C. The high frequency of ionizations along a high LET track assures the occurrence of the requisite number of events within the DNA molecule provided that just one track passes through it.

energy deposition events (ionizations) along the tracks of various types of radiation. Radiations of low LET (250 KV X-rays, Co-60 X-rays, 10 MeV linac photons) are called *sparsely* ionizing; radiations of high LET (accelerated α-particles, accelerated neon nuclei) are called *densely* ionizing. In the intermediate LET region (e.g. fast neutrons) we properly should speak of 'intermediate density radiations,' but by common consensus these radiations are loosely designated as '*high LET.*'

Figure 5 also illustrates the influence of LET on the generation of biologic damage for a 'four-hit' process, i.e. four ionizing events are required within the critical molecule for its inactivation. With low LET radiation two conditions must be fulfilled for an inactivation: not only must four separate charged particle tracks cross the target, but they must each undergo an ionization either within the target or very close to it. It would be extremely unlikely for one charged particle to transverse the target and undergo four successive interactions over the short target distance. In contrast, with high LET radiation only one condition is necessary for inactivation: the charged particle must cross or pass close by the target. When this occurs four successive interactions within the target volume are virtually guaranteed by virtue of the high frequency of ionizations. This is essentially the mechanism for the greater efficiency of high LET compared to low LET radiation on a dose-for-dose basis. There is an upper limit to this efficiency which occurs at LET values so high that more than the minimum requisite number of ionizations occur within the target leading to an 'overkill' effect with decline in efficiency.

Efficiency, however, is not the main virtue of high LET radiations and it might even be regarded as a nuisance. Their crucial characteristics of potential therapeutic value is an 'insensibility phemonemon.' Whereas the induction and expression of low LET-induced biologic damage is very substantially modulated by metabolic repair processes and by extraneous agents (such as oxygen, sensitizers and protectors), the induction and expression of high LET-induced damage is relatively insensible to all these factors. Apparently the high ionization density generates such high local concentrations of chemically reactive intermediates that externally added agents have little chemical scope for action. Furthermore, the induction of multi-hit lesions by single tracks largely does away with sublethal repairable damage. As might be expected, this insensibility to modulation is not all-or-none, but increases as LET increases to about 200 KEV/micron beyond which no external modulation is demonstrable and survival curves are strictly experimental [9, 10].

2.2.2. Relative Biologic Effectiveness (RBE)

Although efficiency may not be a biologically virtuous quality (it merely saves energy), it must be explicitly quantitated for accurate biologic dosimetry. *Relative biologic effectiveness (RBE) is the term used to compare the efficiency of different types of radiation in producing a given biologic effect.* The RBE of any test radiation is defined as follows:

$$RBE = \frac{\text{Dose of standard radiation required to produce a given effect}}{\text{Dose of the test radiation required for the same effect}}.$$

The standard radiation is usually taken to be orthovoltage X-rays (200–500 KVP). Any radiation more efficient than this will have an RBE greater than 1.0. Megavoltage beams have an RBE of approximately 0.85 and high LET radiations can reach an RBE of 8.0.

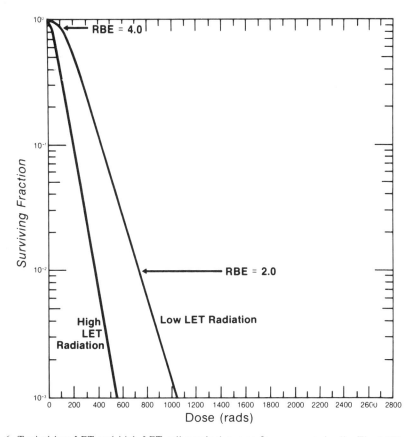

Fig. 6. Typical low LET and high LET cell survival curves for oxygenated cells. The LET curve has a smaller shoulder and sleeper slope than the low LET curve. RBE is a function of the survival fraction (SF) desired and increases as SF decreases. At an SF of 10^{-2} RBE is 2.0; at an SF of 0.85, RBE is 4.0.

In reality, RBE is a complex parameter and general statements about the RBE of a particular radiation beam may well go into the domain of dangerous error. Fig. 6 illustrates typical low and high LET, all survival curves, and highlights the importance of dose as determinant of RBE. The high LET survival curve has a much smaller shoulder and a steeper slope than the low LET curve. The shapes of the two curves are not the same and so the ratios of doses will vary with the surviving fraction. *For high LET radiations, RBE increases as dose decreases.* Table 1 lists additional factors which determine RBE and ideally each must be specified whenever an RBE value is quoted.

2.2.3. The Relationship Between LET, RBE and OER

If the modulating factors outlined in Table 1 are kept constant but the average LET is increased, then RBE rises (at first slowly, but beyond

Table 1. Determinants of RBE.

(1) Linear energy transfer of radiation.
(2) Radiation dose.
(3) Fractionation pattern.
(4) Dose rate.
(5) Biological test system.
(6) Endpoint under study.
(7) Oxygenation status.
(8) Presence or absence of sensitizer or protector.

10 KEV/micron very rapidly) to reach a peak value at about 200 KEV/micron. At higher LET values radiation efficiency decreases due to the overkill phemonemon. There is an important relation between LET and OER: for LET up to about 10 KEV/micron, OER remains between 2.5 and 3.0; but as LET rises further, OER falls dramatically and at about 200 KEV/micron an oxygen effect is no longer evident. *As LET rises so the cellular protective effect of hypoxia diminishes and at sufficiently high ionization densities oxygen exerts no sensitizing effect.* Clearly, high LET radiations provide one approach to the abrogation of hypoxic cell effects in clinical radiotherapy.

The diminution of oxygen effect is not totally lost when high LET radiations are combined with low LET radiation (mixed beam therapy)[9]. Whereas, the overall RBE for such mixed treatments varies linearly with the neutron percentage of the total dose, the variation of OER is an interesting function of the proportion of total dose given as low LET radiation[16]. OER falls rather dramatically as a small proportion of neutron therapy is added to Co-60 irradiation[16]. When half of the dose is given as photons and half as neutrons the OER is essentially indistinguishable from full neutron therapy. This is a rationale for the use of mixed beam therapy.

2.2.4. The Therapeutic Gain Factor (TGF)

The fact that some radiation may be more efficient than another is in itself of little therapeutic value. What is required is that there be some selectivity of this enhanced efficiency toward tumors. If the efficiency of tumor cell kill is enhanced more than the efficiency of normal cell kill, then we may speak of a therapeutic gain. For high LET radiation we may conceptualize this very simply by means of the therapeutic gain factor (TGF)[10].

$$TGF = \frac{RBE\ tumor}{RBE\ normal}.$$

If RBE for a tumor is greater than RBE for the critical complication-determining tissue in the radiation field, then a therapeutic gain has been achieved. Unfortunately, the complexity of the determinant factors of RBE

(Table 1) precludes any simple a priori statement as to whether TGF will be favorable in any given circumstance and it may be unreasonable to expect that it will be favorable in all situations. The only clear factor operating to selectively increase tumor RBE is the oxygen effect. Since the oxygen effect is reduced at high LET, it follows that the ratio of RBE hypoxic/RBE oxygenated cells will be greater than 1.0. Other factors being equal, this should extrapolate to tumors with hypoxic fractions and yield a TGF greater than 1.0. In practice, it has been demonstrated that in mice, lung tissue has an RBE smaller than any other normal tissue or tumor at all dose levels[29]. This suggests an advantage for high LET radiations in the treatment of lung lesions.

3. RADIATION ONCOLOGY INNOVATIONS FOR LUNG CANCER THERAPY

In an attempt to cure or palliate lung cancer patients, the main goal of radiation therapy is to obtain the best possible *local-regional tumor control* with minimal normal tissue toxicity. There are some physical limitations frustrating efforts to achieve this goal: (1) Bulky tumors containing enormous loads of tumor cells such that a radiation dose yielding a high probability of killing all cells cannot be attained within normal tissue tolerance; (2) Tumors located in sites involving or contiguous with critical dose-limited normal tissues (i.e. spinal cord, normal lung, heart and esophagus) where delivering higher doses of radiation would exceed the tolerance of these tissues; and (3) Tumors which have by extensive invasion so damaged the normal structures that subsequent healing would result in unacceptable normal tissue sequelae (i.e. tracheo-esophageal or bronchio-esophageal fistulae). There are also some major biological tumor limitations which make conventional irradiation for lung cancer ineffective: (1) A high propensity for distant spread; (2) a high hypoxic fraction of radioresistant cells; (3) A great capacity to repair sublethal radiation damage leading to decreased effectiveness of conventional daily small-dose fractionated irradiation; (4) Rapid proliferation such that repopulation occurs between fractions; (5) Cell cycle kinetics such that there will always be a large number of cells in radiation-insensitive cell cycle phases.

There are three general approaches to developing a more effective radiation therapy strategy for lung cancer which could overcome major limitations of the past: (1) increase the tumor responsiveness relative to that of normal tissue; (2) improve the dose distribution, that is, increase the radiation dose in tumor tissues relative to the dose in adjacent normal tissues; and (3) attempt to use radiation systemically for the control of distant metastatic spread. These approaches are based on radiobiological principles discussed in the previous section; this section is limited to consideration of those innovative radiation approaches which have been, are, or could soon be used in the therapy of bronchogenic carcinoma. There are other approaches which will not be discussed because they still are considered experimental or have not been tested in lung cancer patients.

3.1. Hyperbaric Oxygen (HBO) Therapy

The most direct line of attack against radioresistant hypoxic cells is through the use of hyperbaric oxygen (high pressure oxygen, HPO). However, since oxygen is largely transported in blood as oxyhemoglobin, it is relevant to note the possible influence of hemoglobin concentration on local tumor control under ambient atmospheric conditions. Evidence for the thesis that hypoxic cells are one limitation to radiotherapy was recently presented in a retrospective study of patients with cervical carcinoma Stages II-B and III [30]. Those women with hemoglobin levels below 12 gm% had significantly poorer pelvic control by radiation than women whose hemoglobin was above 12 gm%. This same report also showed on a prospective study basis that maintenance of hemoglobin above 12 gm% by transfusion during fractionated therapy improved local control above the results achieved when hemoglobin was allowed to drop to between 10 and 12 gm%. Hyperbaric oxygen attempts to deliver adequate oxygen to hypoxic tumor regions by substantially increasing the concentration of dissolved oxygen in plasma and circumventing to some degree the limitation imposed by fully saturated hemoglobin.

The use of hyperbaric oxygen requires complicated and expensive set-ups which include especially made pressure chambers and allowance for proper decompression. The early HBO experience indicated that large doses of 400–500 rad per fraction should be employed; Van den Brenk demonstrated that when a single dose exceeded 500 rad, the incidence of radiation-induced necrosis rose rapidly [31]. Therefore, there was a need to reduce the number of fractions which became even more appealing for technical considerations. The majority of the HBO trials have employed large fractions of 500–600 rad delivered twice per week for total doses of 3600–5000 rad. The use of these unconventional radiation schedules will be discussed separately in this section.

Despite a large number of human studies using HPO, the clinical usefulness and even the very demonstration of an oxygen effect have not been definitely settled [30–38]. Unfortunately, many of the reported studies have been poorly, if at all, controlled. All too often survival has been the sole endpoint without separate analysis of local control – the rational radiation therapy endpoint. Thus, Cade and McEwen [36] having explored HPO radiation therapy in bronchogenic carcinoma – a tumor with high metastatic propensity – conclude that survival was not improved over that achieved in air, but they present no analysis of local control. Local control was indeed improved in advanced head and neck cancer without a corresponding gain in survival [34]. The Medical Research Council trials of HPO in the United Kingdom demonstrated significant improvement in local control of advanced carcinoma of the cervix treated under HPO and provided perhaps the most definitive evidence for an oxygen effect in this group of human tumors [37]. However, it must remain fair to say that this line of treatment has not fulfilled its early expectations and that the technical problems in setting up a hyperbaric unit more than ofset any demonstrable gains in the eyes of many investigators.

Perhaps the most significant detractor to HPO radiation therapy has been the observation that oxygen breathed under high pressure may still remain inadequate in concentration to reach critical hypoxic foci. Suit *et al.* [38] were unable to demonstrate an oxygen effect in mouse mammary tumors using single radiation doses, i.e. the probability for local control using single doses was unaffected by irradiating at 4 atmospheres oxygen. Only when fractionated doses were given, and when presumably some reoxygenation was occurring, could any oxygen enhancement be demonstrated. Under HPO a significant proportion of human tumors remained at average Po_2 values in the radioresistant range [31]. Evidently, actively respiring perivascular tumor cells impose a substantial barrier to oxygen delivery to more peripheral hypoxic regions.

3.2. Carbogen Breathing

The same principles and connotations discussed for hyperbaric oxygen therapy apply to breathing atmospheric *carbogen* [a mixture of 95% oxygen (O_2) plus 5% carbon dioxide (CO_2)] in conjunction with radiotherapy. DuSault compared the radiocurability of spontaneous mammary carcinoma in C3H mice breathing 100% O_2 at atmospheres of pressure with mice breathing carbogen at atmospheric pressure; the results were similar for hyperbaric oxygen and carbogen breathing [40]. It was found that the addition of a small amount of CO_2 to the gas breathed by an animal caused hyperventilation, a rise in blood pressure, capillary dilatation and an exchange of gases across the endothelial wall – all indicative of an increased oxygen availability [40].

The Radiation Therapy Oncology Group (RTOG) has attempted to compare conventional irradiation with or without carbogen breathing in a number of randomized prospective protocols for a variety of tumors other than lung cancer (oral cavity, head and neck, esophagus and uterine cervix). The vast majority of these studies did not reveal improved results with the use of carbogen breathing. Certain impracticalities were identified with the use of carbogen, the most important of which were: the need in some patients to breath pure oxygen prior to breathing carbogen to avoid nausea; and the fact that all breathing had to be done through a mask with a non-rebreathing valve for 10–20 minutes (before and during the actual time of irradiation) which caused major inconveniences, fear and technical difficulties in many patients.

Although there is little experience in this country with carbogen breathing and radiation therapy for bronchogenic carcinoma, some clinical experience exists in Japan which deserves mention. Abe *et al.* from Kyoto, Japan conducted a randomized trial in 48 consecutive lung cancer patients with clinically inoperable but locally advanced tumors: one half of the patients were treated in air, the other half with carbogen breathing[41]. These investigators did not use conventional radiation therapy but rather adopted a treatment schedule for both groups of patients which was previously used in hyperbaric oxygen trials: two fractions of 500 rad per week for 4–6 weeks delivering doses of 4000–6000 rad. The survival results were 46% and 38% at one year, 17% and 13% at two years, 10% and 9% at 3 years, 6% and 5% at 4 and 5 years for patients treated with carbogen and in air respectively[41]. It was concluded that carbogen breathing had only a temporary effect on survival which was not maintained beyond 2 years. Unfortunately, no mention was made of complications and local tumor control. Judging by the authors' retrospective experience with conventional fractionation schedules of radiation in over 200 locally advanced lung cancer patients (which yielded survival estimates of 28%, 12%, 5%, 3% and 3% from 1–5 years), neither carbogen nor the unorthodox fractionation used yielded an improved cure rate[41].

3.3. Hypoxic Cell Sensitizers

As mentioned earlier, the problem of hypoxic cells is a problem of the transport of oxygen respiring tumor cell masses and its delivery in adequate concentration to non-vascularized but clonogenic cells. The recent discovery of a number of chemical compounds that behave radiobiologically as oxygen-mimetic agents has opened a totally new avenue for the potential exploitation of hypoxic cells in radiation oncology. Indeed, the electron-affinic hypoxic cell radiosensitizer concept has led to one of the most comprehensive, systematic and integrated scientific-clinical research programs in radiation oncology[42]. The impetus for this program was almost unimaginably remote from the clinic: in 1963 Adams and Dewey theorized that the solvated electron produced during water radiolysis was the critical radiochemical species involved in radiosensitization phemonema observed when irradiating dilute suspensions of micro-organisms in the presence of certain organic compounds[13]. The solvated electron was regarded as an important radical-ion in the genesis of biologic damage by virtue of its interaction with critical cell targets (e.g. DNA). Such electrons liberated by ionization-excitation of intracellular water along primary particle tracks would diffuse from their site of production and, either interact with critical biologic molecules or recombine with water to form hydrogen. Clearly, if these solvated electrons could be temporarily and reversibly captured by some molecule, then their chances for recombination would decrease and correspondingly their sphere of action would increase. Such electron carrier molecules should behave as radiosensitizers – this was the new hypothesis, the germination of the idea of electron-affinic radiosensitization. It soon became clear that *electron-affinic sensitization was limited to hypoxic cells*. Since oxygen itself is a highly electron-affinic molecule, oxygen radiobiology becomes unified under the electron affinity concept.

What advantages might compounds other than oxygen have to encourage their exploration as hypoxic cell sensitizers? If a drug is not substantially metabolized by respiring cells, if it diffuses freely through poorly-vascularized cell masses, if it is acceptably non-toxic and if it sensitizes hypoxic cells only,

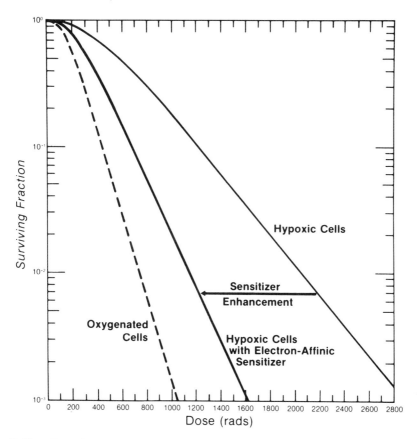

Fig. 7. The effect of electron-affinic hypoxic cell sensitizers on the survival curve of a hypoxic cell population irradiated with single radiation doses. For comparison, the fully oxygenated curve is also illustrated. The sensitizer does not alter the shape of the survival curve, but shifts it toward the oxygenated curve. At adequate sensitizer concentrations (Fig. 8), the hypoxic curve would be superimposed on the oxygenated curve.

then it should effectively reach areas inaccessible to oxygen itself. Large numbers of electron-affinic sensitizers effective in vitro have been identified [43, 44], but only a few possess the additional properties required of a clinically useful drug. Two agents, Metronidazole (Flagyl) and Misonidazole (RO–07–0582) are undergoing clinical trials. A number of new and perhaps more efficient drugs are expected in the clinical area within a short time.

Fig. 7 shows the typical modification of hypoxic cell survival curves produced by irradiation in the presence of a sensitizer. These sensitizers do not in general alter the shape of the hypoxic cell survival curve, but merely shift it to the left by a constant factor, the sensitizer enhancement ratio (SER). *SER is the ratio of radiation dose in the absence of sensitizer to dose in the presence of sensitizer to produce the same biologic effect.* Since these agents behave as

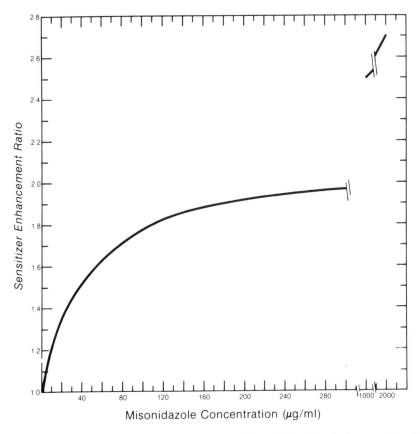

Fig. 8. The relation between sensitizer enhancement ratio and Misonidazole concentration. This curve is qualitatively similar to the oxygen sensitization curve, Fig. 3. While Misonidazole in large concentrations can abolish the protective effect of hypoxia, clinically attainable levels up to about 120 γ/ml achieve only partial sensitization. Relatively little enhancement is gained by doubling drug concentration from 100 to 200 μg/ml. (data from Fowler *et al.* [43].

oxygen-mimetics, they display characteristics qualitatively similar to oxygen and *SER is analogous to OER*. Just as oxygen sensitization is a function of oxygen concentration (Fig. 3), so too, SER depends on sensitizer concentration (Fig. 8). Similarly, sensitizer enhancement decreases for intermediate density radiations (15 MeV neutrons) and is absent with high density radiation. There is, however, one phenomenon which appears to be unique to these agents: *specific cytotoxicity for hypoxic cells* [45]. This effect depends on drug concentration and duration of exposure and is significantly potentiated by modest hyperthermia. Quantitatively the cytotoxic effect is small relative to radiosensitization, but if low drug levels are maintained over many hours this chemotherapeutic effect may be an important reinforcement to radiosensitization. Indeed, a study is being developed at the University of Rochester to evaluate the clinical effectiveness of 5-Fluorouracil (effective against oxygenated cycling cells) combined with Misonidazole (effective against hypoxic non-cycling cells).

The full exploitation of currently available sensitizers is limited by their toxicity. Misonidazole, the most powerful clinically used sensitizer, is limited by acute gastrointestinal toxicity to about 5 g/M^2 as a single oral dose and by peripheral and central neuropathy to about 15 g/M^2 total dose when given in fractions over 4 to 6 weeks [46–48]. Though virtually full oxygen-equivalent sensitization can be achieved by Misonidazole at concentrations of 2000 μg/ml (Fig. 8), such levels are well beyond clinical reach. Typical safe human blood levels for multi-fraction administration range between 50 and 120 μg/ml and one would not expect the single radiation dose SER to exceed 1.80 at best. Fig. 9 illustrates the implications of limited hypoxic cell sensitization in a mixed oxygenated-hypoxic tumor exposed to single doses of X or γ rays. Any hypoxic cell sensitizer can only shift the mixed-cell survival curve to the left within the shaded zone. At low radiation doses there is little scope for demonstrable sensitization; at high radiation doses the relative importance of sensitizer increases. Also shown is a theoretic (multi-target, single hit) curve for a sensitizer achieving an SER of 1.80. Clearly, the relative gains of this agent increase as radiation dose increases. Below 300 rad there is only minute enhancement. A number of in vivo experimental systems have verified this prediction: when tested on mouse tumors, giving single large radiation doses, Misonidazole yields very significant sensitization; multifractionated dose schedules with single doses less than 300 rad produce little or no enhancement [43]. These observations are one reason why Misonidazole in clinical protocols has been used with relatively large radiation fractions (400 to 600 rad).

Misonidazole is the most powerful nitromidazole sensitizer that has received clinical evaluation [46–52]. Misonidazole is a small and readily diffusible molecule which binds only minimally to plasma proteins. Its absorption

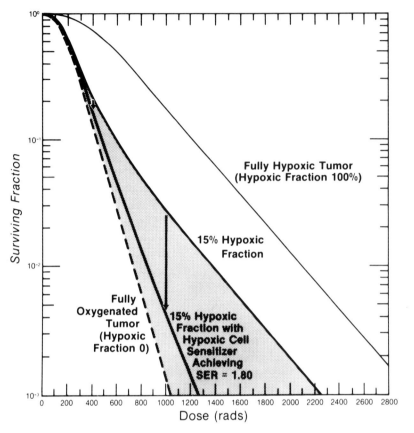

Fig. 9. Theoretic multi-target, single-hit cell survival curves for tumors with various hypoxic fractions showing the influence of hypoxic cell sensitization. A hypoxic cell sensitizer modifies the 15% hypoxic fraction survival curve by moving it into the shaded zone progressively closer to the fully oxygenated curve as sensitizer concentration (or SER) rises. The survival curve of the 15% hypoxic tumor in the presence of a sensitizer concentration achieving an SER of 1.80 illustrates that relatively greater therapeutic effects are expected at higher radiation doses (vertical arrows). At 1000 rad survival of tumor cells is reduced by a factor of 6.5 in the pressure of sensitizer; at 400 rad, the gain is only by a factor of 1.3. This has been one of the reasons for using large radiation dose fractions in clinical radiosensitizer studies.

from the gut is complete and rapid with peak plasma concentrations occurring 1 to 2 hours after oral intake. The drug is cleared slowly from the circulation with a half-life of about 12 hours. The pathways of excretion remain to be fully delineated, though direct urinary filtration, demethylation, hepatic break-down and gut flora metabolism are involved. Oral phenytoin sodium (Dilantin) seems to enhance drug clearance and in our patients Misonidazole half-lives were significantly shorter in those receiving phenytoin (8 hours versus 13 hours). However, hepatic enzyme induction by Misonidazole itself has not been observed in humans. Tumor biopsies show tissue concentrations varying between 14% and 120% of corresponding blood values, with most estimated around 80% [43, 47, 49]. Concentrations in the critical hypoxic regions of solid tumors have not been evaluated. Although peak plasma levels occur 1 to 2 hours after oral administration, it is tacitly assumed that time must be allowed for drug penetration into tumors and *radiation is usually given about 4 hours after oral intake*. The 4 hour plasma concentration (μg/ml) is approximately 38 times the oral dose (g/M^2), though relatively wide variations occur.

The toxicity of Misonidazole is now well-delineated. Anorexia, nausea, vomiting and occasional diarrhea occur with doses in excess of 2.5 g/M^2. This immediate toxicity limits single oral doses to a maximum of about 5 g/M^2 – at this level nausea and vomiting can be severe, intractable and prolonged. The major dose-limiting toxicity is peripheral neuropathy [46–48, 51, 52]. This syndrome is observed with multi-fractionated, high total dose Misonidazole schedules and commences 2 to 6 weeks after beginning treatment. The neuropathy is largely sensory with paraesthesia of hands and feet and objective sensory findings in a glove and stocking distribution. Occasionally the paresthesiae are severe. The symptoms gradually subside and motor deficits are uncommon. The neuropathy is of axonal degeneration type and its pathogenesis is obscure [52]. It is however, clearly related to total Misonidazole dose: the higher the total dose, the higher is the incidence and the greater is the severity of the neuropathy [47, 48]. Total doses in excess of 15 g/M^2 given over 3 to 6 weeks will produce significant neuropathy in 80% or more of patients. Doses of 12 g/M^2 or less given over 17 days produce about a 30% incidence of neuropathy [47]. Quite apart from total dose, tissue exposure is another parameter correlated with neuropathy [47]. For the same total dose administered those patients achieving unusually high peak concentrations or having especially prolonged half-lives have a higher incidence of neuropathy [47].

A number of other toxicities have been recorded. Ototoxicity due to cochlear damage leading to high-frequency tone deafness has occurred [46, 48]. Grand mal convulsions are infrequently encountered, mainly in elderly, debilitated and dehydrated patients [48]; transient organic psychosyndromes may occur [46]; and rarely skin rashes have been seen.

Given these clinical toxicity limitations, we are faced with the question of how best to administer the maximal Misonidazole allowance. A number of rational approaches are available and comparative (Phase III) clinical trials are in process in a number of centers to evaluate various schedules for a number of tumor sites. Each approach has theoretic advantages and disadvantages and only further clinical and laboratory investigation will provide firm answers. The idea illustrated in Fig. 9 argues for the use of a relatively few large-dose radiation fractions combined with maximal tolerated Misonidazole doses, e.g. 600 rad $\times$ 6 with 2.0–2.5 g/M^2 Misonidazole with each irradiation. The main detractor to this approach comes from the empiric observation of clinical radiotherapy that protracted fractionated treatment is the optimal mode for highest local control [53]. Short, sharp courses of radiation have been generally regarded as yielding disappointing results with high complication rates. Nevertheless, reduced fractionation schedules using concentrated radiation doses have been and are being tested at the present time. The subject of unconventional fractionation schedules will be discussed later on in this chapter.

Whether Misonidazole can 'rescue' some of these unconventional fractionation schedules and even increase their effectiveness above standard treatment patterns, remains to be seen. The Radiation Therapy Oncology Group (RTOG) selected an unconventional fractionation schedule of delivering fractions of 600 rad twice per week for three weeks in combination with Misonidazole for a Phase I–II study on locally advanced non-small cell bronchogenic carcinoma [54]. This study has recently closed and results are not yet available. The alternate approach of adding low dose Misonidazole to each of a large number of standard radiation fractions, attempts to enhance the favorable factors inherent in such fractionation by adding only small hypoxic enhancements to each dose. The RTOG has selected this approach for its Phase II–III protocol for locally advanced bronchogenic carcinoma [55]. This protocol has just been opened and it will take several months before results can be obtained; whether demonstrable overall enhancement will be obtained remains to be seen. It is also possible to take advantage of the relatively long half-life of Misonidazole by giving a number of radiation fractions with each drug dose; the radiations are spaced to allow for repair of sublethal radiation damage (intervals of 3–4 hours), or RT can be given on a continuous low dose-rate basis as advocated by Pierquin [56]. Finally, a relatively standard course of radiation might be punctuated by a number of large fractional doses combined with Misonidazole and utilizing cone-down, boost techniques.

The current standard hypoxic cell sensitizer is Misonidazole (RO–07–0582). As clinical and laboratory investigation delineate further the virtures and limitations of this agent, new and potentially better radiosensitizers will be developed. The demethylated metabolite of Misonidazole, RO–07–9963, (desmethylmisonidazole) is expected to reach the clinical arena by the time this publication is released [42]. The major advantage expected of 9963 is its short plasma half-life due to its higher water solubility and rapid renal filtration [42]. This short half-life and lower octanol water partition coefficient, imply less nervous tissue exposure and lower neurotoxicity. A number of other newer agents with promising pharmacokinetic parameters are being developed: RO–05–9963; SR–2508; SR–2555.

3.4. Radioprotective Agents

It has been known for many decades that compounds containing sulfhydryl groups (SH) are radioprotective [57]. The clinical usefulness of the commonly known radioprotectants such as cysteine and cysteamine has been curtailed by the toxicity of doses required to produce significant radioprotection. However, the United States Army Medical Research and Development Command has carried out an extensive screening program for radioprotective agents and a number of thiophosphate derivatives of cysteamine (Table 2) have been singled out as potentially useful [42]. In 1969, one of these substances, aminopropylaminoethylphosphorothioic acid (WR 2721) was reported to selectively protect normal tissues with little effect on tumor response [58]. Since then, steady progress in analyzing this compound has brought it close to the clinical arena [42].

The mechanism for the radioprotection afforded by sulfhydryl compounds has long been a matter of debate with the favored hypothesis being that they act as 'radical scavengers' and reduce the yield of biologically damaging radiochemical species [10]. More recent insights [59–63] have revealed a *fundamental relation between the oxygen effect and sulfhydryl protection*. On the whole, sulfhydryl agents have little, if any, effect on the radiation response of hypoxic cells. Their protective effect seems to consist in the negation of oxygen sensitization. Accordingly, the OER in the presence of a radioprotector is 1.0 and hypoxic cell sensitization by electron affinic drugs is abolished by adequate concentrations of a radioprotector [60, 62]. This relation to the oxygen effect also seems to underly the pattern of radioprotection with radiations of different LET: protection is pronounced for low LET radiations and is absent with very high LET radiations, having an intermediate role for intermediate density radiations such as fast neutrons [10, 64].

WR–2721:

WR–2721 is a thiophosphate derivative of cysteamine and has a phosphate group covering the SH moiety. To become an active radioprotector this compound must undergo hydrolytic dephosphorylation to uncover the sulfhydryl; the active compound is WR–1065 (Table 2). WR–2721 enters cells by passive or facilitated diffusion and is dephosphorylated within the cell by a number of hydrolase enzymes [59]. The permeability of cell membranes to the

Table 2. Chemical structure of thiophosphate derivatives of cysteamine.

Cysteamine	$H_2NCH_2CH_2SH$
WR-2721	$H_2N(CH_2)_3NHCH_2CH_2SPO_3H_2$
WR-1065	$H_2N(CH_2)_3NHCH_2CH_2SH$

drug is very restricted and greatly modulated by membrane changes such as occur during the explantation of cells into culture. In vitro most cells are almost impermeable to WR-2721 and little protection is demonstrable [59, 63]. Oral absorption is poor and when administered parenterally to rodents, WR-2721 localizes in various tissues: kidneys, liver, skin, intestinal mucosa, bone marrow and salivary glands; relatively little is found in skeletal muscle and brain shows essentially no uptake [65]. The pattern of tissue uptake is probably species and strain specific. Some mouse strains show poor pulmonary uptake with a corresponding low protection against pulmonary radiation death [65], while other strains show high lung concentration with substantial pulmonary protection [66]. Tumor uptake of the compound has been uniformly low though with some variations. The actual amount absorbed into a lesion may be a characteristic of each tumor type [65]. These variations in tissue distribution probably depend on variations in vascularity, cell membrane structure and intracellular dephosphorylase activity.

Radioprotection is quantitated as a Dose Reduction Factor (DRF). *DRF is the ratio of radiation dose in the presence of a protector to the dose in the absence of a protector to produce a given biologic effect.* Loosely speaking, DRF may be thought of as the factor by which the radiation dose is effectively reduced because a radioprotectant is present. In all in-vivo animal systems studies, WR-2721 has demonstrated substantial radioprotection for a variety of normal tissues at drug doses well below toxicity. Doses of 400–500 mg/Kg protect rodents against hematopoietic death (DRF 2.7), against gastrointestinal radiation death (DRF 1.8), against skin damage (DRF 2.4), against esophageal and renal death (DRF 1.5) and in some strains, against lung damage (DRF 1.7) [65–67]. The drug is ineffective in modulating the CNS radiation syndrome [66]. Corresponding to the whole-animal protective phenomena, in-vivo cell survival curves have shown a DRF of 3.0 for bone marrow colony forming units (CFUs) and a DRF of 2.1 for intestinal crypt cell survival [67]. In contrast, a variety of hypoxic normal tissues show little or no protection when WR-2721 is added [61]. The DRF for hypoxic CFUs was reduced to 1.6 [58].

Though normal tissues are efficiently protected against radiation damage, WR-2721 has little effect on tumors in the same animals which show DRF's of 1.0 to 1.2 [58, 59, 61, 67, 68]. For example, 400 mg/Kg WR-2721 protected RFM mice against pulmonary radiation death with a DRF of 1.7 with no effect on the radiation response of urethan-induced pulmonary adenomas [66]. This *selective normal tissue protection* seems to depend on the specific exclusion of drug from tumor tissue. However, quite apart from selectivity of drug distribution (which may not be reliable qualitatively for human cancer), WR-2721 provides a potential mode for abrogation of the oxygen effect. Since the drug protects only oxygenated cells and can reduce OER to approximately

1.0 [61], it eliminates the differential resistance of hypoxic tumor fractions and permits the use of large radiation doses to effectively destroy hypoxic cells.

Since WR–2721 is a poorly diffusible molecule that fails to penetrate tumors but protects normal tissues while Misonidazole, being freely diffusible, sensitizes hypoxic cells of tumors only, it is rational to attempt simultaneous (or sequential) administration of both. The use of both drugs simultaneously requires the achievement of a very fine balance in the concentrations and tissue distributions of each, since they may totally antagonize each other under some conditions. Misonidazole can completely reverse the ability of WR–2721 to radioprotect hematopoietic tissues [68]. Similarly, both the radio-sensitization and cytotoxicity of hypoxic cells due to Misonidazole can be prevented by appropriate concentrations of sulfhydryl protectants [62]. However, careful control of Misonidazole and WR–2721 dosage has achieved very substantial therapeutic gain in some mouse tumors, far greater than observed when using either agent alone [68]. The simultaneous use of these agents does not seem to be a realistic clinical goal for the immediate future, but their sequential use is anticipated in the near future.

3.5. Unconventional Fractionation Schedules

Emerging in a rather empirical fashion as most approaches in oncology and allowed to mature after interplay with a scientific rationale, unconventional fractionation schedules have been steadily added to the radiation oncology armamentarium. In this section, by 'conventional' fractionation schedules, is implied the continuous delivery of radiation treatments with a single daily dose of 150–200 rad, given 5–6 times per week, until the total intended tumor dose is reached. Any planned major deviation from this normal practice can be regarded as an 'unconventional' radiation therapy schedule. There are basically three main unconventional types of fractionation approaches: the *Split-Course* schedules employing one equal single daily dose of 200–400 rad, 5–6 times per week, until half of the total intended tumor dose is reached and after a rest period of 2–4 weeks the whole treatment cycle is repeated until the total tumor dose is delivered; the *Uneven Fractionation* schedules employing different single daily radiation doses, which usually include one large weekly fraction of 400–600 rad with or without smaller doses on subsequent days, in a continuous or interrupted fashion; and the *Super or Hyperfractionation* schedules delivering more than one daily fraction continuously or interruptedly until the intended total dose has been delivered.

3.5.1. Split-Course Schedules

A practical need to interrupt or accelerate treatment in some patients who were either too ill to continue their conventional radiation therapy or had to travel large distances to receive daily and prolonged radiation treatments, gave rise to the split-course therapy schedules. It was observed from the very early experience that patients whose therapy had to be temporarily interrupted, exhibited a better tolerance to the radiation program and attained similar treatment results as did patients who were able to receive continuous conventional radiation schedules [8]. Since then, the use of split-course therapy has expanded and several variations have been added to this therapeutic concept. Presently, split-course schedules are the most commonly utilized unconventional radiation therapy schedules. This therapeutic strategy has been employed for a variety of tumors and in particular, it has been widely used in the treatment of lung cancer.

One of the advantages of split-course radiation therapy is its potential to achieve a higher therapeutic ratio than continuous schedules delivering similar total doses. This is possible by: an increase in the fractional dose, a reduction in the total number of fractions, and using a rest period which allows for a better normal tissue repair and tumor reoxygenation. One of the few ways available to radiation oncologists to analyze and compare various treatment schedules delivering different fractional and total doses is to utilize the Ellis' concept of the *Nominal Standard Dose (NSD)* [69]. NSD doses are expressed in *ret* and result from a mathematical computation which incorporates several important parameters: the total dose delivered in rad, the total number of radiation fractions employed, and the total time (in days) taken to deliver the radiation [70]. The NSD concept is indeed one of 'dose-time-relation'; in general, the higher the ret dose, the higher the biological dose. Although the NSD concept has not been universally accepted, and may not even be applicable to all circumstances (such as delivering more than one fraction per day, using one large single radiation dose and complex or prolonged treatment interruptions), it certainly represents one of several guiding parameters by which different treatment schedules could be quantitatively compared. Table 3 gives common fractionation schedules employed in lung cancer therapy and presents values in *rad* and *ret* as well as other parameters for conventional and unconventional radiation therapy schedules. It becomes evident that different treatment schedules delivering similar total doses in rad are *not,* in fact, biologically equivalent as represented in their different *ret* doses. These biologic dissimilarities exert profound influence not only on the tumor, but also on the normal tissue and thus affect the therapeutic ratio [7].

With rare exceptions, split-course radiation therapy for lung cancer has yielded equal results and better tolerance than continuous conventional irradiation. Scanlon first advocated split-course radiation therapy in 1960 [71], followed by Sambrook in 1964 [72]; both investigators noted that treatment tolerance improved with mandatory interruptions. In 1967, a randomized trial on 29 lung cancer patients was conducted to compare split-course with con-

Table 3. Fractionation schedules in lung cancer treatment.

Total dose (rad)	Daily fract (rad)	Total no. fract	Total no. days	Total NSD dose (ret)	* Comments; For split-course: fract. dose in rad × No. fract. (rest periods in weeks)
Continuous schedules					
2000	200	10	12	875	
2000	400	5	5	1127	
2500	250	10	12	1094	
3000	200	15	19	1133	
3000	300	10	12	1313	
4000	200	20	26	1360	
4500	180	25	22	1410	
5000	200	25	22	1570	
5500	200	28	38	1654	
6000	150	40	54	1585	
6000	200	30	40	1760	
Split-course					
3000	300	10	26	1281	$300 \times 5 \xrightarrow{(2)} 300 \times 5$
3600	600	6	34	1681	$600 \times 3 \xrightarrow{(4)} 600 \times 3$
4000	200	20	40	1319	$200 \times 10 \xrightarrow{(2)} 200 \times 10$
4000	400 → 250	13	31	1459	$400 \times 5 \xrightarrow{(2)} 250 \times 8$
4000	400	10	33	1623	$400 \times 5 \xrightarrow{(3)} 400 \times 5$
4000	400	10	33	1670	$400 \times 5 \xrightarrow{(2)} 400 \times 5$
4500	300	15	33	1646	$300 \times 10 \xrightarrow{(2)} 300 \times 10$
5000	250	20	40	1650	$250 \times 10 \xrightarrow{(2)} 250 \times 10$
6000	200	30	54	1729	$200 \times 15 \xrightarrow{(2)} 200 \times 15$
6000	300	20	40	1820	$300 \times 10 \xrightarrow{(2)} 300 \times 10$
7000	250 → 200	30	68	1994	$250 \times 10 \xrightarrow{(2)} 250 \times 10 \xrightarrow{(2)} 200 \times 10$
once-a- week					
3672	612	6	36	1615	
4020	670	6	36	1768	
4080	680	6	36	1795	
4305	615	7	43	1790	
5000	500	10	68	1826	
6000	500	12	89	3050	
6300	900 → 500*	12	89	2243	* 900 rad/wk × 2 wks $\xrightarrow{(1)}$ 500 rad/ wk × 9 wks.

Table 3. (Continuation)

Total dose (rad)	Daily fract (rad)	Total no. fract	Total no. days	Total NSD dose (ret)	* Comments; For split-course: fract. dose in rad × No. fract. (rest periods in weeks)
Two RX per wk.					
3600	600	6	18	1710	
4000	500	8	26	1711	
6000	500	12	40	2225	
Decrease dose schedules					
5000	1000 → 200*	14	33	2011	* 1000 rad (day 1 of 1st wk.); 700 rad (days 1 & 5 of 2nd wk); 300 rad (days 1-3-5 of 34d & 4th wk); and 200 rad (days 1 → 5 of 5th wk)
6000	600 → 120	26	36	1967	* 600 rad (day 1 of each wk for 6 wks); 120 rad (days 2 → 4 of each wk for 6 wks).

tinuous radiation therapy: the split-course consisted of 1800 rad in 3 fractions repeated after a 4 week rest period; the continuous therapy consisted of 6000 rad in 6–8 weeks [73]. The authors noted less pulmonary fibrosis and better treatment tolerance with the split-course, but there were no differences in symptomatic relief or survival rates between these two treatment schedules [73]. In 1969 another randomized trial was conducted in Europe in over 200 lung cancer patients: the split-course consisted of 3000 rad in 15 fractions repeated after a rest period of 2–3 weeks, and the continuous therapy consisted of 5500 rad in 5.5 weeks [74]. Although equal daily fractionation of 200 rad were used in both schedules, the rest period in the split-course led to milder treatment reactions and an apparent trend toward better survival and recurrence-free rates [74]. In 1970, Abramson and Cavanaugh reported on 82 patients with locally advanced lung cancer: half were treated with 6000 rad in 30 fractions of continuous radiotherapy, the other half received a short split-course which consisted of 5 fractions of 400 rad each and a rest period of 3 weeks followed by an identical course of irradiation [75]. These investigators were the first to report a significantly higher 1-year survival in patients treated with split-course (43%) than in patients treated continuously (14%). They extended their experience with this short-course split regime and later reported on 271 patients confirming their preliminary findings of an almost 40% 1-year survival which decreased to 7% in 44 patients who were available for a 4-year follow-up analysis [76]. The value of the split-course regime was therefore established.

From 1973 to the present time, newer split-course fractionation schedules have been explored. A randomized study on 74 lung cancer patients in 1973 compared the short split-course of Abramson and Cavanaugh to a new schedule that delivered 3000 rad in 10 fractions followed by a similar course after a 4 week rest period [77]. The median, one-year, and 18-month survival were found to be higher with the newer schedule, which in fact delivered a higher biological dose (Table 3). A different split-course schedule was reported in 1974 on 75 consecutive lung cancer patients employing 3000 rad in 10 fractions followed by a 2 week rest period and then 5 fractions of 300 rad each; the authors reported extremely high 1 and 2-year survival figures without observing serious complications other than transitory esophagitis [78]. In the same year, another report compared retrospectively 2 different split-course regimens: a short split-course for less advanced lung tumors which consisted of 5 treatments of 400 rad each followed by a two week rest period and 8 fractions of 250 rad and a longer split-course for more advanced lesions consisting of 10 treatments of 200 rad each repeated after a 2 week rest period [79]. The shorter split-course yielded better 1 and 2-year survival results than the longer course, but these results could have been influenced by the more advanced tumors treated by the latter. In 1976, the University of Rochester published its results on split-course radiation therapy for lung cancer: three different split-courses were retrospectively compared to several continuous courses of therapy and the results confirmed the experience of Abramson and Cavanaugh that a better treatment tolerance, but more importantly, improved survival results could be achieved by interrupted therapy schedules [8]. Unfortunately, 19 patients treated with the short split-course of Abramson and Cavanaugh (4000 rad) were analyzed together for survival results with 31 patients treated with a more protracted 5000 rad split-course schedule (delivering 10 fractions of 250 rad which was repeated after a 2-week rest period) and with a small group of 9 patients treated with the same 5000 rad split-course which was followed after another rest period of 2 weeks with a boost of 2000 rad in 10 fractions. When the three types of split courses were compared separately, it was found that the one delivering 5000 rad gave the highest rates of complete tumor resolution (35%) and the lowest incidence of fibrosis and pneumonitis; the high-dose split-course (7000 rad) yielded a higher incidence of complications with no improvements in the results over the other two split-course schedules; and the short-course (4000 rad) schedule yielded results which were similar to those previously reported by Abramson and Cavanaugh [8].

The convenience of using rest periods in the middle of concentrated radiation therapy courses arouse considerable interest to use this therapeutic approach with chemotherapy for small cell bronchogenic carcinoma (SCBC). Over 1000 patients with SCBC have been treated with combined modality approaches employing split-courses of irradiation [4, 5]. It is important to mention that, unfortunately, some of the split-courses employed for SCBC have delivered smaller biological doses than what has been estimated to be tumoricidal for this particular entity (≥ 1400 ret)[80].

The Radiation Therapy Oncology Group (RTOG) challenged the short split-course of Abramson and Cavanaugh against several courses of continuous therapy schedules (4000, 5000 and 6000 rad) in a randomized group-wide protocol for localized non-small cell bronchogenic carcinoma[81]. The outcome was disappointing since no major differences in survival were found among the different schedules and the 4000 rad split-course yielded the lowest percentage of complete responses and a high incidence of treatment-related complications[81]. However, the RTOG experience constitutes the only major setback for this particular split-course schedule and may be a reflection of many participating institutions using a technique which requires judicious implementation and protection of vital structures.

Recently, Holsti detailed long-term results from Helsinki with split-course irradiation [82]. The tumor doses employed in this randomized trial were 5000 rad in the continuously treated group and 5500 rad for the group receiving split-course therapy: no differences in absolute or disease-free survival were apparent between the two treatment regimens; no significant differences were found by all four major histologic types; in patients with localized disease, survival results were somewhat better in the split-course group for 6 months and a year, but not later; the continuously treated responders survived slightly better than the split-course responders. It became evident from this article that the results achievable with split-course therapy were similar to those with continuous treatment but the former yielded milder acute side effects and fibrosis than the latter.

One must conclude that there seems to be no major differences in survival when split-courses are compared to continuous therapy schedules although reactions to the radiation program seem somewhat lessened in the former. It must be emphasized that there are many split-course schedules which are in use and the biological dose delivered may vary considerably among them (Table 3). Failure to demonstrate superiority of *one* split-course schedule over continuous therapy regimens in *one* study does not constitute solid grounds to discard altogether this therapeutic approach.

There are certain advantages to both the patient and the therapist with the use of split-courses of irradiation: (1) higher biological doses which could have a more pronounced effect on the oxic tumor cells and allow for more reoxygenation of the hypoxic fraction as the primary tumor mass reduces in size; (2) rest periods which could convey a better reassessment of tumor resonse in mid-therapy allow, a better field reduction tailored to the response achieved, and allow more time for a proper reassessment of disease extent before further radiation is delivered to the patient; (3) a concentrated and mandatorily interrupted radiation therapy delivery which translates into a more convenient and economic approach for large patient loads; and (4) a convenient design which facilitates pulsing of cytotoxic agents in combined modality approaches.

However, there are some intrinsic problems with the use of split-course irradiation which really pivot around the protection of vital structures in the treatment field. Protection of the spinal cord is of paramount concern since radiation myelopathy is a delayed treatment complication[7]. It has been estimated that the tolerance dose of the spinal cord is around 1550 ret[83]. With continuous schedules delivering 200 rad per fraction, protection of this structure is recommended at 4500 rad. Nevertheless, most split-course schedules yield biological doses higher than 1550 ret which implies that spinal cord protection is mandatory early in the treatment plan; this also represents protecting disease in the mediastinum. Nevertheless, when a shrinking field technique is employed and careful treatment planning is performed for lung cancer patients, split-course schedules can be safely and conveniently employed yielding rewarding local results without severe morbidity.

3.5.2. Uneven Fractionation Schedules

The early German practice of radiation therapy consisted in actually delivering the whole tumor dose at one time[84]. After careful clinical observations, the French school began promoting daily radiation treatments since investigators felt that better results were being obtained when the total dose was fractionated many times over several weeks[84]. Fractionation schedules using 2 or 3 fractions per week were used for technical convenience during radiotherapy under hyperbaric oxygen. Attempts to reduce even more the number of treatments given has been tried for patient convenience and hoping to reduce excessive work loads on radiation centers. This took a more important overtone with the advent of radiosensitizers since in order to obtain maximum advantage of their effect and reduce the toxicity associated with their administration, fewer number of radiation fractions delivering higher doses constitute an appealing approach. This treatment strategy has important radiobiological connotations and ways to intensify the degree of reoxygenation by varying the fraction size and the faction intervals have been presented by Elkind et al. [85].

Most of the experience with uneven fractionation schedules of radiation therapy for lung cancer has emerged from countries other than the United States. Three main categories of uneven fractionation schedules can be distinguished: schedules using once-a-week treatments, schedules using 2–3 treatments per week, and schedules using decreasing individual doses.

3.5.2.1. Once-A-Week Treatment

The practice of radiation therapy in many countries often faces severe shortage of trained personnel, standard equipment, sophisticated machines and economic resources to confront excessive loads of cancer patients. In one part of Colombia, South America, where there was one Cobalt unit for nearly 3 million people, employing a single dose of 500 rad once a week for a total dose of 5000 rad (1826 ret) made it possible to treat many patients who otherwise would have gone untreated [86]. An identical approach was used in the 1950's for cancer patients from outlying Ohio farms who could not come or could not be brought for radiotherapy often [84]. In a cancer hospital in India, in order to cope with the work load using continuous conventional fractionation regimes, its only Cobalt unit had to be used around the clock. As a consequence, six fractions of 670 rad each were delivered at weekly intervals (1768 ret) for patients with a variety of epithelial tumors yielding good tolerance and ⊥atisfactory treatment responses [87]. These investigators then proceeded to challenge this unconventional approach against continuous fractionation schedules in a prospective randomized study; they found comparable treatment results but a better tolerance by the patients receiving the weekly fractionation schedule [87]. After a retrospective analysis of their experience, Greenberg *et al.* gathered 17 patients who were treated with one weekly fraction of 612–680 rad repeated for 6 weeks (1615–1795 ret) and concluded that local tumor control and normal tissue reactions in these patients were comparable to those with conventional fractionation [88].

Realizing that one treatment per week constitutes one of the most convenient schedules for many cancer patients who do not require hospitalization and/or who live a great distance, Ellis *et al.* explored this approach for 35 advanced cancer patients at Memorial Hospital in New York City [84]. These investigators employed 7 fractions of 615 rad delivered at weekly intervals (1780 ret). Among their reported cases were some lung cancer patients and their results corroborated previous experiences with this approach. Perhaps the most solid experience with this technique comes from Berlin (Germany) where Schumacher attempted to improve local control and survival in bronchogenic carcinoma using high dose fractions of radiation delivered at weekly intervals with a 35 MeV betatron [89]. Schumacher found that large, single fractions of 500 rad delivered weekly over 12 weeks (2050 ret) appeared to improve survival. More than 1000 lung cancer patients were treated: Over 50% were squamous cell carcinomas, 18% small cell and 15% large cell and adenocarcinomas. Schumacher reported survival figures of 63%, 29%, 16%, 9% and 8.1% at one to five years [89]. His experience constituted the basis for a protocol by the Lung Working Party which actually was never completed. Nevertheless, the Berlin experience indicated that this approach had acceptable toxicity and responses were apparently at least as good as with conventional fractionation schedules.

Ellis has mentioned that a small number of large-dose fractions, delivering similar NSD ret doses as curative conventional fractionation regimes, convey the same cell-killing effect on cells with low extrapolation number (such as the normal connective tissue) and a greater cell-killing effect on cells with high extrapolation number (such as those of the more radioresistant tumors)[90]. Slow-dividing malignant cells which die as a result of radiation damage in subsequent mitosis require considerable damage and time before significant amounts of cell lysis and reoxygenation occur[90]. Since a substantial tumor cell-killing seems to be a prerequisite towards obtaining a better degree of oxygenation and therefore radiosensitivity, the use of large single doses at weekly intervals constitute a sound radiobiological approach to the problem of hypoxia. On the other hand, a better normal tissue tolerance may be expected from this approach since more time is allowed between fractions to maximize repair of sublethal radiation damage in normal tissues. In fact, Ellis mentions in his review of the subject that reactions to this unorthodox therapeutic approach seem to be equal or even less than to conventional fractionation schedules[84].

3.5.2.2. Two or Three Treatments per Week

A technical convenience to employ fewer radiation treatments per week with hyperbaric oxygen therapy propulsed exploration of unconventional fractionation schedules[91]. Their scientific and practical rationale is identical to the one previously discussed for treating patients only once a week. The use of 2–3 fractions of radiation per week has been tested in head and neck tumors, breast cancer and gynecologic malignancies[84], but little experience has been reported for lung cancer.

Abe et al. from Kyoto, Japan treated 24 locally advanced, unresectable lung cancer patients with two fractions of 500 rad per week for 4–6 weeks (total doses of 4000–6000 rad, 1711–2225 ret)[41]. As a control, the authors used their retrospecive experience with conventional fractionation in over 200 equally advanced lung cancer patients. The survival results were 38% and 28% at one year and 13% and 12% at two years for the shorter and the conventional fractionation schedule respectively[41]. Unfortunately, local tumor control or treatment reactions was not mentioned in their report. Perhaps the most solid available information comes from the hyperbaric oxygen trial for lung cancer patients at Portsmouth, England[36]. In this trial, some of the control patients received treatment only twice per week. Of 135 lung cancer control patients treated in air, two-thirds of whom had squamous cell carcinoma, 96 patients were treated with 600 rad fractions twice per week for three weeks (total dose of 3600 rad or 1710 ret); the remaining 39 patients were treated with a continuous conventional fractionation schedule employing 150 rad fractions over 8 weeks (total dose of 6000 rad or 1585 ret). It must be emphasized that this was not a prospective comparison of fractionation schedules nor constituted the main purpose of that particular study; nevertheless, there were no significant differences in survival for both groups, and again, no mention was made in this report on local tumor control or treatment-related complications [36]. With the need to use fewer radiation treatments for the new radiosensitizing compounds, the Radiation Therapy Oncology Group (RTOG) adopted the Portsmouth schedule of treating twice per week with fractions of 600 rad for a total dose of 3600 rad when it launched a Phase I–II protocol with Misonidazole for locally advanced lung cancer [54]. This RTOG study has recently closed and results are not yet available.

3.5.2.3. Decreasing Dose Schedules

The increasingly closer relation and interaction between radiation oncologists and radiation biologists has stimulated the development of uneven fractionation schemes based not on empiricism or convenience, but actually on sound scientific laboratory experience. As was mentioned earlier, a significant amount of cell-killing might be required before sufficient tumor cell lysis and reoxygenation occur. This suggested that using large radiation fractions might be best to destroy most of the oxic tumor population, spacing these fractions long enough to allow tumor reoxygenation and normal tissue repair. Nevertheless, the hypoxic tumor fraction will remain constant (despite apparent rapid reoxygenation) until the tumor begins macroscopic regression. Spacing large radiation fractions 4 or more cell-cycle times away could delay this process by allowing for some tumor *repopulation*. One way to obtain ineffective contributions from repopulation would be to use shorter intervals between large fractions. This led to the use of decreasing dose schedules of radiation therapy. This approach is in fact not new, but a revival of an old concept mentioned by Pfahler in 1926 termed 'a saturation method' of delivering treatment, and consisted in giving maximum radiation in the shortest period of time with a large dose and continuing this maximum effect with smaller doses thereafter [92]. Two groups have used decreasing-dose schedules recently and deserve mentioning in this section.

The group from Helsinki, Finland used radiotherapy with decreasing individual tumor doses in the treatment of 25 patients with primary lung carcinomas or lung metastases [93]. This was actually the clinical implementation of a research schedule proposed by Elkind [85]. A single fraction of 1000 rad was given on Monday of the first week, 700 rad and 500 rad on Monday and Friday of the second week, three fractions of 300 rad each given weekly for the next two weeks, and finally, 5 fractions of 200 rad were given daily during the fifth week [93]. The total tumor dose was 5000 rad delivered in 14 fractions over 33 days (2011 ret). Eight other patients received 5000 rad in 5 weeks of conventional daily radiotherapy (1570 ret); they served as the control group. The authors quantitated tumor regressions and plotted these against time to obtain regression slopes. Interestingly, in both the unconventional fractionation schedule (UFS) and the conventional one (CFS), two types of curves were identified: one corresponding to well-responding or rapidly regressing tumors and another with a flatter slope belonging to poorly-responding or slowly shrinking neoplasms [93]. A number of important observations were made: the UFS achieved 50% higher number of rapid regressions; responses in the UFS began to occur immediately after the first dose fraction while in the CFS shrinkage started 2–4 weeks after the first fraction; most of the tumor responses in the UFS were complete; the regression slope of the poorly responding tumor to UFS was similar to the regression slope of the well responding tumors to CFS; the incidence of pulmonary fibrosis was milder in the CFS; the average time for the appearance of fibrosis was 4.5 and 3.5 months for the UFS and CFS respectively. Since the total dose and overall time was the same for both the UFS and the CFS, the fraction size and the actual fewer fractions of the UFS appeared to have been responsible for the larger biologic effect. The authors are now trying to reduce the initial large dose in an attempt to ameliorate somewhat the degree of resultant fibrosis. Nevertheless, these investigators are convinced that the first dose has to be large enough to cause sufficient tumor damage to initiate shrinkage, so that succeeding doses have reoxygenated cells to work on.

The group from Kyoto, Japan approached the problem of tumor repopulation from a different angle: these investigators believed that large doses are required to destroy most of the oxic tumor cells, but also thought that a series of small-dose fractions may be required between large-dose fractions to inflict damage on the remaining anoxic tumor cells [41]. They postulated that during this series of small-dose fractions, the anoxic tumor cells could accumulate the radiation damage without recovery and repopulation, while the normal tissues could be spared because of their capacity to repair and recover from the radiation damage in the presence of oxygen. When vascularization conditions improved and reoxygenation of hypoxic tumor cells became possible, irradiating once again with a large-dose fraction followed by a series of smaller-dose fractions appeared to be a logical treatment approach. Subsequently, this hypothesis was tested in 52 locally advanced lung cancer patients treated with 6 fractions of 600 rad given the first day of each consecutive week followed by 4 small fractions of 120 rad during the remaining 4 days of each week for 5 weeks [41]. The total dose was 6000 rad delivered in 26 radiation fractions over 36 days (1967 ret). Their results yielded a 37% 1-year survival and a 30% 2-year survival which was better than their retrospective series of patients treated with conventional radiation which yielded a 1-year survival of 28% and a 2-year survival of 12% [41]. In a recent update of their experience, it was mentioned that with their uneven fractionation schedule there was a slightly higher incidence of pulmonary fibrosis which was more pronounced and had a shorter onset (around 4.5 months) than in patients who received conventional treatment [94]. This group of investigators have been encouraged by their preliminary results and continue to explore this innovative treatment approach.

3.5.3. Super or Hyperfractionation Schedules

The use of 2 or more daily fractions of radiation is not new for radiation oncologists. This approach has been termed 'superfractionated or hyperfractionated' irradiation. It poses certain impracticalities for outpatients or departments treating heavy patient loads since one patient is brought to the treatment unit several times in one day. The ultimate superfractionated regime consists in the continuous administration of low-dose radiotherapy for several hours as advocated by Pierquin [56]. Little has been done with this superfractioned regimens for lung cancer patients. One of the best known experiences was that of the National Cancer Institute – Radiation Oncology Division using superfractionation schedules in conjunction with intensive chemotherapy for small cell bronchogenic carcinoma; the effort yielded unacceptable high treatment related complications [95].

The advent of radiosensitizers may popularize using 2 or more daily radiation fractions per day to take advantage of high blood concentration of these agents which may persist for several hours. The new experimental intravenous administration of Misonidazole could lead to the continuous administration of this agent while continuous low-dose rate irradiation is delivered to patients. Further discussion of this therapeutic approach in this chapter would be futuristic and highly speculative.

3.6. Hemibody (Half-Body) Irradiation (HBI)

The HBI technique developed empirically to meet the need of treating patients with advanced cancer in multiple sites confined to one half of the body. It provided an appealing convenience to both patients and physicians to encompass most of the lesions in a relatively short period to time. The sequential irradiation of both halves of the body represented an attempt to employ radiation as a systemic agent; consequently, this therapeutic technique has been called 'Systemic Irradiation' [96].

Total body irradiation (TBI) is the best known form of systemic irradiation and was first used in the treatment of disseminated cancer over half a century ago [97]. TBI has been used in a number of hematologic malignancies (chronic lymphocytic leukemia, acute myelocytic leukemia, lymphomas, lymphosarcoma, and multiple myeloma) because of their known radiosensitivity [96].

Recently, TBI was used as an adjuvant in management of patients with Ewing's sarcoma because of the high incidence of distant metastases in these patients after local RT [98]. In the majority of instances when TBI has been used, the maximum doses that could be given to patients never exceeded 300 rad in a single or fractionated doses. Severe bone marrow depression constituted the major dose-limiting toxicity. A significant contribution in this respect has been achieved by radiation oncologists at the Princess Margaret Hospital in Toronto who, for the last 18 years, have been using the hemibody irradiation technique [99]. When using HBI, these investigators were able to use higher single doses (600, 800, and 1000 rad) delivered sequentially to both halves of the body [100]. Severe bone marrow depression was no longer observed and radiation pneumonopathy became the major dose-limiting toxicity. Reasons why the bone marrow was able to tolerate higher doses with sequential HBI applications than with TBI have to be sought in the kinetics and radiobiology of this important dose-limiting organ:

3.6.1. Bone Marrow Kinetics and Radiobiology

Radiation effects on bone marrow are critically dependent on: (1) the proportion of total marrow exposed and (2) the radiation dose. Exposure of the entire human marrow has a low LD 50/30 (lethal dose achieving 50% mortality within 30 days) of approximately 500 rad. Shielding of even relatively small portions of the bone marrow organ has a dramatic protective effect against hematologic death and marrow failure is no longer the dose-limiting event in large segment irradiation. Active marrow in the adult has a dominantly axial distribution: skull 13%; upper limb girdle 8%; sternum and ribs 10.5%; cervical vertebrae 3.5%; thoracic vertebrae 14%; lumbar vertebrae 11%; sacrum 14%; and pelvic girdle 26% [9]. A typical upper hemibody field encompasses about 55% of active marrow leaving close to half of the whole marrow organ as a reserve.

The dose necessary to render an irradiated segment of marrow permanently aplastic has not been accurately defined, but fractionated doses of about 4000 rad are associated with in-field regeneration though at delayed times of 1–5 years [101, 102]. Single doses in the range of 500–1000 rad would not be expected to permanently depopulate and fibrose marrow spaces. Indeed, clinical [103] and experimental [101, 104] studies have shown rapid local regeneration of irradiated marrow segments following single doses up to 1000 rad. The mechanism for this recovery very probably involves several processes: (1) the proliferation of surviving local stem cells; (2) the migration of circulating stem cells from unirradiated segments; and (3) the heterotopic conversion of local radioresistant uncommitted mesenchymal stem cells [101]. Irradiated marrow of rabbits given 1000 rad hemibody irradiation shows a profound depletion of committed stem cells (CFU$_c$) one week following treatment, with a return to normal at 4 weeks[101]. This rapid repopulation may depend on colony stimulating activity (CSA) perhaps generated by peripheral leukopenia or monocytosis. In addition to rapid proliferation of surviving stem cells, migration of uncommitted stem cells (CFUs) from irradiated segments may be important and CFUs are present in peripheral blood and do increase following radiation[105]. Finally, marrow behaves as a functional unit and depletion in one area is sensed by other areas which respond by compensatory hyperplasia to blunt the expected peripheral depletion[101, 106]. These mechanisms account for the hematologic safety of hemibody irradiation.

In almost 400 patients with advanced, progressive and symptomatic cancer, Fitzpatrick and Rider found that the use of higher single doses of HBI were capable of achieving dramatic relief of cancer pain, often within 24 hours after the procedure[99, 100]. In this early experience of Toronto, systemic HBI was utilized primarily in terminally-ill patients after all other therapeutic modalities had failed. Survival time varied from a few weeks to a few months; this often prevented assessment of the objective tumoricidal effect of the technique. A later high-risk Phase I–II pilot study conducted at the University of Rochester Cancer Center for the Radiation Therapy Oncology Group (RTOG) using HBI in advanced cancer patients[96] and subsequent analysis of the Toronto data[107] yielded the needed response-toxicity information with the use of this technique.

3.6.2. HBI: Tumor Responses

Treatment responses with HBI in advanced cancer patients have yielded important information. If the relief of pain from metastatic disease is utilized as a criterion of *subjective tumor responses,* this therapeutic technique has proven to be a very effective one since over 80% of all patients achieve relief of their cancer pain[96, 99, 100]. Moreover, the pain relief is dramatic, often complete, and occurs within the first 48 hours in more than 70% of the patients[96, 99, 100]. In those terminally ill cancer patients (many of whom had lung tumors) who survived HBI for more than two months, *objective tumor responses,* most of which were partial, occurred in nearly 80% of the instances[1, 4, 5]. Moreover, the search for *pathologic tumor responses* in autopsied HBI patients demonstrated marked radiation damage of tumor cells located within the treatment field[96].

Nevertheless, despite documentation of a tumoricidal effect with single large doses of HBI on bulky metastatic disease, only *short-lived responses* (median of 12 weeks) could be demonstrated. This was a clear indication that a *limited cell kill* could only be achieved by the use of this technique[96]. Overt disease implies tumor collections of 10^9 to 10^{12} cells since clinical metastases need to be of at least 2 cm to be detectable (10^9 cells) and life is probably incompatible with tumor burdens greater than 10^{12} cells. Based on this, the early HBI experience in advanced metastatic patients lent itself to speculative thoughts that single doses of 600–1000 rad accomplished less than 4 logs of cell kill since most of the observed tumor responses were partial [96]. Experimental systems in the laboratory indicated that such doses delivered with orthovoltage equipment (250 KVP) were capable of achieving only 1–3 logs of cell kill [23]. Later clinical studies with HBI in NSCBC patients corroborated these early observations and established that *a single dose of 800 rad was as effective as 1500 rad of conventional continuous irradiation* [6]. It became evident that *if HBI is to be used with other than a palliative intent, supplementary local RT booster doses were needed.*

Since the early HBI experience in advanced cancer patients demonstrated that the technique could reduce massive tumor growths, alleviate related cancer pain, and show pathologic evidence of tumor cell destruction, it was reasonable to expect that this modality could be used more effectively in less advanced cancer patients with tumors characterized by a high tendency to disseminate. Lung cancer management became the most promising testing grounds because of the overall poor survival results so far achieved for bronchogenic carcinoma. Consequently, a research logic was conceived and put into effect for the use of HBI in patients with lung cancer and other tumors [96, 108].

3.6.3. The Delivery of HBI

Irradiation of large sections of human anatomy is a relatively simple procedure. All that is needed are: (1) a megavoltage photon or a high-energy electron unit (preferably with adjustable dose-rate) and (2) a well-shielded treatment room that would allow for sufficient treatment distances (≥ 180 cms) to encompass the desired target volume. The patient (who lies on the floor, inches from the floor on a small couch, or against the wall) is irradiated with anterior-posterior (parallel-opposed) field arrangements aimed at the target volume; irradiation is usually given with dose-rates of 35–55 rad/minute until the prescribed dose is reached.

Essentially, there are three basic field arrangements for HBI (Fig. 10): (1) *Upper Half-Body Irradiation (UHBI):* This is irradiation from the top of the iliac crest (bottom of the 4th lumbar vertebrae (L-4) or usually the umbilicus) all the way up including the skull. Included in this field arrangement are: the brain, lungs, heart, liver, adrenal, kidneys, pancreas, stomach, intestines, 55% of th adult bone marrow, plus corresponding bones and lymph nodes; (2) *Lower Half-Body Irradiation (LHBI):* This is irradiating from the top of the iliac crest to the ankle level. Included in this field arrangement are: the pelvic organs, 45% of the adult bone marrow, plus corresponding bones and lymph nodes; and (3) *Mid-Body Irradiation (MBI):* This is basically irradiating the entire abdominal cavity from the top of the diaphragm to the bottom of the

Half-body Irradiation

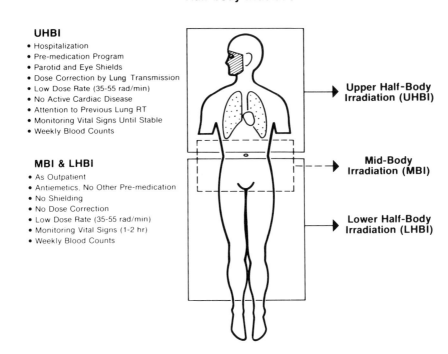

UHBI
- Hospitalization
- Pre-medication Program
- Parotid and Eye Shields
- Dose Correction by Lung Transmission
- Low Dose Rate (35-55 rad/min)
- No Active Cardiac Disease
- Attention to Previous Lung RT
- Monitoring Vital Signs Until Stable
- Weekly Blood Counts

MBI & LHBI
- As Outpatient
- Antiemetics. No Other Pre-medication
- No Shielding
- No Dose Correction
- Low Dose Rate (35-55 rad/min)
- Monitoring Vital Signs (1-2 hr)
- Weekly Blood Counts

Upper Half-Body
Irradiation (UHBI)

Mid-Body
Irradiation (MBI)

Lower Half-Body
Irradiation (LHBI)

Fig. 10. The *Half-Body Irradiation Program*. On the right, the three different field arrangements with the HBI technique. On the left precautions and corrections with HBI delivery. The *premedication program with UHBI* consists of: (1) Prednisone, 10 mg P.O. q.i.d. (24 hours before); (2) nothing per mouth (6 hours before); (3) Prochlorperazine (Compazine) 10 mg P.O. (4 hours before); (4) 1000 cc 5% Dextrose in 0.5 normal saline solution with 20 meq. KCL., I.V. (Started 2 hours before and set to run in 4 hours); (5) Prochlorperazine 10 mg I.M. (1 hour before); 100 mg of Hydrocortisone Sodium Succinate (Solu-Cortef) in 100 cc of IV fluid by Soluset (to run 30 min. before UHBI). UHBI requires hospitalization with close monitoring of vital signs every 30 minutes until stable after delivery of irradiation. MBI and LHBI do not require hospitalization and can be performed on outpatients as long as they can be observed for 1–2 hours after irradiation for monitoring of vital signs. UHBI and LHBI can be applied sequentially after bone marrow revovery. MBI should not be used prior or subsequent to UHBI or LHBI.

obturator foramina. Included in this field arrangement are: the entire abdominal organs, 60% of the adult bone marrow, plus corresponding bones and lymph nodes.

3.6.4. HBI: Toxicity and Corrections

The principal toxicity and main limitation of HBI is radiation pneumonopathy. For reasons mentioned earlier, irradiation of one half of the body with single doses ≤1000 rad is hematologically a relatively safe procedure which allows subsequent treatment of the other half of the body once bone marrow recovery has occurred. Other acute toxic reactions previously seen with the HBI have now been reduced to a minimum after several corrective measures are applied. A discussion of the toxic effects of HBI and corrective measures currently in use has been published [96]. A brief overview on the subject follows and has been summarized in Fig. 10.

The *'Acute Radiation Syndrome'*: It became evident from the early experience that the principal toxic manifestations with HBI mainly occurred when the upper half of the body was irradiated. An 'acute radiation syndrome' developed shortly after UHBI and subsided within 4–10 hours; it consisted of intractable nausea and vomiting, increases in basal temperatures and pulse rate, tremors, shaking chills, and a concomitant drop in blood pressure [96]. As a result of these acute symptoms, two early fatalities occurred in elderly cardiac patients due to hypotension leading to hypovolemia and decreased coronary perfusion, consequently, UHBI was no longer recommended for patients older than 75 years or with active cardiac disease. Nevertheless, the 'acute radiation syndrome' was severe enough in other patients that corrective measures were needed. The syndrome was not of a central origin since it persisted in patients in whom brain irradiation was purposely deleted from the UHBI field. Actually, the syndrome resembled the 'stress reaction syndrome' from a lack of adrenal reserve and based on the type of symptoms observed in the first irradiated patients, a comprehensive premedication program under close observation of the patients was initiated [96]. Ths premedication program is outlined in Fig. 10; it consisted of hydration, antiemetics, oral as well as intravenous cortisone administration, and hospitalization prior to UHBI. The premedication program has been tested in more than 100 consecutive patients; it has minimized the acute toxicity of UHBI to only scanty episodes of nausea and an average of 1.35 episodes of vomiting per patient.

The *'Dry-mouth Syndrome'*: This interesting syndrome was identified with the early UHBI clinical experience: it was characterized by a dry-mouth, pasty saliva and a 'metalic' taste of food. It occurred in 1–2 weeks after UHBI and in many patients, most of whom were chronically debilitated by illness, led to a decrease in appetite and severe weight loss. It was felt that this was a direct radiation effect on the major salivary glands and taste buds; it has been totally minimized by adding a protective lead shield to encompass the mouth and parotid glands. When UHBI began to be used in less advanced patients, the shield was extended to cover the eyes but care was taken not to protect the brain or upper cervical nodes (Fig. 10).

Other subacute toxicity seen with UHBI include: *partial (transitory) alopecia* with hair falling 2–3 weeks after the procedure and regrowing in 2–4 months; one intance of acute mastitis in a pre-menopausal female occurring one day

Hematologic Toxicity of Half-Body Irradiation

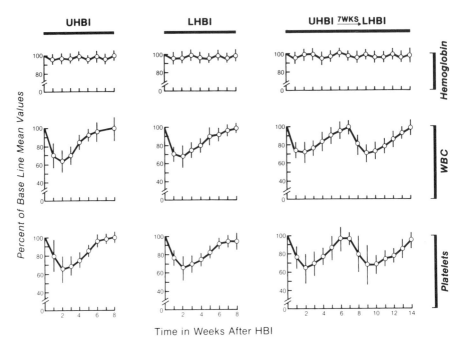

Time in Weeks After HBI

Fig. 11. *Hematologic Toxicity of Half-Body Irradiation (HBI):* The separate effects on peripheral counts by upper half-body irradiation (UHBI) and lower half-body irradiation (LHBI) are presented in the first two diagrams. The sequential application of UHBI and LHBI separated by a rest period of 7 weeks is presented in the third diagram. This represents the experience of the University of Rochester in over 200 HBI applications on cancer patients. Hematologically, HBI is a safe technique. All counts are expressed as percentage of baseline counts prior to HBI. The hemoglobin (Hg) is unaffected; white blood cell (WBC) and platelet counts are depressed with nadir counts at 1–2 weeks with subsequent recovery in 4–6 weeks.

after UHBI and totally subsiding in one week; and complaints of 'weakness' and 'tiredness' 1–2 weeks after the procedure which was in fact related to a transitory bone marrow depression.

The *Hematologic Toxicity:* Hematologically HBI is a safe technique. Peripheral blood counts are depressed with a nadir at 1–2 weeks after the procedure and total recovery to pre-irradiation levels occurs in 4–6 weeks (Fig. 11). This allowed for the sequential irradiation of the contralateral half of the body [6, 96] and the safe administration of UHBI after induction chemotherapy with subsequent allowance of maintenance CT in SCBC [109].

The *Pulmonary Toxicity:* The pulmonary toxicity with UHBI constitutes the main limitation of the technique. It consists of an acute radiation pneumonitis occurring 2–4 months after the procedure which is almost invariably, irreversible and fulminating. On chest X-rays, this pneumonitis appears as a diffuse bilateral infiltrate throughout the lungs and consequently does not resemble the classic picture of pneumonitis following fibrosis within the confines of a local chest RT field. The Toronto experience indicated that *there is a very sharp threshold dose for the production of fatal radiation pneumonitis with UHBI* [107]. The latest update of the Toronto data yields an incidence of 2%, 12.5%, 19% and 52% with less than 600 rad, 600 rad, 800 rad and 1000 rad doses of UHBI respectively [107]. The early experience of the University of Rochester indicated a 15% incidence of fatal radiation pneumonitis with a single dose of 800 rad of UHBI [96]. The explanation and the actual incidence of this complication had to be searched in the radiation biophysics of normal lung tissue. After subsequent corrections for an increase of dose transmission in air, the incidence of this complication has been reduced to acceptable levels.

3.6.5. Radiation Pathology and Biophysics of the Normal Lung Tissue

There has been recent efforts to qualitate and quantitate radiation effects on pathologic and normal lung tissues after fractionated RT schedules or single doses of UHBI [110, 111]. The procedure is complex but mainly consists of: (1) removal of the lungs *en bloc* at autopsy; (2) re-inflation of the lungs in formaline; (3) slicing the lungs in thin (0.5 cm) sections; (4) fixation and staining of these sections; (5) superimposing the patient's 3-dimensional computerized dosimetry plans over the stained sections; (6) identification of the dose delivered to several points in each specific section; (7) ultrastructural analysis of these points to quantitate thickness of the alveolar walls and increased cellularity of the normal lung tissues. A dose-dependent increase in alveolar wall thickness and cellularity was found [110]; this corroborated previous dose-dependent increase in pulmonary fibrosis after RT [7]. Recently, elegant laboratory investigations have served to identify *the lesion of radiation pneumonitis* as being *a direct radiation damage on the type II pneumocyte cells of the alveoli which are responsible for the production of surfactant* [112]. The decreased production of surfactant (a phospholipid which coats, soothes and reduces tension of the alveolar walls) by these damaged cells, leads to the increased thickness and acute inflammatory reaction of the alveolar septae characteristic of radiation pneumonitis; then a subsequent loss of tension and of expansion in the alveolar septae supervenes, culminating in a type of alveolar-capillary block which is reminiscent of the respiratory distress syndrome seen in infants.

Previous clinical experience with several doses of continuous and split-course RT schedules for lung cancer patients served to identify a proportional increase of radiation fibrosis with an increase in the total dose and a sharp threshold dose for radiation pneumonitis occurring around 1600 ret [7]. These observations were made in fractionated radiation dose-schedules and would not predict for single-dose schedules such as that of UHBI. Nevertheless, a series of laboratory experiments carried out in dogs with UHBI at the University of Rochester delivered single (mid-air) doses of 970 rad, 1215 rad, 1750 rad and 2125 rad with a 1000 KVP X-ray unit [113–115]. It was found that pulmonary manifestations did not occur with single doses less than 1200 rad and were only 25% with 1750 rad [115]. All evidence seemed to indicate that delivery of single doses of 600 rad to 1000 rad to the upper-half of the body should not have resulted in significant pulmonary toxicity. This in fact was not the case with human subjects [107] and the subtle differences in incidence of pulmonary complications between Toronto [107] and Rochester [96] led to a search for suitable explanations.

It was thought that the dose-rate had some influence since the Toronto group delivered UHBI at 100 rad/minute and the Rochester group at 35–55 rad/minute. Nevertheless, the total dose was the same and the higher dose-rate probably had no other influence than to accentuate the 'acute radiation syndrome.' The only other difference between both groups was the energy source employed: in Toronto a Co-60 unit was used, in Rochester a 10 MeV linear accelerator was employed. A well-known radiation physics concept was invoked: the lungs, being filled with air, demonstrate *an increased transmission of the radiation dose as it traverses the lungs due to their relative less denseness when compared to other tissues and this increase in dose within the lungs is energy and thickness dependent.* Detailed radiation physics investigations conducted at the University of Rochester served to establish a series of dosage correction factors resulting from increased lung transmission [116]. Based on these experiments, percentages of dose increase in the lungs as a result of increase transmission were estimated for large fields irradiated with different energies and transversing several lung tissue thicknesses [116]. An abbreviated version appears in Table 4 where it can be appreciated that delivery of a single dose of 800 rad (calculated at mid-field of UHBI) given to an emphysematous patient with a lung thickness of 20 cm could represent an actual increase of 15% (920 rad) if a Cobalt-60 unit was employed and of 7% (856 rad) if a 10 MeV photon unit was used. This would explain some of the differences in pneumonitis incidence between Toronto and Rochester. As a result, all UHBI doses began to be corrected for lung transmission in order to establish comparative data. When these corrections were made, the incidence of fatal pneumonitis with 800 rad UHBI was 9% [6] and with 600 rad was 0% [109]; this brought the level of toxicity into more acceptable grounds and certainly comparable to the toxicity of some intensive chemotherapeutic approaches for SCBC [4]. Nevertheless, realizing that very subtle differences in dose could trigger this fatal complication, smaller (corrected) doses of UHBI

Table 4. Absorbed dosage in lung as a result of increase lung transmission of X and γ irradiation*.

Energy (MeV)	A-P lung thickness (cm)	% increase in dose mid-lung
Co^{60}	10	3
	15	8
	20	15
Co^4	10	3
	15	8
	20	14
Co^6	10	2
	15	7
	20	10
Co^8	10	1
	15	5
	20	8
Co^{10}	10	"0"
	15	2
	20	7

* From reference (116).

(700 rad) were recommended for primary therapy and even smaller doses of 600 rad when the technique was going to be used for consolidation after a primary treatment had been given.

3.6.6. The Use of HBI in NSCBC

A series of high-risk pilot studies exploring HBI for the treatment of micrometastases were conducted for the Eastern Cooperative Oncology Group (ECOG) in locally advanced, unresectable, non-metastatic, non-small cell bronchogenic carcinoma (NSCBC)[6]. Twenty of such patients were treated with local (split-course) chest irradiation (LCI) plus TBI (UHBI followed by LHBI); thirty equally advanced, non-metastatic patients who were treated with only localized split-course chest irradiation were matched and served as a retrospective control group. The first 11 patients received LCI followed by HBI protecting the previously irradiated local chest fields (Pilot Study No. 1), but 5 patients (45%) had evidence of distant metastases before UHBI could be delivered. This was not different from the control group where 11 patients (37%) had evidence of distant dissemination in less than 2.5 months from the onset of local treatment. Trying to overcome this pattern of early metastases, in the remaining 9 patients UHBI was given before LCI (LCI was given at reduced doses without protection), and then LHBI followed (Pilot Study

**Hypothesis for the Evolution of Metastatic Disease as a Function
of Tumor Burden and Kinetics for Unresectable NSCBC
Confined to the Thorax**

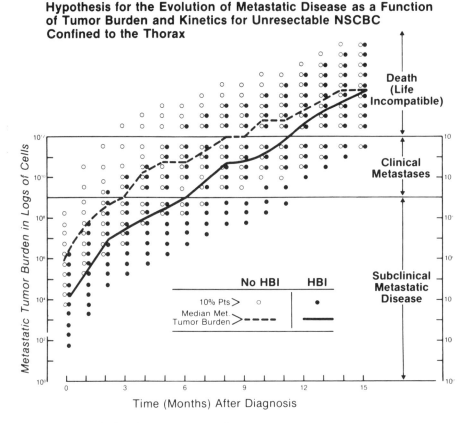

Time (Months) After Diagnosis

Fig. 12. Hypothesis for the development of clinical distant metastases in locally advanced, unresectable, non-small cell bronchogenic carcinoma (NSCBC). Two groups of patients are presented: (1) the control group consisting of patients receiving local chest irradiation (LCI) and no elective HBI, and (2) the HBI patients consisting of patients receiving LCI plus elective HBI for micrometastases. Each circle represents 10% of the patients in each group. Transition from clinical metastases to death was obtained from clinical data (6); extrapolation of this data into the subclinical metastatic disease status was performed. The lines connect the median metastatic tumor burden at each time interval. The circles at the extremes of the median metastatic tumor burden for each time interval represent the range of metastatic tumor burden.

No. 2); only one patient (11%) had evidence of distant metastases in the first 2.5 months.

The use of elective HBI for subclinical metastases yielded a significant prolongation of the median recurrence-free survival (43 weeks vs 13 weeks), a significant increase in the median time to develop metastases (10 months vs 3 months) and a decreased incidence in liver metastases (1 in 13 patients vs 10 in 29 patients) when compared with the control group. There was also a significant increase in local tumor control when single doses of 800 rad of

UHBI were supplemented with doses of LCI in Pilot Study No. 2 [6]. However, *although elective HBI seemed to delay the appearance of distant metastases, it did not prevent their occurrence, alter patterns of first relapse or significantly improve the overall survival of patients.* Nevertheless, a therapeutic gain was achieved and its potential exploitation requires some discussion.

Based on the data obtained in these pilot studies [6], a hypothesis was constructed for the development of distant metastases in these locally advanced NSCBC patients (Fig. 12). It can be appreciated that for the control patients who did not receive elective systemic HBI, there was a rapid transition from subclinical metastatic status to overt metastases and subsequent death. The important compartment is the *subclinical metastatic compartment* which by definition encompasses a broad range of 10^0 to 10^8 cells (median of 10^6 cells) and only one doubling was required to make some of the subclinical metastatic disease clinically evident. If the same data-extrapolation is done for patients receiving elective systemic HBI, the median subclinical metastatic load was 10^4 cells (range of 10^2 to 10^6 cells). This indicated a net effect of *2 logs of cell kill by HBI* which corroborated previous observations [23]. The transition from subclinical to clinical metastases and death in these HBI patients was delayed by that same factor and it became evident that the technique was limited in attaining cure or a significantly better overall survival. Nevertheless, the transitory delay for the clinical detection of metastatic disease with HBI constitutes a significant therapeutic gain which conceivably could allow today's ineffective CT in NSCBC to become more effective by reducing the subclinical metastatic burden that needs to be treated and allowing more time for cytotoxic drugs to act. Chemotherapy for instance, could be given after hematologic recovery from HBI has occurred (4–6 weeks) without a significant increase in the subclinical metastatic burden which was effectively reduced by the systemic irradiation (Fig. 12). This hypothesis remains to be tested clinically; at the present time HBI supplemented with LCI is being tested against LCI alone and LCI plus CT in a randomized protocol of the ECOG (EST–3578).

3.6.7. The Use of HBI in SCBC

SCBC is a radiosensitive tumor and perhaps becomes a more suitable target for systemic irradiation. However, since effective CT is available for these tumors, UHBI has been only explored as a consolidative approach after induction CT for extensive disease patients [109]. It was hoped that the combination of standard CT with UHBI (supplemented with local chest irradiation) would have the same results as more intensive CT approaches which are associated with considerable morbidity [4]. In a two-institution pilot study for the ECOG this concept was tested [109]: nineteen extensive disease patients were induced with standard ECOG CT with Cyclophosphamide and

CCNU; responders to this induction therapy were to be consolidated with 600 rad of UHBI followed one week later with 2000 rad in one week of localized chest irradiation. Only 9 patients responded to induction CT; all responses were partial. RT consolidation was used in these 9 patients: 7 patients (78%) became complete responders in the chest, of these 5 (63%) became overall complete responders, of these 3 survived over one year, of these 2 are alive disease-free over 70 weeks from the initiation of treatment. Only one of the RT consolidated patients had his first clinical recurrence in the chest; this reinforced the value of RT for controlling intrathoracic disease. No major complications were observed with the use of consolidation RT and no serious delays or interruptions in maintenance CT was necessary in these patients [109]. We were encouraged that the use of this RT consolidation did not increase toxicity and may have actually improved survival when patients treated by both participating institutions with identical CT without RT were used as retrospective controls. A new pilot study for the ECOG (PB–579) explores intensive CT induction with this type of RT consolidation in extensive SCBC, hoping to be able to consolidate a higher percentage of complete responders. Corroboration of results obtained in this pilot study [109] is being attempted in Canada [117] and in Italy [118]. If results are corroborated in extensive SCBC patients, the application of this technique in limited SCBC patients should be further investigated.

3.6.8. The Future Uses of HBI in Lung Cancer
Several ideas need to be tested: (1) using HBI with CT for locally advanced NSCBC; (2) using HBI and the radiosensitizers with and without CT; (3) fractionating HBI into 2 or 3 doses rather than one single application. Further discussion at this point would be highly speculative.

3.7. Increasing the Tumor Dose
Local chest irradiation is an effective treatment for the local-regional control of lung cancer. There are many recent publications and review articles which support this position [1, 4, 5, 81, 119, 120]. When the regional nodes are included in the treatment portals, the ONLY way to assess the effectiveness of thoracic irradiation is to examine closely its degree of local control. Patterns of failure and spread must be thoroughly established. Documenting at the time of the first recurrence whether it occurred within or outside previous treatment bounderies is of major clinical importance because it will establish the true incidence of local-regional failure after thoracic RT; this can be accomplished in most cases by superimposing simulation and beam films over diagnostic X-rays or CAT scans which demonstrate the tumor recurrence. Utilizing survival as the sole criterion for response and/or RT effectiveness, is

misleading and totally inadequate since most lung cancer patients will exhibit and die of distant metastases.

If tumor sterilization is used as the criterion for response, the use of preoperative RT with doses of 5000–6000 rad in potentially operable candidates have yielded sterilization rates of 40–60% for the primary tumor [121–123] and almost 90% for mediastinal lymph nodes [123]. For inoperable candidates treated curatively with similar doses of radiation, the autopsies of some patients, dying of causes other than their tumors shortly after treatment ended, have yielded similar sterilization rates in the local-regional areas [124]. If tumor resolution in diagnostic films is used as the criterion of response for unresectable patients, an average response rate of 50–55% can be achieved with 5000–6000 rad with a range of 30% to 80% for doses of 4000–7000 rad respectively [1, 8, 81, 119, 120]. Nevertheless, it becomes crucial to quantify objective tumor responses by histology since SCBC is more sensitive to RT than NSCBC. It is also equally important to quantifiably relate complete tumor responses with tumor size to obtain the range of tumor cell kill that can be achieved.

A recently completed study of the RTOG comparing continuous fractionated RT schedules delivering various doses (4000, 5000 and 6000 rad) for locally advanced NSCBC demonstrated that better local tumor control was achieved with the higher doses [81]. The information available in the literature strongly suggests that to achieve a higher degree of local tumor resolution, the total dose to be delivered with conventional continuous fractionated schedules must be *higher than 6000 rad* [1, 8]. Indications also exist that optimum regressions are achieved with doses of 6500 rad; beyond this range, the dose-response curve flattens out and one enters a zone of obvious overkill [1, 8, 119, 125]. The use of doses as high as 7500 rad delivered with split-course fractionation have yielded severe complications with no apparent increase in therapeutic results [8].

Thoracic RT is limited by the toxicity to vital organs that unavoidably lie in the treatment field. It is the tolerance of these organs which prevents delivery of higher doses of radiation. The main complications of thoracic irradiation: pneumonopathy, myelopathy and to some extent, cardiomyopathy, are all time-dose-volume related phenomena [7]. The dose of RT delivered with conventional continuous fractionated schedules that would yield the minimum number of complications appears to be *less than 4000 rad* [1, 7, 8]. Doses as low as 2500 rad will induce pulmonary fibrosis and doses as high as 6000 rad will lead to severe radiation fibrosis (with or without effusion) and/or pneumonitis, which could or will threaten the patient's life [7]. Doses higher than 4500 rad delivered continuously or doses higher than 1550 ret can lead to chronic irreversible radiation myelopathy [7]. It comes to mind that, if the best tumoricidal dose of radiation that can be delivered with conventional fractionation is greater than 6000 rad, but the dose which yields minimum toxicity is below 4000 rad, the traditional treatment of 5000 rad in 5 weeks is a suitable compromise.

There have been recent developments which have helped radiation oncologists understand and attempt to overcome the limitations imposed by the normal irradiated tissues: (1) computerized axial chest tomograms (CAT scans) have given a more precise definition of the target volume that needs to be boosted; (2) lung pathophysiologists have indicated that the apical areas of both lungs will tolerate higher doses since they are less vascularized (i.e. more hypoxic) and thus less susceptible to radiation damage; (3) radiobiological and biochemical studies have served to identify the lesion leading to the development of pneumonitis as being radiation damage to the alveolar type II pneumocyte with a corresponding decrease of surfactant production[112]; (4) surgical training of radiation oncologists has allowed interstitial implantation techniques to flourish; (5) a team-work approach of radiation physicists, dosimetrists and technicians with radiation oncologists have helped to refine treatment planning and deliver sophisticated and extremely accurate irradiation; and (6) a closer relation between radiation oncologists and surgical oncologists has allowed for operative assessment and intraoperative action.

Several ways by which a higher tumoricidal dose could be delivered without significant compromise of the normal tissues include: *treatment planning, intraoperative interstitial implantation* and *intraoperative external high energy irradiation*. Careful treatment planning tailored to a better target volume definition can allow delivery of higher RT boosted doses by the use of multiple field arrangements[119]. Exposing the target volume after collapsing the lung at thoracotomy could allow using intensive concentrated external irradiation to the tumoral tissue with high energy electrons during the actual operative procedure; this would spare some of the vital normal tissues from irradiation. Finally, the interstitial implantation technique which has matured through many years of experience by dedicated workers in specialized centers allows delivery of very high tumoral doses. This deserves special mention in this section.

Interstitial implants deliver only a small dose outside the implanted volume and consequently, minimal damage to the surrounding tissues occurs. The actual technique of implanting lung tumors has been discussed by Henschke[126, 127]. The experience with this technique in hundreds of lung cancer patients has yielded very acceptable results[128, 129]. There are certain advantages for lung tumor implants: (1) can be performed at the time and under the anesthesia of the exploratory thoracotomy; (2) can be tailored to the actual tumor volume; (3) can deliver tumoral doses as high as 33,000 rad; and (4) the dose to the surrounding tissues is minimal. The main disadvantages of the technique are requiring: (1) special trained personnel; (2) maximum cooperation with the surgical team; and (3) supplemental external irradiation to the mediastinum and supraclavicular areas with 3000-4000 rad.

Of the many isotopes that can be used for lung cancer implantation, radon, Iridium-192 (Ir^{192}) and Gold-198 (Au^{198}) are the most popular. All of these isotopes are γ-emitters and of the three, Ir^{192} seems to be the best. Ir^{192} delivers protracted irradiation since its half-life is 74.5 days as compared to a half-life of 2.7 days and 3.8 days for Au^{198} and radon respectively[128]. In addition, Ir^{192} can be given with an after loading technique and because the sources are smaller than radon, several sources can be loaded into a thinner needle resulting in less bleeding, less air-leakage and less trauma to the lung[128]. Ir^{192} is also more economical and actually delivers the same depth dose up to 6 cm as the other two isotopes.

3.8. Hyperthermia

The recent remissance in hyperthermia has provided *in vitro* [130], *in vivo* [130] and clinical data [130–134] that encourage the systematic investigation of hyperthermia in clinical oncology. Though heat alone has some anti-tumor effect, its main potential will be in an adjuvant role for radiation or chemotherapy. The physical nature of this modality makes it a natural choice for the radiation oncologist to adopt and investigate.

In vitro studies have provided a rationale for combining radiation with localized hyperthermia by delineating a number of mechanics through which heat could produce a therapeutic gain[135]. There is a pronounced complimentarity between the cell populations most susceptible to the cytotoxicity of radiation or hyperthermia: hypoxic, acidic and poorly nourished cells are strikingly sensitive to heat[135, 136] in contrast to their radiation resistance; similarly, radioresistant S-phase cells are particularly sensitive to hyperthermia[137]. The dove-tailing of susceptible cell populations is a powerful argument for combining the two modalities and promises yet another approach to the elimination of therapy-limiting hypoxic cells. Exploitation of this complimentary cytotoxic effect makes no theoretic demand for a close temporal ralation between radiation and heat. However, the development of thermal tolerance may require relatively prolonged time intervals between thermal doses. Thermal tolerance, the acquisition of cellular resistance to subsequent thermal doses[138], develops either during prolonged low temperature (41–42°C for 2 hours) exposure[139] or after high temperature (42–45°C) exposure[140] and persists for 24–72 hours[141]. Hyperthermia during this thermotolerant phase has little cytotoxicity and thermal fractionation to achieve optimal cell-killing requires cognizance of this phenomenon.

The time course for extinction of thermal resistance is likely to vary between tumors and no human data are available though most clinical studies have employed 48 to 72 hours between successive heat treatments [131].

In addition to the cytotoxicity of hyperthermia, significant radiosensitization occurs when heat is applied in close temporal relation to radiation [135, 142, 143]. The magnitude of this synergism is determined by many factors: (1) the time interval between heat and radiation; (2) the sequence of the two modalities; (3) the thermal dose (temperature and time); (4) radiation dose; (5) radiation dose-rate; (6) radiation LET; (7) cell cycle phase; and (8) oxygenation status. Only a few of these factors will be discussed here.

In general, the greatest synergism between heat and radiation is observed when both are administered simultaneously [130]. Logistically this is not a feasible clinical approach and the alternatives are heating immediately before or immediately after radiation. It seems probable, though not certain, that with the relatively low thermal doses achievable clinically (41–43 °C for 1/2 to 1 hour), *greater synergism occurs when heating is applied immediately after radiation* rather than in the opposite sequence [130, 143]. Higher thermal doses (44–45 °C) appear to sensitize most, if given just prior to radiation. *Increasing the time interval between the two modes reduces the synergism and spacings in excess of 3 hours largely abolish any interaction* [130]. Interestingly, thermally tolerant cells remain susceptible to the radiosensitizing effect of heat despite their enhanced resistance to heat-induced death [144]. Therefore, a combination of radiation-hyperthermia on a daily basis may be a rational approach to exploit thermal radiosensitization rather than thermal cytotoxicity. This approach would avoid the added complexity of novel radiation fractionation schedules.

Thermal radiosensitization increases as thermal dose increases though relatively little effect occurs up to 41 °C for one hour. In going from 41 °C to 43.5 °C for one hour, a twofold reduction in radiation dose is necessary to achieve the same effect as obtained at 37–41 °C. Sensitization is greatest for hypoxic, acidic and undernourished cells [136], resulting in a reduced OER. This reduction in the protective effect of hypoxia against radiation may be one of the most important aspects of hyperthermic radiosensitization and is the clearest a priori factor suggesting that tumors may be more sensitized than normal tissues. Recent studies have also shown that many tumors achieve higher temperatures than surrounding normal tissues when heat is applied regionally [145] due to their lower perfusion rate [146]. This higher thermal exposure will produce greater sensitization.

Any potential clinical exploitation of hyperthermia is critically contingent on the availability of adequate technology to produce controlled hyperthermia. The major obstacle to clinical evaluation of heat has been the lack of an effective method to generate localized deep hyperthermia and to monitor the temperatures achieved. Hot water bath immersion and heated vascular perfusion are limited to the extremities while ultrasound and electromagnetic energy coupling have their own limitations [147]. Ultrasound though capable of useful penetration does not pass through bone or air cavities and produces preferential bone heating [131]. Radiofrequency energy applied via electrodes couples readily to fat tissue resulting in preferential fat heating, while microwave frequencies have low penetration [148]. However, recent advances in the technology of these methods [147] have considerably improved their clinical prospects and multiple-applicator low-frequency microwave systems may allow useful heating of deep human tumors including bronchial carcinoma. In parallel with advances in temperature generation, a number of invasive temperature-increasing probes have been developed and electromagnetically nonperturbing devices are available for use in microwave fields [149]. Non-invasive ultrasound temperature tomography, which maps tissue temperature by measuring changes in the velocity of sound within heated tissue, is an appealing though as yet unavailable technique.

Due to the technical limitations of local heat delivery, relatively few well-documented clinical studies have been recently reported [134, 145, 148, 150] and only one group has reported a significant number of lung cancer patients [132, 151]. They applied radiofrequency energy to several bronchogenic carcinomas and though temperature measurements were not performed, regressions were observed. More importantly, in three cases thoracotomy and resection followed radiofrequency heating and the pathologic specimens revealed considerable tumor necrosis with relatively little normal lung changes [151]. This provides direct clinical support for the continued evaluation of hyperthermia in bronchogenic carcinoma.

3.9. High LET Radiation

Particle beams constitute new and very important radiation sources of clinical potential benefit. These beams have high-linear energy transfer (High LET) characteristics and offer either or both a greater biological effect on tumoral tissues or a better dose distribution which avoids unnecessary irradiation of normal tissues.

Inactivation of tumor cells by High-LET radiation differs from that by photon irradiation in that: (1) cell sensitivity is less dependant on cellular oxygen concentration at the time of radiation, thus a more effective cell-kill is achieved; (2) less radiation energy is required for cell inactivation, thus a more efficient cell-kill is obtained; (3) cells submitted to High-LET radiations are less capable of repairing the induced radiation damage, thus tumor repopulation is decreased; (4) cell sensitivity is not as dependent upon the position of the cells in the replication cycle; and (5) cells of high ploidy are relatively more sensitive than euploid cells [152]. This indicates that the biological effectiveness of High-LET radiations is higher than that of low-LET radiation.

The particle beams which are of interest for clinical testing at the present time are: fast neutrons, negative pions, alpha particles (helium), heavy ions (carbon, neon, argon), and protons[152]. The radiobiological characteristics of fast neutrons, negative pions and heavy ions are similar and result because each is a densely ionizing radiation beam. The dose distribution patterns achieved by using negative pions, heavy ions and protons are qualitatively similar and far more favorable than those obtained by using X-rays, photons or neutrons[152]. This more favorable dose distribution is due to the fact that with the latter particles, the dose decreases exponentially with tissue thickness while for negative pions, heavy ions and protons, a low entrance dose with a deeper high-rate energy deposition at the end of a finite range can be achieved[152].

During the last decade, there have been active programs to characterize fast neutrons, pions, helium and heavy ions by radiation physicists and radiobiologists. These programs have provided enough scientific basis to initiate clinical studies with these High-LET particles[152]. Highly specialized and expensive facilities are necessary to produce and apply most of these particles. Since there are very few centers throughout the world especializing in the clinical usefulness of any one High-LET particle beam, and since most of the clinical experience with these particles is still in a gestational phase, further discussion in this section will be limited to the use of fast neutrons.

Fast Neutron Irradiation for Lung Cancer

Large, rapidly-growing tumors tend to outgrow their blood supply resulting in necrotic areas surrounded by hypoxic cells which tend to be resistant to conventional low-LET megavoltage photon irradiation[153]. A characteristic of High-LET radiation is a low OER and a high RBE which make this type of radiation of interest for treating lung cancer, a disease which is still difficult to control locally by conventional megavoltage photon irradiation[81]. Fast-neutrons constitute one of the most popular High-LET radiations and since neutron facilities are increasing in the United States, comprehensive clinical trials with these particles have been launched for a variety of tumors by the Radiation Therapy Oncology Group (RTOG).

The radiobiology of fast neutrons has been discussed earlier in this chapter. The clinical experience with this form of radiation originated with tumors other than lung cancer. A higher rate of local control for fast neutrons over conventional megavoltage photon irradiation has been demonstrated in malignant gliomas[154, 155] and in cervical adenopathies from advanced squamous cell carcinomas from the head and neck regions[156, 157]. Subsequently, fast neutron therapy has been used in sarcomas[158], epidermoid carcinomas of the aerodigestive tract [159], and carcinoma of the major salivary glands [160]. Although major accomplishments have been obtained with the use of fast neutrons, such as sterilization of glioblastoma mutliforme [154, 155], considerable toxicity has also been reported [154–156, 159]. This toxicity is dose-dependent and definitely related to normal tissue damage (i.e. myelitis and brain damage).

Laboratory experiments have indicated that combining fast neutrons with conventional photon irradiation ('mixed beam therapy') achieves an enhanced therapeutic ratio compared with fast neutrons alone [161, 162]. Clinical pilot studies have substantiated these laboratory findings by yielding an equal [154] or higher [156, 163] local control rate for the mixed beam mode when compared with neutrons alone. The mixed beam approach also appears to cause less morbidity than fast neutrons alone [156, 162].

The RTOG has recently activated a Phase III protocol for localized, inoperable, NSCBC in institutions with neutron facilities [164]. This protocol compares conventional megavoltage photon irradiation (6000 rad in 30 fractions over 6–7 weeks) with fast neutrons alone (1800 rad in 24 fractions over 6–7 weeks) and with mixed beam (neutron-720 rad in 12 fractions with photon-3600 rad in 18 fractions, over 6–7 weeks). Patients will be treated 5 times a week on the photon arm, 4 times a week on the neutron only arm, and on the mixed beam arm will receive neutrons twice a week and photons three times a week. The smaller dose for neutron arms represents correcting for the increased RBE of the neutron beam which depends upon the energy spectrum of the neutron beam and will vary among facilities.

3.10. Combined Modality Therapy Approaches

Bronchogenic carcinomas constitute a group of tumors for the vast majority of which, it could be stated that each main therapeutic modality (surgery, radiotherapy and chemotherapy) alone, simply cannot offer an effective curative treatment. Most lung tumors fail in all compartments (T, N and M) and aside from being most of the time unresectable and submitted to various forms of aggressive therapy, patients ultimately die of uncontrolled local disease as well as nodal and distant metastases. For several decades, lung cancer treatment has constituted one of the most frustrating experiences in Oncology despite the significant gains achieved in the management of small cell tumors. However, the mere acceptance of the limitations that each therapeutic modality has, constitutes a forward step towards achieving the ultimate curative goal. Disappointments of the past have led to a total reassessment of the available options, and ways to combine therapeutic efforts without compromising the quality of the patient's life will constitute the backbone of future approaches for lung cancer.

After more than two decades in which surgery, radiotherapy and chemotherapy have been available, there is an urgent need to establish a better rationale for their integration. Perhaps a new concept is needed more urgently than new modalities, new drugs and new forms of radiation. Steel and Peckham [165] have attempted to provide this concept and with it a new terminology under the heading of exploitable mechanisms in combined modality approaches. The object of any of such approaches is to achieve an improvement in therapeutic results and not simply a greater tumor cell kill which could lead to greater treatment toxicity. A modification of their concepts as applied to clinical trials follows, since their intention was to sharpen laboratory and experimental models applied to the clinical setting [166]. There seem to be four basically different forms of combining therapy modes:

3.10.1. Independent Toxicity

When one combines without dose curtailment, partially effective modalities with different toxic endpoints to obtain an improvement in therapeutic results. An example would be elective (prophylactic) brain irradiation used in conjunction with systemic CT for SCBC where the toxic endpoint for RT is the normal brain tissue and for CT other organ systems.

3.10.2. Spatial Cooperation

When one modality fails to affect disease in some particular anatomical site, the addition of a second agent that does deal with it will improve results. Examples would be: local RT affecting the T and N compartments and CT affecting the metastatic compartment; surgery for the T compartment and local RT for regional nodal disease (N compartment); interstitial implants plus supplementary external RT for the T and N compartments respectively.

3.10.3. Therapeutic Additivity and Synergism

When the combination of two agents acting through different mechanisms can enhance cell kill. There are several processes which may be exploited in principle to achieve such enhancement: (a) modification of the initial radiation damage; (b) inhibition of repair of sublethal radiation damage in tumor cells; (c) exploitation of induced cell synchrony; (d) reoxygenation of the hypoxic tumor fraction; (e) improved drug access following RT; (f) improved oxygenation following drug treatment and before RT; (g) tumor reduction after RT leading to more rapid proliferation and greater chemosensitivity of tumor cells; (h) tumor reduction after CT allowing the use of smaller radiation treatment portals and higher RT doses. All these processes usually require interaction between modes at the biochemical or cellular level. Examples of therapeutic additivity are many of the new RT approaches discussed in this chapter (i.e. sensitizers, radioprotectors, hyperbaric oxygen therapy, carbogen breathing, and hyperthermia) when combined with local RT. Another example of therapeutic additivity would be using hemibody irradiation followed by systemic CT for subclinical distant metastases in NSCBC.

3.10.4. Temporal Consolidation

When one modality is used to induce maximum regression and is followed immediately by a second modality to eradicate the residual or microscopic disease. This implies capitalizing in the gains of one modality to ensure results; it also allows for a reduction in the dose and aggressiveness of the consolidating modality. An example would be CT induction followed by hemibody consolidation for extensive SCBC.

Most of the new RT approaches previously discussed in this chapter have been aimed to make local RT more effective and/or less toxic. As mentioned earlier, many of these innovations when combined with local RT constitute in themselves combined modality approaches of the therapeutic additivity type. Other innovations such as unconventional fractionation schedules, increasing the tumor dose and high-LET irradiation, constitute variations of the same treatment modality. In either circumstance, when these new innovations are used with or as local RT, the goal is to improve the local-regional control of lung cancer. Even if this could be achieved, it will be unlikely that the effort will yield an effective curative approach for lung tumors because of their exquisite tendency for early distant metastases. The introduction of hemibody irradiation constitutes an attempt to use RT systemically to attack the problem of distant metastases but, as mentioned in earlier sections, this approach has a self-limiting toxicity and achieves only temporary gains. There is absolutely no question that in a curative attempt for locally advanced lung cancer, a systemic treatment such as CT should be added to an effective local therapy, such as RT.

Accepting the premise that the treatment of most lung tumors requires in addition to an effective local treatment a systemic form of therapy, constitutes a mere surface scratch to a large problem. The core of this problem is how to best combine these two modalities to yield significant therapeutic gains. Most combined modality approaches for lung cancer have been employed for SCBC for which there is effective systemic CT available; combined approaches are beginning to emerge for NSCBC for which there have been no effective combinations available [167–169]. Although the goal in all these attempts has been to enhance results, quite frequently the opposite occurs, particularly when each modality is given with full conventional doses and worse yet, when each is intensified. That is, an increase in toxicity often supervenes from the additive attempt and this toxicity requires dose reduction and/or treatment interruptions which curtails the efficacy of one or both modes. Combining more than two modalities increases the possible permutations of administration and intensifies the problem. *The way to effectively combine RT and CT is far from being defined.* Without a firm scientific basis for combining modalities, research progress has been slow, ideas remain untested, conflicts arise and competition for clinical cases occurs.

A logical approach to use combined-modality therapy for lung cancer is to identify priorities and the nature of the impending problem. Patients with limited disease have the main tumor burden (10^9–10^{12} cells) in the local-regional areas while systemic disease is still subclinical (10^0–10^8 cells). Patients with extensive disease have large tumor burdens (10^9–10^{12} cells) both in local-regional areas and in distant sites. Rationally, the approach should be to attack the heaviest tumor burden with the most effective modality and to utilize with moderation the second modality until the first one has accomplished its task. Nevertheless, *the optimal timing of drugs and RT for lung cancer is also far from being defined.*

Although the most effective way to combine RT and CT for lung cancer therapy is not known, the fact that this combination can lead to an undesired increase in treatment-related complications has been thoroughly documented [4]. The well-established concepts of Rubin and Cassarett [170] regarding the 'tolerance-dose' of certain vital organs affected in the radiation treatment of lung cancer (bone marrow, lung, esophagus, spinal cord, heart, and to some extent skin) will no longer apply when CT is combined with, precedes and sometimes even when it is given after RT. There are many drugs which are currently used for lung cancer which are by themselves toxic to many of these vital organs and/or will become toxic or even more toxic when com-

Table 5. Combined chemotherapy and radiotherapy treatment of lung cancer: End-Organ toxicity*.

Drugs	Bone marrow	Lung	Esophagus	Heart	Spinal cord	Skin
Adriamycin	●	○	●○	●○	○	○
Bleomycin	(○)	●○	●○			●○
Mitomycin C	●	●		(●)		
Cyclophosphamide	●	●○		(●)		
Methotrexate	●	●○	●			●
CCNU	●	(●)				
Vincristine			○		(●)	
Procarbazine	●		○			
VP-16	●					
Cis-Platinum	●					○
Hexamethylmelamine	●					

* ● = Toxicity caused by drug per se.
 ○ = Toxicity reported with CT + RT.
 ( ) = Potential toxicity.

bined with RT. Table 5 lists some of these drugs with their respective end-organ toxicity. There have been attempts to define and quantitate these modifications of radiation injury to normal tissues by chemotherapeutic agents [171–174]. The problem attains even greater proportions when some of the new RT innovations (such as unconventional fractionation schedules, hypoxic cell sensitizers and hyperthermia), which by themselves can modify radiation injury, begin to be combined with CT.

The large investment in cooperative group clinical trials attempting to employ combined modalities in lung cancer requires establishment of a research logic with criteria for an orderly flow of ideas from the laboratory into the clinical Phase I and II studies. The optimal timing of drug and RT relative to cell cycle kinetics is not defined but continues to be investigated in the laboratory [175]. There is a need for relevant data on which such cell renewal kinetics, particularly when it has been perturbed by radiation (such as bone marrow), can be effectively utilized. In this regard, it is also essential that there be direct comparative data between malignant and normal tissue systems so that kinetic differences can be applied when combining treatment modalities which differentially affect various end-organs and specific cell-cycle kinetics.

4. CONCLUSIONS

At the present time there is no predictable curative therapy for the majority of lung cancer patients. All therapeutic modalities are limited in several ways from reaching by themselves significant long term survival results. Intensifying present therapies (whether CT or RT), attempting to achieve a higher percentage of responses, could lead to a significant increase in fatal and life-threatening toxicity which would defeat the intended purpose. *The morbidity of the therapeutic approach and its compromise of the patients' quality of life should not and cannot outweigh the therapy benefits.* If it were possible to achieve a higher number of complete responders with minimal toxicity, the clinical disappearance of all visible tumor (complete response), even when corroborated radiologically, chemically or surgically (by bronchoscopy and rebiopsy), does not imply that the disease will not recur [19]. There is a large undetected subclinical tumor burden which becomes the greatest limitation and the main cause of all past frustrations.

The major contribution of thoracic RT to the primary management of lung cancer patients has been and is the local-regional tumor control. Most RT innovations are geared to increase its local effectiveness and/or decrease its toxicity. However, most forms of lung cancer, even when only locally advanced, can be regarded as disseminated disease requiring systemic therapy.

Table 6. An optimally timed treatment strategy.

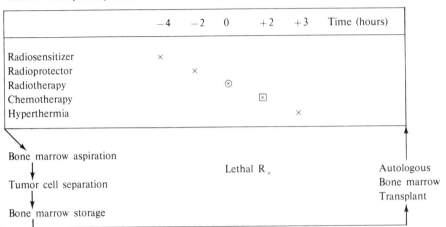

RT has proven effective in decreasing the incidence of brain metastases (a sanctuary site) when used electively. Other forms of RT such as HBI, when supplemented with thoracic irradiation, are beginning to emerge as helpful and hopeful consolidation approaches after systemic CT induction in SCBC and perhaps as an adjuvant systemic therapy in NSCBC.

The empiricism of the earlier years has been surpassed by scientific notions adopted from the basic sciences. Many of the RT innovations such as hypoxic cell sensitizers and hyperthermia could be used with systemic CT hoping to enhance its effect. This opens up large number of permutations and combinations in a new era of combined modality approaches. How to best combine an effective local therapy such as RT with CT and other enhancing modes will become the challenge of the next decade. It may well be that the day for an optimally-timed combined modality treatment strategy such as the one outlined in Table 6 will not be far off. A sensitizer and a radioprotector could be given prior to RT so that when this is delivered, these substances would be at peak concentrations; the RT could consist of mixed high LET and photon beams given in an unconventional fractionation; the sensitizers would still be at high concentrations to conceivably enhance systemic CT when given after RT; and finally, hyperthermia could enhance both RT and CT. Conceivably, one could even consider autologous bone marrow storage and transplantation embracing a lethal enhanced treatment for this devastating disease.

ACKNOWLEDGEMENT

The authors acknowledge with gratitude the help of Doris Commons for the typing of the manuscript.

REFERENCES

1. Salazar OM, Rubin P, Brown JC, Feldstein ML and Keller BE: Predictors of Radiation Response in Lung Cancer – A Clinico-Pathological Analysis. Cancer 37:2636-2650, 1976.
2. Manual for Staging of Cancer of Cancer 1978 of the American Joint Committee for Cancer Staging and end-results (AJCCS). Chicago, Illinois: Whiting Press, 1978. pp 59-64.
3. Greco FA and Oldham RK: Current concepts in Cancer: Small-Cell Lung Cancer. New Engl J Med 301:355-358, 1979.
4. Salazar OM and Creech RH: Small Cell Bronchogenic Carcinoma – 'The State of the Art' – Towards defining the role of Radiation Therapy in the Management of this disease. Int J Rad Onc Biol Phys 6:1103-1117, 1980.
5. Salazar OM: Moments of Decision in Lung Cancer. (ed) Rubin P, Chevy Chase, American College of Radiology, Chicago Illinois. In press 1980.
6. Salazar OM, Scarantino CW, Rubin P, Feldstein ML and Keller BE: Total (Half-Body) Systemic Irradiation for Occult Metastases in Non-Small Cell Lung Cancer: An Eastern cooperative Oncology Group Pilot report. Proc Am Soc Ther Radiol Int J Rad Oncol Biol Phys 5:59, 1979 and submitted to Cancer for publication, 1980.
7. Salazar OM: Tumor Control and Radiation Toxicity in the Treatment of Lung cancer: An Analysis of Time-Dose-Volume Factor. In: Lung Cancer: Progress in Therapeutic Research, Muggia F and Rozencweig (eds), Raven Press, New York, 1979, p 267-278.
8. Salazar OM, Rubin P, Brown JC, Feldstein ML and Keller BE: The Assessment of Tumor Response to Irradiation of Lung Cancer: Continuous versus Split-Course Regimens. Int J rad Oncol Biol Phys 1:1107-1118, 1976.
9. Andrews JR: The Radiobiology of Human Cancer Radiotherapy. 2nd Edition, Baltimore, University Park Press, 1978.
10. Hall EJ: Radiobiology for the Radiologist. 2nd Edition, Maryland, Harper and Row, 1978.
11. Thomlinson RH, Gray LH: The Histological Structure of some Human Lung Cancers and Possible Implications for Radiotherapy. Brit J Cancer, 9:539-549, 1955.
12. Ling CC: Time Scale of Radiation-Induced Oxygen Depletion and Decay Kinetics of Oxygen-dependent Damage in cells Irradiated at Ultrahigh dose rates. Radiat Res 63:455-467, 1975.
13. Adams GE, Dewey DL: Hydrated Electrons and Radiobiological Sensitization. Biochem Biophys Res Commun 12:473-477, 1963.
14. Lohmann W: The Molecular Mechanism of Radiation Protection and Sensitization. In: Advances in Chemical Radiosensitization, Vienna, Intern Atomic Energy Agency, PL-544/11, P 115-121, 1974.
15. Barendsen GW, Walter HMD, Fowler JF, Dewley DK: Effects of Different Ionizing Radiations on Human Cells in Tissue Culture III, Experiments with Cyclotron Accelerated Alpha Particles and Electrons. Radiat Res 18:106-119, 1963.
16. Katz R, Sharma SC: Cellular Survival in a Mixed Radiation Environment. Int J Radiat Biol 26:143-146, 1974.
17. Tannock IF: Oxygen Diffusion and the Distribution of Cellular Radiosensitivity in Tumors. Brit J Radiol 45:515-524, 1972.
18. Kolstad P: Intercapillary distance, Oxygen Tension and Local Recurrence in cervix cancer. Scand J Clin Lab Invest 22:145-157, 1968.
19. Evans NTS, Naylor PFD: The Effect of Oxygen Breathing and Radiotherapy upon the Tissue Oxygen Tension of Some Human Tumors. Brit J Radiol 36:418-425, 1963.
20. Jamieson D, Van den Brenk HAS: Oxygen Tension in Human Malignant Disease under hyperbaric conditions. Brit J Cancer 19:139-150, 1965.

21. Thomlinson RH: Oxygen Therapy: Biological Considerations. In: Modern Trends in Radiotherapy, Deely TF, Woods CAP (eds), Butterworths, London, p 52-72, 1967.
22. VanPutten LM, Kallman RF: Oxygenation Status of a Transplantable Tumor During Fractionated Radiotherapy. J Natl Cancer Inst 40:441-451, 1968.
23. Sutherland RM and Durand RE: Radiation Response of Multicell Spheroids – AN in vitro Tumor Model. Curr Topics Rad Res Quarterly 11:87-139, 1976.
24. VanPutten LM: Reoxygenation of Hypoxic Tumor Cells. Strahlentherapie 153:380-386, 1977.
25. Kallman RF: The Phenomenon of Reoxygenation and its Implications for Fractionated Radiotherapy. Radiology, 105:135-142, 1972.
26. VanPutten, LM: Tumor Reoxygenation during Fractionated Radiotherapy. Studies with a Transplantable Osteosarcoma. Eur J Cancer 4:173-182, 1968.
27. Withers, HR: The Four R's of Radiotherapy. Advances Radiat Biol 5:241-271, 1975.
28. Kellerer AM, Rossi HH: The Theory of Dual Radiation Action. Curr Topics Radiat Res 8:85-158, 1972.
29. Field, SB: An Historical Survey of Radiobiology and Radiotherapy with Fast Neutrons. Curr Topics Radiat Res 11:1-86, 1976.
30. Bush RS, Jenkin RDT, Allt WEC, Beale FA, Bean H, Dembo AJ, Pringle JF: Definitive Evidence for Hypoxic Cells Influencing cure in Cancer Therapy. Brit J Cancer 37: Suppl III 302-306, 1978.
31. VandenBrenk HAS: Hyperbaric Oxygen in Radiation Therapy. An Investigation of Dose-Effect Relationships in Tumor Response and Tissue Damage. Am J Roentgenol 102:8-26, 1968.
32. Fletcher GH, Lingberg RD, Cardarao JB, Wharton JT: Hyperbaric Oxygen as a Radiotherapeutic Adjuvant in Advanced Cancer of the Cervix. Cancer 39:617-623, 1977.
33. Glassburn JR, Brady LN, Plenk HP: Hyperbaric Oxygen in Radiation Therapy. Cancer 39:751-765, 1977.
34. Henk JM, Kunkler PB, Smith CW: Radiotherapy and Hyperbaric Oxygen in Head and Neck Cancer. Final Report of First Controlled Trial. Lancet ii:101-103, 1977.
35. Henk JM, Smith CW: Radiotherapy and Hyperbaric Oxygen in Head and Neck Cancer. Interim Report of Second Clinical Trial. Lancet ii:104-105, 1977.
36. Cade IS, McEwen JB: Clinical Trials of Radiotherapy in Hyperbaric Oxygen at Portsmouth. Clin Radiol 29:333-338, 1978.
37. Watson ER, Halnan KE, Dische S, Saunders MI, Cade IS, McEwen JB, Wierwik G, Perrins DJD, Sutherland I: Hyperbaric Oxygen and Radiotherapy: A Medical Research Council Trial in Carcinoma of the Cervix. Brit J Radiol 51:879-887, 1978.
38. Dische S: Hyperbaric Oxygen: The Medical Research Council Trials and Their Significance. Brit J Radiol 51:888-894, 1978.
39. Suit HD, Maeda M: Hyperbaric Oxygen and Radiobiology of a C3H Mouse Mammary Carcinoma, J Natl Cancer Inst 39:639-652, 1967.
40. DuSault LA: The Effect of Oxygen on the Response of Spontaneous Tumors to Radiotherapy. Brit J Radiol 36:749-754, 1963.
41. Abe M, Yabumoto E, Mishidai T and Takahashi M: Trials of New Forms of Radiotherapy for Locally Advanced Bronchogenic Carcinoma. Irradiation under 95% O_2 plus 5% CO_2 Inhalation, Uneven Fractionation and Intraoperative Irradiation. Strahlentherapie 153:149-158, 1977.
42. ROCS: The Radiation Oncology Research Program. Recommended Research Proposals. Int J Rad Oncol Biol Phys 5:593-773, 1979.
43. Fowler JF, Adams GE, Denekamp J: Radiosensitizers of Hypoxic Cells in Solid Tumors. Cancer Treat Reviewes 3:227-256, 1976.

44. Adams GE, Clarke ED, Flockhart IR, Jacobs RS, Sehmi DS, Stratford IJ, Wardman P, Watts ME, Parrick J, Wallace RG, Smithen CE: Structure-Activity Relationships in the Development of Hypoxic Cell Radiosensitizers. I. Sensitization Efficiency. Int J Radial Biol 35:133-150, 1979.

45. Sutherland RM: Selective Chemotherapy of Noncycling Cells in an *in vitro* Tumor Model. Cancer Res 34:3501-3503, 1974.

46. Kogelink HD, Meyer HJ, Jentzsch K, Szepesi T, Karcher KH, Maida E, Manoli B, Wessely P, Zaumbauer F: Further Clinical Experiences of a Phase I Study with the Hypoxic Cell Radiosensitizer Misonidazole. Brit J Cancer 37: Suppl III:281-285, 1978.

47. Dische S, Saunders MI, Flockhart IR, Lee ME, Anderson P: Misonidazole – A Drug for trial in Radiotherapy and Oncology. Int J Rad Oncol Biol Phys 5:851-860, 1979.

48. Wasserman TH, Phillips TL, Johnson RJ, Gomer CJ, Lawrence GA, Sadee W, Marques RA, Levin VA, VanRaalte G: Initial United States Clinical and Pharmacologic Evaluation of Misonidazole (RO-07-0582), A Hypoxic Cell Radiosensitizer. Int J Rad Oncol Biol Phys 5:775-786, 1979.

49. Dische S, Saunders MI, Lee ME, Adams GE, Flockhart IR: Clinical Testing of the Radiosensitizer RO-07-0582: Experience with Multiple Doses. Brit J Cancer 35:567-579, 1977.

50. Phillips TL, Wasserman TH, Johnson RJ, Cauer CJ, Lawrence GA, Levine ML, Sadee W, Penta JS, Rubin DJ: The Hypoxic Cell Sensitizer Program in the United States. Brit J Cancer 37: Suppl III 276-280, 1978.

51. Saunders MI, Dische S, Anderson P, Flockhart IR: The Neurotoxicity of Misonidazole and its Relationship to Dose, Half-Life and Concentration in Serum. Brit J Cancer 37:Suppl III 268-270, 1978.

52. Urtasun RA, Chapman JD, Feldstein ML, Band RP, Rabin HR, Wilson AF, Marynowski B, Starreveld E, Stritka T: Peripheral Neuropathy Related to Misonidazole: Incidence and Pathology. Brit J Cancer 37: Suppl III 271-275, 1978.

53. Fletcher GH: The Evolution of Basic Concepts Underlying the Practice of Radiotherapy from 1949 to 1977. Radiology 127:3-19, 1978.

54. Radiation Therapy Oncology Group (RTOG) Protocol 78-14: Phase I/II Protocol to Study the Value of Misonidazole Combined with Radiation in the Treatment of Locally Advanced Lung Cancer. Activated on August 15, 1978. Available from the RTOG Operations Office, Thomas Jefferson University Hospital, 1015 Walnut Street, Philadelphia, Pennsylvania 19107, USA.

55. Radiation Therapy Oncology Group (RTOG) Protocol 79-17: Phase III Protocol Study to Compare Misonidazole Combined with Irradiation or Radiation Therapy Alone in the Treatment of Locally Advanced (stage III) Non-Oat Cell Lung Cancer. Activated on September 4, 1979. Available from the RTOG Operations Office, Thomas Jefferson University Hospital, 1015 Walnut Street, Philadelphia, Pennsylvania 19107, USA.

56. Pierquin BM, Mueller WK, Baillet F: Low Dose Rate Irradiation of Advanced Head and Neck Cancers: Present Studies. Int J Rad Oncol Biol Phys 4:565-572, 1978.

57. Patt HM: Protective Mechanisms in Ionizing Radiation Injury. Physiol Rev 33:35-96, 1953.

58. Yuhas JM, Storer JB: Differential Chemoprotection of Normal and Malignant Tissues. J Nat Cancer Inst 42:331-335, 1969.

59. Harris JW, Phillips TL: Radiobiological and Biochemical Studies of Thiophosphate Radioprotective Compounds Related to Cysteamine. Rad Res 46:362-379, 1971.

60. Chapman JD, Reuvers AP, Borsa J, Greenstock CL: Chemical Radioprotection and Radiosensitization of Mammalian Cells Growing *in vitro*. Radiat Res 56:291-306, 1973.

61. Utley JF, Phillips TL, Kane LF, Wharman MD, Wara WM: Differential Radioprotection of Enoxic and Hypoxic Mouse Mammary Tumors by a Thiophosphate Compound. Radiology 110:213-216, 1974.

62. Hall EJ, Aster M, Geard C, Biaglow J: Cytotoxicity of RO-07-0582; Enhancement by Hyperthermia and Protection by Cysteamine. Brit J Cancer 35:809-815, 1977.

63. Purdie JW: A Comparative Study of the Radioprotective Effects of Cysteamine, WR-2721 and WR-1065 in Cultured Human Cells. Rad Res 77:303-311, 1979.

64. Utley JF, Phillips TL, and Kane WJ: Protection of normal Tissues by WR-2721 during Fractionated Irradiation. Int J Rad Oncol Biol Phys 1:699-703, 1976.

65. Utley JF, Marlowe C and Waddell WJ: Distribution of ^{35}S-Labelled WR-2721 in Normal and Malignant Tissues of the Mouse. Rad Research 68:284-291, 1976.

66. Yuhas JM and Storer JB: Chemoprotection Against Three Modes of Radiation Death in the Mouse. Int J Rad Biol 15:233-237, 1969.

67. Phillips TL, Kane L, Utley JF: Radioprotection of Tumor and Normal Tissues by Thiophosphate Compounds. Cancer 32:528-535, 1973.

68. Yuhas JM, Yurconic M, Kligerman MM, West G, Peterson DF: Combined use of Radioprotective and Radiosensitizing Drugs in Experimental Radiotherapy. Rad Res 70:433-443, 1977.

69. Ellis F: Dose, Time and Fractionation: A Clinical Hypothesis. Radiol 20:1-7, 1967.

70. Dixon RL: General Equation for the Calculation of Nominal Standard Dose. Acta Radiol Ther Phys Biol 11:305-311, 1972.

71. Scanlon PW: Initial Experiences with Split-dose Periodic Radiation Therapy. Am J Roentgenol 84:632-644, 1960.

72. Sambrook DK: Split-Course Radiation Therapy in Malignant Tumors. Am J Roentgenol 91:37-45, 1965.

73. Levitt SH, Bogardus CR and Ladd G: Split-dose Intensive Radiation Therapy in the Treatment of Advanced Lung Cancer: A Randomized Study. Radiol 88:1159-1161, 1967.

74. Holsti LR: Clinical Experience With Split-Course Radiotherapy. A Randomized Clinical Trial. Radiol 92:591-596, 1969.

75. Abramson N and Cavanaugh PJ: Short-course Radiation Therapy in Carcinoma of the Lung. Radiol 96:627-630, 1970.

76. Abramson N and Cavanaugh PJ: Short-course Radiation Therapy in Carcinoma of the Lung: A Second Look. Radiol 108:685-687, 1973.

77. Guthrie RT, Ptacek JJ and Hass AC: Comparative Analysis of Two regimens of Split-Course Radiation in Carcinoma of the Lung. Am J Roentgenol 117:605-608, 1973.

78. Hazra TA, Chandrasekaran MS, Colman M, Prempree T and Inalsingh A: Survival in Carcinoma of the Lung After a Split-Course of Radiotherapy. Br J Radiol 47:464-466, 1974.

79. Scruggs H, El-Mahdi A, Marks RD and Constable WC: The Results of Split-Course Radiation Therapy in Cancer of the Lung. Am J Roentgenol 121:754-760, 1974.

80. Cox JD, Byhardt RW, Wilson JF, Komaki P, Eisert DR and Greenberg M: Dose-Time Relationship and Local Control of Small Cell Carcinoma of the Lung. Radiol 128:205-207, 1978.

81. Perez CA, Stanley K, Rubin P, Kramer S, Brady L, Perez-Tamayo R, Brown S, Concannon J, Rotman M and Seydel HG: Prospective Radnomized Study of Various Irradiation Doses and Fractionation Schedules in the Treatment of Inoperable Non-Oat Cell Carcinoma of the Lung. Preliminary Report by the Radiation Therapy Oncology Group. Cancer 45:2744-2753, 1980.

82. Holsti L: Long Term Results of Split-Course Radiation Therapy of Lung Cancer: A Randomized Study Presented at the EORTC Symposium on Progress and Prospectives in

Lung Cancer Treatment, Brussels, Belgium, May 3-5, 1979 Int J Rad Oncol Biol and Phys 6:977-981, 1980.

83. Keller BE, Salazar OM, Rubin P: Radiation Myelitis in the Treatment of Lung Cancer. Accepted for publication in Cancer 1979.

84. Ellis F and Goldson AL: Once a Week Treatments. Int J Rad Oncol Biol Phys 2:537-548, 1977.

85. Elkind MM, Withers HR and Belli JA: Intracellular Repair and The Oxygen Effect in Radiobiology and Radiotherapy. Front Rad Ther Oncol 3:55-58, 1968.

86. Aristizabal S: Discussion Remarks. In: Proceedings of Conference on the Time-Dose Relationship in Clinical Radiotherapy. Caldwell WL and Middleton DD (eds) Madison Printing and Publishing, Middleton, Wisconsin 1977, p 189.

87. Dvivedi M and Prahdan DG: Immediate Results of Weekly Fractionation in external Radiotherapy. Int J Rad Oncol Biol Phys 4:573-578, 1978.

88. Greenberg M, Eisert DR and Cox JD: Initial Evaluation of Reduced Fractionation in the Irradiation of Malignant Epithelial Tumors. Am J Roentgenol 126:268-271, 1976.

89. Schumacher W: The Use of High-Energy Electrons in the Treatment of Inoperable Lung and Bronchogenic Carcinoma. In: High Energy Photons and Electrons. Kramer S (ed) John Wiley and Sons, New York 1976, p 257-284.

90. Ellis F: Letter: The NSD Concept and Radioresistant Tumors. Br J Radiol 47:909, 1974.

91. Churchill-Davidson I: Oxygen Therapy Clinical Experience. In: Modern Trends in Radiotherapy. Deeley TJ and Woods APC (eds) Butterowrth, London 1967, p. 73-91.

92. Pfahler GE: The Saturation Method in Roentgentherapy as Applied to Deep-Seated Malignant Disease. Br J Radiol 31:45-58, 1926.

93. Holsti LR, Salmo M, and Elkind MM: Unconventional Fractionation in Clinical Radiotherapy. Br J Cancer 37:307-310, 1978.

94. Abe M: Improved Radiotherapy with Fractionation Irradiation. Presented at the 5th Joint Meeting on Lung Cancer of the United States-Japan Cooperative Research Program. Miami, Florida, February 1-2, 1979.

95. Brereton HD, Kent CH and Johnson RE: Chemotherapy and Radiation Therapy for Small Cell Carcinoma of the Lung: A Remedy for Past Therapeutic Failure. In: Lung Cancer: Progress in Therapeutic Research. Muggia FN and Rozencweiz M (eds). New York Raven Press, Progress in Cancer Research And Therapy Volume II: 575-586, 1979.

96. Salazar OM, Rubin P, Keller BE and Scarantino CW: Systemic (Half-Body) Radiation Therapy: Response and Toxicity. Int J Rad Oncol Biol Phys 4:937-950, 1978.

97. Chaoul H and Lange K: Verber. Lymphogranulomatose and Behandlung Mit Rotengestrahlen. Much Med Wochenschr 70:725-727, 1923.

98. Jenkin RDT, Rider WD and Sonley MJ: Ewing's Sarcoma: A Trial of Adjuvant Total Body Irradiation. Radiology 96:151-155, 1970.

99. Fitzpatrick PJ and Rider WD: Half-Body Radiotherapy of Advanced Lung Cancer. J Can Assoc Radiol 27:75-79, 1976.

100. Fitspatrick PJ and Rider WD: Half-Body Radiotherapy. Int J Rad Oncol Biol Phys 1:197-207, 1976.

101. Rubin P, Scarantino CW: The Bone Marrow Organ: The Critical Structure in Radiation – Drug Interaction. Int J Radiol Biol Phys 4:3-23, 1978.

102. Sacks EL, Goris ML, Glatstein E, Gilbert E, Kaplan HS: Bone Marrow Regneration Following Large Field Radiation. Cancer 42:1057-1065, 1978.

103. Sykes MP, Chu FCH, Savel H, Bonnadonna G, Mathis H: The Effects of Varying Dosages of Irradiation Upon Sternal Marrow Regeneration. Radiology 83:1084-1087, 1964.

104. Knospe WH, Blorn J, Crosby WH: Regeneration of Locally Irradiated Bone Marrow. 1 Dose-dependent, Long-term Changes in the Rad with Particular Emphais upon Vascular and Stromal Reaction. Blood 28:398-415, 1966.

105. Lajtha LG: Haemopoietic Stem Cells. Brit J Haematol 29:529-535, 1975.
106. Rubin P: Regeneration of Bone Marrow in Rabbits Following Local Fractionated Irradiation. Cancer 32:847-852, 1973.
107. Fryer CJH, Fitzpatrick PJ, Ricer WD and Poon P: Radiation Pneumonitis: Experience following a Large Single Dose of Radiation. Int J Rad Oncol Biol Phys 4:931-936, 1978.
108. Rubin P: The Radiotherapeutic Approach: Reappraisal and Prospects In: Lung Cancer: Progress in Therapeutic Research. Muggia F, and Rozencweig M (eds). New York Raven Press, 1979, p 33-340.
109. Salazar OM, Creech RH, Rubin P, Bennett JM, Mason BA, Young JJ, Scarantino CW and Catalano RB: Half-Body and Local Chest Irradiation as Consolidation following Response to Standard Induction Chemotherapy for Disseminated Small Cell Lung Cancer – An Eastern Cooperative Oncology Group Pilot Report. Proc Am Soc Ther Radiol Int J Rad Oncol Biol Phys 5:60, 1979. Int J Rad Oncol Biol Phys 6:1093-1102, 1980.
110. Moosavi H, McDonald SC, Rubin P, Cooper R, Stuart ID and Penny D: Early Radiation Response in Lung: An Ultrastructural Study. Int J Rad Oncol Biol Phys 2:921–932, 1977.
111. Rubin P: Radiation Toxicology: Quantitative Radiation Pathology for Predicting Effects. Cancer 39:729-736, 1976.
112. Rubin P, Shapiro DL, Finkelstein JN and Penny DP: The Early Release of Surfactant Following Irradiation of the Alveolar Type II Cells. Proc Am Soc Ther Radiol Int J Rad Oncol Biol Phys 5:58, 1979.
113. Michaelson SM and Schreiner BF: Cardiopulmonary Effects of Upper Body X-Irradiation in the Dog. Rad Res 47:168-181, 1971.
114. Schreiner BF, Michaelson SM and Yuile CL: The Effects of Thoracic Irradiation Upon Cardiopulmonary Function in the Dog. Am Rev Resp Dis 99:205-218, 1969.
115. Weir GS and Michaelson SM: Pulmonary Radiation Reactions. Springfield Illinois, Charles C Thomas, 1971, p 36-41.
116. McDonald SC, Keller BE and Rubin P: Method for Calculating Dose Where Lung Tumor Lies in the Treatment Field. Med Phys 2:210-216, 1976.
117. Urtasun Raul, Personal Communication on 8/27/79 – 'A Pilot Study for the Comparison of the Use of Systemic Radiation Therapy versus a Course of Simultaneous Polychemotherapy with Debulking of Gross Disease in Oat Cell Carcinoma of the Lung Studying in those Patients Receiving Systemic Radiation, The Effects of using or not the Radiosensitizer Misonidazole (RO-07-0582).' Edmonton, Alberta, Canada.
118. Veronessi V, Bonadonna G and Ravasi G (Study Coordinators). Instituto Nationale Tumori, Milano, Italy. NCI registered Protocol No. 7705. 'Protocol for the Treatment of Small Cell Bronchogenic Carcinoma (Limited and Minimal Extensive Disease).' Milan, Italy.
119. Rubin P, Perez CA and Keller B: The Logical Basis of Radiation Treatment Policies in the Multidisciplinary Approach to Lung Cancer. In: Lung Cancer Natural History, Prognosis and Treatment. Israel L and Chahinian AP (eds) Academic Press, New York 1976, p 160-199.
120. Phillips TL and Miller RJ: Should Asymptomatic Patients with inoperable Bronchogenic Carcinoma Receive Immediate Radiotherapy? Yes – An editorial Am Rev Resp Dis 117:405-410, 1978.
121. Bromley LL and Szur L: Combined Radiotherapy and Resection of Carcinoma of the Bronchus: Experience with 66 Patients. Lancet 2:937-941, 1955.
122. Bloedorn FG, Cowley RA, Cuccia CA, Mercado Jr, R, Wizenberg MJ and Linberg FJ: Preoperative Irradiation in Bronchogenic Carcinoma. Am J Roentgenol 92:77-87, 1964.
123. Collaborative Study: Preoperative Irradiation of Cancer of the Lung: Preliminary Report of a Therapeutic Trial. Cancer 23:419-429, 1969.

124. Rissanen PM, Tikka V and Holsti LR: Autopsy Findings in Lung Cancer Treated with Megavoltage Radiotherapy. Acta Radiolog 7:433-442, 1968.
125. Pereslegin IA: Radiotherapy of Lung Cancer, Moscow: Meditsena, 1963.
126. Henschke VK: Techniques for Permanent Implantation of Radioisotopes. Radiology 68:256,1957.
127. Henschke VK: Interstitial Implantation in the Treatment of Primary Bronchogenic Carcinoma. Am J Roentg Rad Ther and Nucl Med 79:981-987, 1958.
128. Hilaris BS, Henschke VK and Holt JG: Clinical Experience with Long Half-Life and Low-Energy Encapsulated Radioactive Sources in Cancer Radiation Therapy. Radiology 91:1163-1167, 1968.
129. Hilaris BS and Martini N: Interstitial Brachytherapy in Cancer of the Lung: A 20-year experience. Accepted for publication Int J Rad Oncol Biol Phys (1980).
130. Dewey WC, Hopeood LE, Sapareto SA, Gerweck LE: Cellular Responses do Combinations of Hyperthermia and Radiation. Radiology 123:463-474, 1977.
131. Marmor JB, Pounds D, Postic TB, Habin GM: Treatment of Superficial Human Neoplasms by Local Hyperthermia Induced by Ultrasound. Cancer 43:188-197, 1979.
132. LeVeen HH, Wapnick S, Piccone V, Falk G, Ahmed N: Tumor Eradication by Radiofrequency Therapy. Response in 21 Patients. JAMA 235:2198-2200, 1976.
133. Hornback NC, Shupe R, Shiduia H, Joe BT, Sayoc E, George R, Marshall C: Radiation and Microwave Therapy in the Treatment of Advanced Cancer. Radiology 130:459-469, 1979.
134. Stehlin JS, Giovanella BC, deIlpolyi PD, Anderson RF: Results of Eleven Years Experience with Heated Perfusion for Melanoma of the Extremities. Cancer Res 39:2255-2257, 1979.
135. Suit HD, Gerweck LE: Potential for Hyperthermia and Radiation Therapy. Cancer Res 39:2290-2298, 1979.
136. Overgaard J, Bictrel P: The Influence of Hypoxia and Acidity on the Hyperthermic Response of Malignant Cells in Vitro. Radiology 123:511-514 1977.
137. Westra A, Dewey WC: Variation In Sensitivity to Heat Shock During the Cell Cycle of Chinese Hamster Cells in vitro. Int J Radiat Biol 19:467-477, 1971.
138. Gloner EW, Boone R, Connor WG, Hicks JA, Boone MLM: A Transient Thermotolerant Survival Response Produced by Single Thermal Doses in He La cells. Cancer Res 38:1035-1040, 1976.
139. Harisiadis L, Sung D, Hall EJ: Thermal Tolerance and Repair of Thermal Damage by Cultured Cells. Radiology 123:505-509, 1977.
140. Henle KJ, Leeper DB: Interaction of Hyperthermia and Radiation in CHO Cells: Recovery Kinetics. Rad Res 66:505-518, 1976.
141. Henle KJ, Dethlefsen LA: Heat Fractionation and Thermotolerance: A Review. Cancer Rec 38:1843-1851, 1978.
142. Leith JT, Miller RC, Gerner EW, Boone MLM: Hyperthermic Potentiation: Biological Aspects and Applications to Radiation Therapy. Cancer 39::766-779, 1977.
143. Henle KJ, Leeper DB: The Modifications of Radiation Damage in CHO Cells by Hyperthermia at 40° and 45 °C. Radiat Res 70:415-424, 1977.
144. Nielsen OS, Overgaard J: Hyperthermic Radiosensitization of Thermotolerant Tumor Cells in vitro. Int J Radiat Biol 35:171-177, 1979.
145. Storm FK, Harrison WH, Elliott RS, Merton DL: Normal Tissue and Solid Tumor Effects of Hyperthermia in Animal Models and Clinical Trials. Cancer Res 39:2245-2251, 1979.
146. Mantyla MJ: Regional Blood Flow in Human Tumors. Cancer Res 39:2304-2306, 1979.
147. Atkinson ER: Assessment of Current Hyperthermia Technology. Cancer Res 39:2313-2324, 1979.

148. Mendecki J, Friedenthal E, Botstein C, Sterzer F, Paglione R, Newogrodzki M, Berek E: Microwave-induced Hyperthermia in Cancer Treatment: Apparatus and Preliminary Results. Int J Radiat Oncol Biol Phys 4:1095-1103, 1978.

149. Christensen DA: Thermal Dosimetry and Temperature Measurements. Cancer Res 39: 2325-2327, 1979.

150. Kim JH, Hahn EW, Tokita N: Combination Hyperthermia and Radiation Therapy for Cutaneous Malignant Melanoma. Cancer 41:2143-2148, 1978.

151. Sugaar S, LeVeen HH: A Histopathologic Study on the Effects of Radiofrequency Thermo-therapy on Malignant Tumors of the Lung. Cancer 43:767-783, 1979.

152. The Radiation Oncology Research Program – Recommended Research Proposals by the Radiation Oncology Coordination Subcommittee (ROCS) U.S. Dpt H.E.W. Int J Rad Oncol Biol Phys 5:757-773, 1979.

153. Whithers HR: Biological Basis for High-LET Radiotherapy Beam. Med Phys 4:379-386, 1977.

154. Laramore GE, Griffin TW, Gerdes AJ and Parker RG: Fast Neutron and Mixed (Neutron/ Photon) Beam Teletherapy for Grades III and IV Astrocytomas. Cancer 42:96-103, 1978.

155. Catteral M, Bloom HJG, Ash DV, Walsh L, Richardson A, Uttley D, Gowing NFG, Lewis P and Chaucer B: Fast Neutrons with Supratentorial Glioblastomas: A Control Pilot Study. Int J Rad Oncol Biol Phys (In press) 1980.

156. Griffin TW, Laramore GE, Parker RG, Gerdes AJ, Hevard DW, Blasko JC and Groudine M: An Evaluation of Fast Neutron Beam Teletherapy of Metastatic Cervical Adenopathy from Squamous Cell Carcinomas of the Head and Neck Region. Cancer (in press) 1979.

157. Catteral M, Bewley DK and Sutherland I: Second Report on Results of a Randomized Clinical Trial of Fast Neutrons Compared with X or Gamma rays in the Treatment of Advanced Tumors of the Head and Neck. Br Med J 1:1642-1652, 1977.

158. Salinas R, Hussey DH, Peters LJ and Fletcher GH: Experience in Treating Sarcomas with 50 MeV$_{d \to Be}$ Fast Neutrons. Proc Am Soc Ther Rad (ASTR) Int J Rad Oncol Biol Phys 4:92, 1978.

159. Herskovic A, Lee S, Scheer, A and Ornitz R: Fast Neutron Experience: Epidermoid Carcinoma of the Upper Aerodigestive Tract. Proc Am Soc Ther Rad (ASTR) Int J Rad Oncol Biol Phys 5:53, 1979.

160. Henry LW, Blasko JC and Griffin TW: Evaluation of Fast Neutron Teletherapy for Advanced Carcinomas of the Major Salivary Glands. Proc Am Soc Ther Rad (ASTR) Int J Rad Oncol Biol Phys 4:95, 1978.

161. Nelson JSR, Caprenter RE and Parker RG: Response of Mouse Skin and the C3HBA Mammary Carcinoma of the CdH Mouse to x-rays and Cyclotron Neutrons: Effect of Mixed Neutron-Photon Fractionation Schemes. Europ J Cancer 11:891-901, 1975.

162. Rasey JS, Carpenter RE, Nelson NJ and Parker RG: Cure of EMT-6 Tumors by x-rays or Neutrons: Effect of Mixed and Fractionation Schemes. Radiology 123:207-212, 1977.

163. Laramore GE, Blasko JC, Griffin TW and Groudine MT: Fast Neutron Teletherapy for Advanced Carcinomas of the Oropharynx. Proc Am Soc Ther Rad (ASTR) Int J Rad Oncol Biol Phys 4:94-95, 1978.

164. Radiation Therapy Oncology Group (RTOG) – Protocol 79-07: Phase III Randomized Proto-col to Study Fast Neutron and Mixed Beam (Neutron/Photon) Radiation Therapy in the Treatment of Localized, Inoperable Non-Oat Cell Cancer of the Lung (Squamous cell, Adenocarcinoma and Large Cell Undifferentiated Type) Activated July 9, 1979 and avail-able from RTOG Operations Office, Thomas Jefferson University Hospital, 1015 Walnut Street, Philadelphia, Pennsylvania 19107, ·USA.

165. Steel GG: Terminology in the Description of Drug-Radiation Interactions. Int J Rad Oncol Biol Phys 5:1145-1150, 1979.

166. Rubin P, Salazar OM: The Research Logic of Radiation Oncology in Combined Modality Therapy. Cancer Treat Rep (in press) 1980.
167. Bitran JD, Desser RK, DeMeester TR *et al.*: Cyclophosphamide, Adriamycin, Methotrexate And Procarbazine (CAMP) – Effective Four Drug Combination Chemotherapy for Metastatic Non-Oat Cell Bronchogenic Carcinoma. Cancer Treat Rep 60:1225-1230, 1976.
168. Bitran JD, Desser RD, DeMeester TR *et al.*: Combined Modality Therapy for Stage III Mo Non-Oat Cell Bronchogenic Carcinoma. Cancer Treat Rep 62:327-332, 1978.
169. Ruckdeschel JC, Baxter DH, McKneally MF, Killam DA, Lunia SL and Horton J: Sequential Radiotherapy and Adriamycin in the Management of Bronchogenic Carcinoma: The Question of Additive Toxicity. Int J Rad Oncol Biol Phys 5:1323-1328, 1979.
170. Rubin P, Cassarett G: Clinical Radiation Pathology, Vol 1 and 2 Philadelphia, Pennsylvania, WB Saunders, 1968.
171. Penny DP, Rubin P: Specific Early Fine Structural Changes in the Lung Following Irradiation. Int J Rad Oncol Biol Phys 2:1123-1132, 1977.
172. Phillips TL and FU KK: Quantification of Combined Radiotherapy and Chemotherapy Effects on Critical Normal Tissues. Cancer 37:1186-1200, 1976.
173. Phillips TL, Wharam MD and Margolis LW: Modifications of Radiation Injury to Normal Tissues by Chemotherapeutic Agents. Cancer 35:1678-1684, 1975.
174. Rubin P: Radiation Toxicology: Quantitative Radiation Pathology for Predicting Effects. Cancer 39 (Suppl 2)::729-736, 1977.
175. The Radiation Oncology Research Program: Recommended Research Proposals. Rubin P, Cowen RB and Rubin DJ (eds). Int J Rad Oncol Biol Phys 5:677-298, 1979.

10. Pathology of Small Cell Carcinoma of The Lung and Its Subtypes. A Clinico-Pathologic Correlation

MARY J. MATTHEWS and ADI F. GAZDAR

INTRODUCTION

Remarkable strides have been made in the past several years in our understanding of the clinical behavior, pathology and cell biology of small cell carcinoma of the lung (SCCL). An increasing number of patients with this disease, treated by multiple variable modalities, have had prolonged disease free survivals and may be considered potentially cured [1–4]. Pathologists have come to appreciate the diverse nature of this tumor. A remarkable degree of consistency in diagnosis of lung cancer has become possible among pathologists who accept basic morphologic criteria of lung cancer types. In spite of this, a small percentage of SCCL tumors provoke widely disparate diagnoses. This has been particularly true of tumors which, although predominantly small cell in type, show features of anaplastic large cell malignancies. There is an awareness, also, that morphologic changes can occur in these tumors following chemotherapy and/or radiotherapy. Changes not only in the histologic subtyping but in the histologic typing of the tumor have been observed in posttherapeutic biopsy and autopsy materials [5–9]. Biochemical markers produced by the tumors can be identified and quantified [10–12]. Evidence suggests that biochemical markers may be lost, *in vivo*, following therapy and that the loss may correspond to alterations in the morphology of the tumor [9]. Similar markers may be found in cell cultures or nude mice heterotransplants of these tumors [13]. Alterations in morphology and loss of biochemical markers are being observed in small cell tumors following multiple passages of the tumor through nude mice [14].

Subjects to be addressed in this chapter include: the morphologic criteria for typing and subtyping of small cell carcinoma of the lung and its distinction from large cell carcinoma; clinical and experimental studies of SCCL, which relate to subtyping of this tumor and the significance of mixed cell components. Problems that persist in the diagnosis of this tumor will be

R.B. Livingston (ed.), Lung cancer 1, 283–306. All rights reserved.

discussed. The significance of morphologic changes that occur following therapy and factors associated with long term survivors of SCCL will be briefly summarized.

MORPHOLOGY OF SMALL CELL CARCINOMA OF THE LUNG

Background

Small cell carcinoma of the lung was distinguished as a carcinoma rather than an 'oat-celled sarcoma' of the mediastinum by Barnard in 1926 [15]. In the subsequent 54 years, it is doubtful that anyone, with the possible exception of Azzopardi [16], has described more precisely the pathology of this tumor. It is worthwhile to briefly summarize Barnard's report to put in perspective the confusion that still exists concerning the subtypes of this tumor.

Concerning the incidence of the disease, Barnard noted that the 'oat-celled' tumor was encountered more frequently than the 'horny' squamous cell type of lung cancer. Twelve of the 19 cases that constituted his report were of the oat cell type. The tumors metastasized widely and, in particular, to the brain, liver, pancreas, adrenals, kidneys and bone. Barnard recognized the malignant oat cells looked like lymphocytes, but clustered and were somewhat larger and slightly more 'oaty' in contour, depending on the plane of the cut. He noted that if the same tumor were cut transversely, cells appeared to have a more fusiform, spindled or polygonal appearance. Some tumors had foci of cuboidal cells which formed discrete tubules. Multinucleated giant cells were also described. The clustering of cells and tubule formation convinced him that the 'oat-celled sarcoma' was, in fact, a carcinoma.

The World Health Organization (WHO) classification of small cell carcinoma of the lung, published in 1967 [17], was faithful to Barnard's microscopic description. Each variable shape was made a subtype, i.e., fusiform, polygonal, lymphocyte-like and others (to include tumors forming tubules, squamous nests or giant cells). There has been skepticism about these subtypes ever since. In three editions of 'Pathology of the Lung' from 1962 through 1977, Spencer has combined the polygonal cell with large cell anaplastic carcinomas, feeling that both probably represent anaplastic squamous cell malignancies [18–20]. In 1973, members of the pathology committee of the Working Party for Therapy of Lung Cancer (WP-L) devised a classification [21], compatible with the 1967 WHO lung cancer classification, as well as the Veterans Administration Lung Study Group (VALG) classification [22]. In the WP-L classification, the lymphocyte subtype was segregated from the three other subtypes. The latter were placed in an intermediate category, implying a possible continuum between the small and large cell anaplastic malignancies.

Table 1. Small cell carcinoma of the lung – WHO (1967, 1977) and WP-L histologic classifications.

WHO		WP-L
II. Small cell carcinoma		20 Small cell carcinoma
1967	1977	1973
II.1 Fusiform	II.1 Oat-cell	21 Lymphocyte-like
II.2 Polygonal	II.2 Intermediate	22 Intermediate
II.3 Lymphocyte-like	II.3 Combined	
II.4 Others		
IV. Large cell carcinoma		40 Large cell carcinoma

WHO = World Health Organization,
WP-L = Working Party for Therapy of Lung Cancer.

It was not known at the time whether, in fact, there was a difference in histogenesis, behavior or response to therapy of this more heterogeneous group of tumors. The 1977 WHO classification of lung tumors has adopted this intermediate subtype [23]. In addition, those rare tumors showing frank small cell carcinoma, admixed with squamous cell carcinoma or adenocarcinoma, have been designated as 'combined' small cell tumors. Table 1 compares the 1967 and 1977 WHO lung cancer classifications. The WP-L version is included to distinguish numerically the subtypes used in this paper.

Histologic Criteria of Small Cell Carcinoma

Small cell carcinomas, regardless of subtype, share multiple common features by light and electron microscopy [24]. The most significant diagnostic features of small cell tumors, by light microscopy, are found in the nucleus. In cells in which nuclear characteristics are preserved, nuclear chromatin is distributed in a uniform fine or coarse stippled pattern throughout the entire nucleus. Nucleoli are small and indistinct. Rare prominent nucleoli may be observed per low power field. Numerous mitoses are present. These nuclear features are present regardless of the size or shape of the nucleus or of the cell itself. The majority of cells have meager cytoplasm, resulting in molding and contouring of adjoining nuclei. Cells are arranged in variable patterns, supported by a thin vascular fibrous stroma. The stroma is usually devoid of significant inflammatory infiltrate. In areas of extensive necrosis, there may be staining of preexisting elastic fibrils, particularly of blood vessel walls, by Feulgen positive DNA material [16, 25]. This phenomenon has rarely been described in any tumor except the small cell carcinoma. It is therefore considered almost diagnostic of this tumor when present. Crushing artifact is frequently seen in small biopsies.

In cytologic specimens, neoplastic cells are 2–3 times larger than lymphocytes, cluster, have oval molded nuclei and indistinct cytoplasmic structures. Nuclear characteristics are similar to those described above. The clustering and molding of cells can be reliably identified in cytologic specimens fixed with Saccomanno solution and processed by direct cytocentrifugation in almost all body fluids except sputa.

In electron micrographs, Mackay was unable to distinguish even subtle differences between subtypes of small cell tumors. Nuclei of either subtype are round or ovoid, have diffuse finely dispersed chromatin particles and inconspicuous nucleoli. Cytoplasm is scant and organelles are sparse. Cell membranes are closely apposed and occasionally adjoined by desmosomes. A relatively small number of cells contain membrane bound granules, usually in the pseudopodal processes of the cytoplasm [24].

Lymphocyte/Oat Cell Subtype (WP-L #21)

In this subtype, neoplastic cells tend to be small, round or oval in shape and arranged in grape-like clusters (Fig. 1). In many tumors, particularly in small biopsies, cells have dense hyperchromatic nuclei devoid of distinguishable characteristics. Cytoplasm is indistinct and nuclei frequently appear naked. Mitoses in this setting are difficult to identify. Cells may form anastomosing cords, sheets or pseudorosettes about small vascular channels. Diagnostic difficulties may be encountered in biopsies which show extensive crushing. Likewise, it may be difficult to exclude lymphomas from small biopsies which show a diffuse infiltration of small lymphocytoid cells which do not nest or mold and which are not supported by a vascular stroma.

Difficulties may also occur in cytologic diagnoses of small cell tumors. Single cells, approximately the size of a lymphocyte, with oval naked nuclei and indistinct nuclear characteristics, cannot be relied upon for diagnostic purposes. Clusters of hyperplastic reserve cells can be distinguished from neoplastic cells. The former cells are smaller, have oval uniform nuclei and show little or no nuclear molding because of intervening distinct cytoplasmic processes.

Intermediate Subtype (WP-L #22)

Cells in this subtype tend to be larger than subtype #21. Nuclear shapes are variable, from oval to rounded to spindled or fusiform in type (Fig. 2, 3). Occasional syncytial giant cells may be identified. Cytoplasm may be moderate in amount, particularly in the polygonal variant. Rarely, these tumors may be associated with a fibrotic stroma. The arrangement of the cells is as varied as the nuclear size and shape, giving the tumors a somewhat pleomorphic rather than monotonous appearance. Cells may be arranged in stratifying sheets or pseudoductal structures, with palisading of nuclei about the periphe-

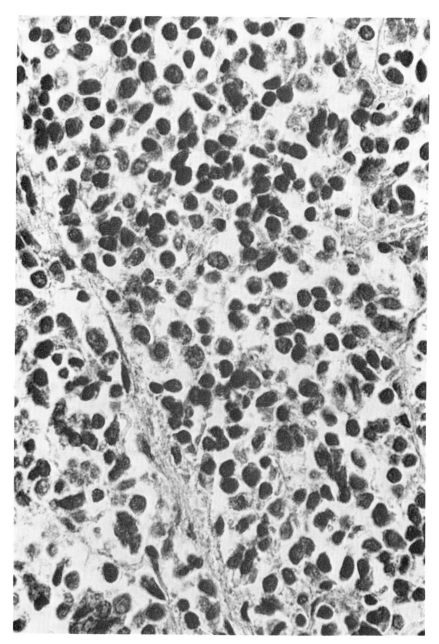

Fig. 1. Small cell carcinoma, lymphocyte-like type. Note vascular stroma, cohesion of cells and molding of nuclei. H & E X400.

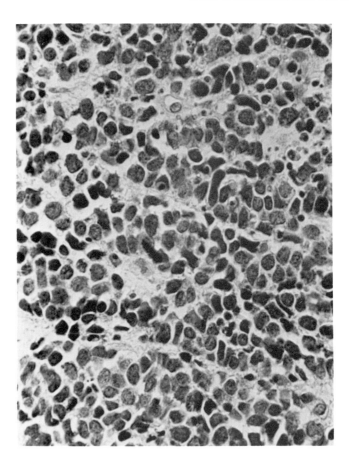

Fig. 2

ry of the sheets and central zones of necrosis. Cells may also be arranged in compact nests, cords, ribbons or trabeculae, separated by vascular or sinusoidal networks. In foci, cells may be cuboidal to columnar in type, form tubules or glands and may rarely secrete intraluminal mucin[16, 20]. Small nests of mature keratinized squamous cells may be identified within small cell tumors, particularly in posttherapeutic materials. The squamous element frequently has a metaplastic rather than neoplastic appearance. Diagnostic difficulties arise in pretreatment materials if tubular or glandular foci, amid a diffuse small cell proliferation, are interpreted as adenocarcinoma, or stratifying pseudoductal structures or squamous nests are interpreted as evidence of squamous cell carcinoma. Tumors predominantly composed of fusiform or polygonal elements with moderate amounts of cytoplasm are, on occasion, interpreted as anaplastic large cell carcinoma. Occasional fusiform tumors may be difficult to distinguish from atypical carcinoids.

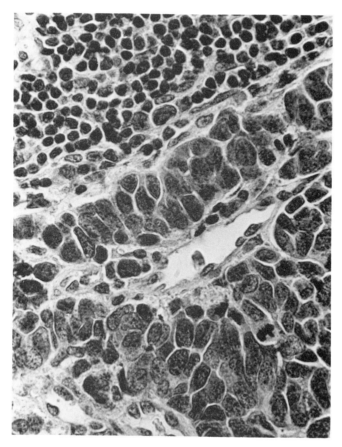

Fig. 3

Fig. 2 and 3. Small cell carcinoma, intermediate type. Note enlarged variable sized vesicular nuclei, diffuse nuclear chromatin distribution, scanty cytoplasm and indistinct cytoplasmic margins. Lymphocytes in stroma of Figure #3 emphasize size of neoplastic cells. H & E X400.

The appearance of polygonal, fusiform and tubular components may be an integral and dimensional aspect of oat cell or lymphocyte like tumors. For this reason, the 1977 WHO lung cancer classification recommends that tumors composed of elements of subtype #21 and #22 be classified as subtype #21 for diagnostic purposes [23].

Large Cell Carcinoma of the Lung (WP-L #40)

Large cell carcinomas of the lung have been defined as anaplastic or undifferentiated epithelial malignancies which show no evidence of maturation to form squamous or glandular structures by light microscopy. Individul cells have enlarged irregular nuclei, show clearing of nuclear chromatin, prominent nucleoli on low power magnification and variable but often abun-

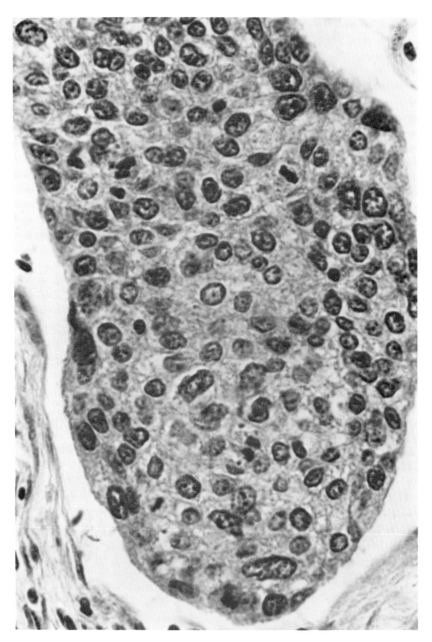

Fig. 4. Large cell carcinoma. Cells have prominent cytoplasm and cytoplasmic membranes, and prominent nucleoli; nuclei show clearing of nuclear chromatin. H & E X400.

dant amounts of cytoplasm. The cells are usually arranged in sheets, solid nests or cords. The stroma is frequently abundant and diffusely infiltrated by lymphocytes and plasma cells (Fig. 4).

Small Cell Carcinoma with Large Cell Component (WP-L #22/40)

A small percentage of small cell lung tumors have, as a component, features of anaplastic large cell carcinoma (WP-L #40). At the National Cancer Institute-Veterans Administration Medical Oncology Branch (NCI-VA MOB), this subset has been designated mixed small cell-large cell carcinoma (subtype #22/40). The tumor is predominantly an intermediate small cell neoplasm, with characteristic nuclear features and molding. Enlarged cells may be recognized with abundant cytoplasm, distinct cytoplasmic margins, enlarged nuclei, irregular nuclear contours and prominent amphophilic nucleoli. They occur as multiple isolated cells or in discrete nodular foci. Nuclei may show clearing or dense clumping of chromatin. As has been mentioned, single cells with prominent nucleoli may be identified infrequently in all small cell tumors. The discrete clustering and the repeated occurrence of these cells through multiple high power fields suggest a significant large cell component (Figs. 5, 6).

Cytologic specimens frequently confirm the mixed nature of these tumors. Numerous single neoplastic cells with enlarged nuclei, prominent nucleoli and distinct cytoplasm can be identified. Clusters of classic small cells are also present.

The 1977 WHO Lung Cancer Classification recognizes the existence of tumors with focal large cell components and has recommended that they be included in the intermediate subtype for diagnostic purposes [23]. Azzopardi also distinguished anaplastic foci in small cell tumors. He felt that they were secondary modifications of the tumor and that they represented squamoid foci [16]. In review of treatment data at the NCI-VA MOB, it was recognized that patients with tumors designated as #22/40 had better objective response rates than patients with non-small cell tumors, but lower response rates and shorter survival times than patients with subtypes #21 or #22. To better understand the natural history and biology of this subset, patients with this diagnosis have been staged and treated on small cell protocols but have been evaluated separately for the past three years [26].

SMALL CELL CARCINOMA: CLINICAL AND EXPERIMENTAL STUDIES

Clinical Studies

In the past 7 years, the NCI-VA MOB has attempted to evaluate the significance of subtyping of SCCL. During this period, approximately 360

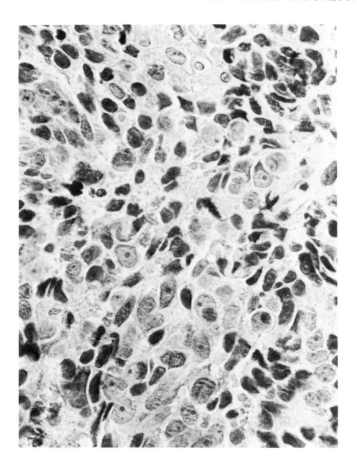

Fig. 5

patients have been staged and treated on various small cell protocols. Subtyping of tumors has been based on the most adequate diagnostic material available. Preference in subtyping has been given to materials obtained from the lung and/or bronchi over tissues taken from metastatic sites [27]. Mediastinal and cervical lymph node biopsies were occasionally considered more optimal for subtyping purposes than needle biopsies of the lung or small crushed bronchial biopsies. Of the classic small cells, 52% were classified as subtype #21; 40% as subtype #22 and 8% as subtype #21/22. The latter groups have been combined with subtype #21 for the purposes of this report. Of the 360 cases, 22 (6%) were classified as #22/40. Of the total number, 121 previously untreated patients, including 18 with a designation of #22/40, were entered on protocols requiring high dose polychemotherapy induction, with or without subsequent radiotherapy, from 1973 through 1977 [28, 29].

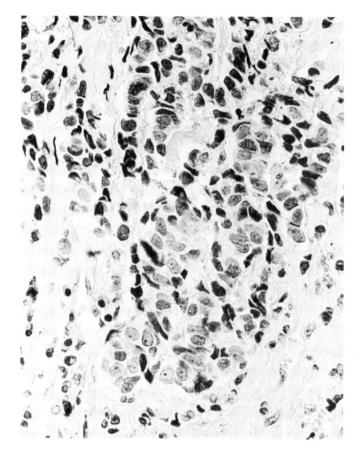

Fig. 6

Fig. 5 and 6. Small cell carcinoma with large cell component. Note cell clusters with oval nuclei, prominent nucleoli and abundant cytoplasm, separated by classic small cells. H & E X400.

Patient characteristics, performance status, extent of disease at presentation and response to therapy have been recorded according to subtype. Extensive staging and follow up procedures were performed on all patients and have been reported elsewhere [28, 29]. Regional disease was defined as tumor confined to the lung, mediastinum and ipsilateral supraclavicular lymph nodes, encompassed by a tolerable radiation port. Extensive disease was defined as tumor in the contralateral lung or other extrathoracic sites. Complete response was defined as absence of identifiable tumor after extensive restaging procedures. Partial response was defined as a greater than 50% decrease in the product of the perpendicular diameters of a measurable tumor. The performance status standards of Zubrod were used [30].

Table 2 enumerates patients' age and sex, performance status, extent of disease at presentation and response to therapy according to cell subtype.

Table 2. Small cell carcinoma of the lung – patient characteristics, performance status, extent of disease and response to therapy, according to cell subtypes.

	Subtype		
	#21 (n-62)	#22 (n-41)	#22/40 (n-18)
Age	56.0 (range 36-74)		52.5 (range 38-63)
Sex	M : F 5.5 : 1		M : F 5 : 1
PS − 1	31 (50%)	23 (56%)	10 (56%)
− 2	21 (34%)	12 (30%)	4 (22%)
− 3	7 (11%)	6 (14%)	4 (22%)
− 4	3 (05%)		
Extent of disease			
LD	20 (32%)	12 (30%)	4 (22%)
ED	42 (68%)	29 (70%)	14 (78%)
Response to therapy			
CR	27 (42%)	20 (50%)	3 (17%)
PR	29 (45%)	17 (41%)	7 (39%)
NC	6 (10%)	4 (09%)	4 (22%)
PD	0	0	4 (22%)

PS – Performance status; LD – local disease; ED – extensive disease; CR – complete response; PR – partial response; NC – no change; PD – progressive disease; # – refers to WP-L designation.

There is no statistical difference in the first three parameters. Although the decrease in objective response rate in patients with subtype #22/40 is statistically significant and striking (56% as compared to 87–91%), this response is clearly better than what may be expected of non-small cell tumors.

Table 3 lists involvement of liver, bone marrow and central nervous system at presentation, according to cell subtype. Again, no significant difference in metastatic behavior can be appreciated. Subtyping of tumors varied frequently

Table 3. Small cell carcinoma of the lung – metastatic sites of tumor at presentation, according to subtype.

Site	Subtype		
	#21 (n-62)	#22 (n-41)	#22/40 (n-18)
Bone marrow biopsy +	12 (20%)	9 (22%)	6 (33%)
Liver biopsy and/or scan +	15 (25%)	14 (34%)	6 (33%)
CNS scan +	7 (11%)	1 (02%)	3 (17%)

NB: Other documented sites of metastases, such as lymph nodes, chest wall, skin or subcutaneous tissues are not included in this table. #-refers to WP-L designation.

Table 4. Small cell carcinoma of the lung – median survival as correlated with performance status, extent of disease, response to therapy and cell subtypes.

Survival	#21 + #22 (n-103)			22/40 (n-18)		
	Median	1 yr	2 yrs	Median	1 yr	2 yrs
Overall	10.2 months	44%	12%	6.6 months	11%	6%
Performance status-1	17.5 months	60%	31%	7.1 months	6	6%
Limited disease	13.7 months	58%	16%	8.1 months	6%	—
Extensive disease	7.8 months	38%	25%	3.7 months	6%	6%
Objective response	11.8 months	48%	23%	7.4 months	11%	6%
Time to progression responders	9.0 months			3.9 months		

#-refers to WP-L designation.

from site to site. Thus, lung, lymph node and bronchial biopsies classified as #22/40 were, on occasion, associated with frank small cell tumors in bone marrow biopsies or in the cytology of bronchial washings [31]. Lung and bronchial biopsies classified as subtype #21 were frequently associated with lymph node, liver or bone marrow biopsies interpreted as subtype #22. In still other instances, patients with bronchial, lung or lymph node biopsies clasified as subtype #22 had bronchial washings or aspirates classified as #22/40.

Median survival times of patients with subtypes #21 and #22 were identical (10.2 months). These 2 subtypes, therefore, have been combined and are compared with subtype #22/40 for evaluation of survival data (Table 4). A decrease in median overall survival (6.6 months as compared to 10.2

Table 5. Small cell carcinoma of the lung – sites of organ involvement at autopsy, according to cell subtype.

Organ site	#21 + #22 (n-21) (%)	#22/40 (n-6) (%)
Lung	100	100
Lymph nodes	95	100
Pleura	62	33
Pericardium	29	33
Liver	81	83
Pancreas	19	33
Adrenals	67	83
CNS	61 (11/18)	33 (1/3)
Bone marrow	57	80 (4/5)

CNS-Central nervous system; #-refers to WP-L designation.

Table 6. Small cell carcinoma of the lung – long term survivors according to subtype.

Subtype	Survivors (n-97) (%)
#21	28
#21/22	16
#22	45
#22/40	10
#22/12*	1

#-WP-L designations; *-WHO-1977 classification II.3.

months) is noted in patients with subtype #22/40. More impressive is the relatively poor survival times of patients with this subtype who presented with good initial performance statuses and/or limited disease. Time to progression was shortened in these patients who showed objective responses (3.9 months as compared to 9 months). On the other hand, 2 patients with subtype #22/40 survived over one year and one of these patients is alive and without evidence of disease 2 1/2 years following onset of therapy.

Autopsy data on 21 patients with classic small cell malignancies and on 6 patients with subtype #22/40 have been compared. Table 5 lists predominant sites of tumor identified at autopsy in the two groups. No appreciable difference can be distinguished in metastatic behavior of the subtypes. Almost one-third of patients with classic small cell tumors showed evidence of anaplastic large cell, syncytial giant cell, occasional tubule, rare carcinoid or squamous cell alterations. In one of these patients, only an anaplastic large cell carcinoma with prominent giant cells could be identified at autopsy. All 6 patients with subtype #22/40 showed focal to diffuse large cell and syncytial giant cell formation. Tubule formation was identified in one and squamous cell proliferation in another. Some residual evidence of small cell tumor was present in all 6 cases.

Over the past 3 years, the National Cancer Institute has sponsored a registry to identify patients with SCCL who have survived over 2 1/2 years [1]. The purpose of the registry has been to identify factors associated with long term survival. To date, 97 patients have been evaluated. Table 6 lists the cell subtypes of these patients. Table 7 lists the modalities of therapy and survival data of the patients. It is apparent that all cell subtypes, including #22/40, are represented in the long term survivors. All modalities of therapy are associated with these survivals.

Experimental Studies

Experimental models have been developed at the NCI-VA MOB to study the biology of SCCL [13, 14]. Tumor materials, mainly from metastatic sites

Table 7. Small cell carcinoma of the lung – effects of therapy on long term survivals.

Treatment modality	Pt ※	Survival	
		5 yrs	10 yrs
Surgery	44	18 (16)*	14 (10)*
Alone	23	8 (6)	6 (6)
+RT	8	3 (3)	4
+CT	11	6 (6)	4
+CT/RT	2	1 (1)	
Radiotherapy	44	10 (6)	1 (1)
alone	19	7 (5)	1 (1)
+CT	25	3 (1)	
Chemotherapy alone	8	1 (1)	
Total	96	29 (23)	15 (11)

RT-radiotherapy; CT-chemotherapy.
* Patients alive and at risk at time of report.

and malignant pleural effusions, have been established as continuous cell lines or heterotransplanted subcutaneously into athymic nude mice. Nude mouse tumors develop at the site of injection and are either simple expansile lesions or show foci of local invasion. Distant metastases do not occur. Tumors are serially transplanted at 1–2 month intervals. Histologic examination is performed at each transplant. Continuous cell lines consist of floating cell aggregates which replicate slowly and clone in soft agarose at low efficiencies. Cytologic examination of the cultured cells is performed every few passages. Injection of cultured cells into nude mice results in tumor formation. The cultures and nude mouse tumors contain neurosecretory granules and have high intracellular levels of the key amine precursor uptake and decarboxylation (APUD) cell enzyme, dopa decarboxylase. Also, the cells fluoresce after exposure to hot formaldehyde vapor, indicating the presence of fluorogenic amines. Many cell lines and tumors release one or more hormones, including ACTH, calcitonin and arginine vasopressin. These studies confirm that the experimental models were derived from SCCL cells.

The initial histology of the nude mouse tumors and cytology of the cultured cells are identical in appearance to that of the intermediate subtype (# 22) of SCCL). Foci of necrosis are present in the larger tumors but DNA staining is rarely observed. The lymphocyte like subtype # 21 or mixed # 21/22 tumors are not observed. However, in ischemic and necrotic foci, obviously degenerating cells resemble the lymphocyte like cells. Foci of large cell carcinoma are not identified in the heterotransplanted tumor, except in the instances in which the patient's primary tumor was classified as #22/40. In experimental models maintained for more than 2 years, some or all of the cells in over half of the transplants have altered and resemble large cell anaplastic tumors (#40). These cells are larger than the average SCCL cell, have large nuclei and lack the stippled chromatin pattern or nuclear characteristics of SCCL cells. One or more prominent eosinophilic nucleoli are usually seen. Moderate amounts of cytoplasm are present and while the nuclear size is larger, its size, relative to the cytoplasmic diameter, is decreased. With continued passage, the percentages of large cells increase and approach 100% in some cases. Such changes suggest that the large cells have had a selective growth advantage over the small cells. Morphologic changes have been accompanied by biological and biochemical alterations. The large cells adhere to the substrate, replicate relatively faster and clone at higher efficiencies than the small cell. The large cells lack the APUD markers, i.e., dopa decarboxylase, neurosecretory granules, formaldehyde induced fluorescence and hormone secretion. Gland formation and squamous cells have not been noted in the experimental model.

DISCUSSION

Strong feelings have existed that there is a difference in behavior and response to therapy of patients with variable subtypes of SCCL. In the past several years, there have been reports suggesting that subtyping of SCCL has no prognostic value in determining patient response to therapy or survival [32–36]. Three early reports noted that prolonged survival times were found in patients with fusiform or polygonal tumor subtypes, as compared to the lymphocyte variant [37–39]. In three more recent reports, the lymphocyte subtype was considered to be more responsive to therapy than other subtypes [40–42].

A number of clinical and pathologic variables can be identified to explain these apparently contradictory results. The most important clinical factors predictive of prolonged survival include patient's performance status and stage of disease at presentation, the effectiveness of chemotherapy and/or radiotherapy protocols and the initial response of the patient to therapy [43–45]. Additional factors important in evaluating the effects of subtyping include the source of diagnostic material (whether surgical lung resection, biopsy or autopsy); type of treatment (whether surgical, chemotherapy and/or radiotherapy or palliative); site of tumor, if surgically resected; and the correlation of objective response and median survival times with subtypes. Only three of the above references clearly included these details so that comparisons can be made of the effects of subtyping from a clinical standpoint [34, 36, 40]. In two of these three reports, subtyping was not considered

Table 8. Small cell carcinoma of the lung – effects of subtyping on clinical response: partial literature review.

Reference	Subtype	Patient % LD*	RX	CR	CR + PR	Median survival
Wheeler [40]		24 (21%)	CT/RT			
	Oat cell	12		42%	77%	9 m
	Non oat cell	12		8%	33%	4.2 m
Burdon [349		46 (17%)	CT/RT			
	Lymphocyte	24		21%	58%	12.2 m
	Fusiform	8		—	63%	8.8 m
	Polygonal	14		21%	64%	8.6 m
Hansen [36]		52	CT (3-drug)			
	Lymphocyte	25		NS	73%	6 m
	Fusiform	8		NS	63%	7 m
	Polygonal	12		NS	75%	5 m
	Other	7		NS	87%	6 m
		53	CT (4-drug)			
	Lymphocyte	21		NS	79%	8.5 m
	Fusiform	13		NS	91%	8 m
	Polygonal	17		NS	65%	6.6 m
	Other	2		NS	100%	5.5 m
Matthews		121 (30%)	CT ± RT			
	Lymphocyte	62		42%	87%	10.2 m
	Intermediate	41		50%	91%	10.2 m
	# 22/40	18		17%	56%	6.6 m

* Numbers in parentheses % of patients with regional disease; RX = therapy; CR = complete response; CR + PR = objective response; NS = not stated; CT/RT = chemotherapy, radiotherapy; m = months.

to have any predictive or prognostic value. Table 8 summarizes data from these three studies, as well as material included in this chapter. In the one report that considered the oat-cell subtype more responsive to therapy [40], the objective response of the non oat cell group was 33%, results much poorer than those reported for subtype # 22/40. This stongly suggests the inclusion of large cell tumors as well as subtype # 22/40 in the non-oat cell group.

In some of the other references cited, post irradiation surgical or posttherapeutic autopsy materials were used for evaluation of subtyping. Such material is not considered reliable. In some reports, patients had received no treatment and tumor was identified at autopsy. Reports noting a better survival of patients with fusiform or polygonal cell subtypes were surgically oriented. It is pertinent that in two studies dealing with subtyping of surgical lung resections [39, 46], there was a predominance of intermediate subtypes in the resected lung specimens (67% and 87%, respectively). This suggests that untreated resectable, usually peripheral small cell tumors are most frequently of an intermediate cell subtype. Interpolation that surgical survival relates to cell subtype seems unjustified. Survival, in such cases, more clearly relates to the resectable location of the tumor. In most biopsy series, to the contrary, there is an approximate 50–50 subdivision of the two subtypes, as noted in this paper and in Table 8.

Pathologic factors that lead to these variable results are both technical and interpretative. Improper handling and fixation of specimens are major factors in discrepant diagnoses. Diagnostic materials, obtained by fiberoptic bronchoscopy or needle biopsy, may be extensively crushed or necrotic and difficult to type, much less subtype. Poor fixation causes artifactual distortion of nuclear detail (vacuolization or watery intranuclear changes) which may preclude a light microscopic diagnosis of SCCL. Tubules and squamous nests are uncommonly seen in bronchial biopsies of SCCL. Their presence in metastatic lesions does not exclude the diagnosis of small cell carcinoma.

Interpretative difficulties persist in evaluation of some small cell tumors. Yesner first drew attention to the difficulty in attaining consistency among observers in the diagnosis of the polygonal cell subtype [47]. Much of this difficulty persists and may be ascribed to the 1967 WHO description of the polygonal cell subtype and the accompanying illustration [17]. Cells in the polygonal subtype were said to or implied to have prominent nucleoli, irregular nuclear contours, showed clearing of nuclear chromatin and modest amounts of cytoplasm. Such a description does not differ from the anaplastic large cell carcinoma. In retrospect, the tumor illustrated is a large cell carcinoma, not a polygonal small cell. The inclusion of such 'polygonal cell tumors' in some statistics assures that all other subtypes would have a better response to therapy and improved survival. Likewise, although it is appreciated that the tumor designated here as #22/40 is a small cell malignancy, inclusion of patients with this subtype in statistical studies may be reflected in a somewhat poorer response and survival of patients in the non lymphocyte or oat-cell subtypes.

In this report, no significant difference could be identified in metastases of the subtypes in staging procedures or at autopsy. There was marked transformation of the tumor to a large cell-giant cell pattern in tumors initially designated #22/40. Similar transformations were seen in one-third of patients with classic small cell tumors. One concludes that there is no valid reason to subtype or segregate classic small cell tumors (#21 or #22). It is apparent, also, that subtype #22/40 is a subset of SCCL and that patients with this subtype should be treated on small cell protocols. While their median survival is shortened, some of these patients are capable of having a prolonged survival. Reports indicating no distinction in subtyping probably exclude this group from their studies, as the NCI-VA MOB has done prospectively for the past 3 years. Reports that indicate a better prognosis for the lymphocyte and/or fusiform variants, on the other hand, apparently include this group (#22/40) as well as polygonal large cell tumors under the intermediate or polygonal small cell subtype.

In materials from the experimental models, it has been noted that the lymphocyte-like subtype is absent. Possibly this may represent, as suggested by Yesner [48], a transition from the lymphocyte-like to intermediate cell form. For unknown reasons, this process would then appear to be accelerated in heterotransplants. An alternate explanation is that the lymphocyte-like cell represents an artifact induced by ischemia and mishandling and that the 'true' SCCL cell is the intermediate form.

The experimental models confirm clinical findings that tumors of mixed histology (#22/40) may be relatively common, particularly in the later stages of disease. In the model systems, SCCL replicate relatively slowly and the large cells have a selective advantage. In contrast, clinical SCCL tumors have a relatively more rapid doubling time [49]. The predominance of large cells at autopsy in some SCCL patients may result from the relative resistance of a minor pre-existing large cell component to therapy. Alternatively, transitions of small cells to large cells may be induced or accelerated by therapy.

Tumors of mixed histology (#22/40) and the changes in morphology identified in posttherapy surgical and autopsy materials [5-9] represent an interesting phenomenon with important clinical and biologic significance. Resistance to therapy, failure to induce complete remission and recurrence after remission may, in part, be due to the large cell component. Tumors that recur following remission may represent another cell type. Treatment must vary accordingly, including the possibility of surgery, if the tumor on restaging appears limited to the lung.

The large cell carcinoma discussed in these pages is indistinguishable from that present in large portions of poorly differentiated adenocarcinoma or squamous cell carcinomas of the lung. The latter tumors are considered of entodermal origin. It is highly probable that SCCL tumors arise from APUD cells of the tracheobronchial tree (Kultchitzky or K-type cells) [12]. Although it was postulated by Pearse that APUD cells arose from the neural crest [50], recent evidence indicates that APUD cells of the gastrointestinal tract are of entodermal origin [51, 52]. In the absence of proof to the contrary, the APUD cells of the respiratory tract may also be presumed to be of entodermal origin. The basal or reserve progenitor cells lying over the basement membrane of the tracheobronchial tree may give rise to all of the mucosal elements and the tumors derived from them. Such an interpretation permits a better understanding of the interrelationship of the major forms of lung cancer and, in particular, the mixed histology types.

SUMMARY

1. Light microscopic criteria of small cell carcinoma subtypes are described. The most important characteristic of all small cell tumors is the nuclear appearance. Chromatin is diffusely stippled through the entire nucleus and nucleoli are small or indistinct. Poor fixation may alter nuclear characteristics and cause discrepant diagnoses. The nuclear size, shape and amount of cytoplasm are of secondary importance in the diagnosis of this tumor.

2. A subset of small cell tumors are characterized by multiple cells, arranged in small nests or at random, with nuclear characteristics of anaplastic large cell carcinoma, i.e., clearing of nuclear chromatin, prominent nucleoli, irregular nuclear contours. This subset has been designated as #22/40.

3. Of 121 patients treated on high dose chemotherapy protocols, with or without radiotherapy, 103 patients had tumors designated as subtype #21 or #22; 18 were subtyped as #22/40. There was no difference in patient characteristics, performance status, extent of disease at presentation or biologic behavior as identified by staging procedures prior to therapy or at autopsy. Patients with subtypes #21 and #22 had objective response rates of 87–91%, respectively; in comparison, patients subtyped as #22/40 had a response rate of 56%. Patients with this latter subset also had a decreased median survival (6.6 months as compared to 10.2 months); a shorter time to relapse in responders; and a relatively decreased median survival, particularly impressive in patients presenting with limited disease and good initial performance statuses. Changes in morphology and typing of the tumors was noted at autopsy.

4. Subtyping was not a prognostic factor in the survival of 97 patients who survived over 2 1/2 years from diagnosis of SCCL. All subtypes, including subtype #22/40 were represented in the survivals. All modes of therapy contributed to these survivals. Because so few patients relapsed after 4 years, it is speculated that patients surviving at least 5 years may be considered potentially cured of the disease.

5. Reports suggesting that the lymphocyte subtype are more responsive to therapy than the polygonal, fusiform or other variants are possibly based on inclusion of patients with subtype #22/40 or frank large cell tumors.

6. Reports suggesting that the fusiform or polygonal subtypes have prolonged survival are from surgical series. These subtypes are more commonly identified in peripheral small cell tumors of the lung. Survival probably relates more to the location and resectability of the tumors than subtype.

7. Although there is evidence to suggest that patients with subtype #22/40 have a poorer prognosis than those with classic small cell tumors, some of these patients are capable of responding to therapy and may survive for prolonged periods. It is important that this group be recognized as a small cell

tumor, regardless of name or terminology, so that patients can be provided with optimal treatment. It is possible that the relatively poor response of patients with this subtype relates to the selecting out and destruction of the sensitive small cells and repopulation by less sensitive large cells.

8. The changes in morphology following chemotherapy and/or radiotherapy, and the transformation of cells to anaplastic large cells, glandular or squamous nests imply that some progenitor cells may function as or be of entodermal origin. The spontaneous occurrence of these transformed cells in some tumors prior to therapy and the loss of biochemical markers in these tumors at autopsy would confirm the altered nature of the cells. The transformation of small cells in nude mice to anaplastic large cells following multiple passages and the simultaneous loss of biochemical and biologic properties in the model tumors affirm, also, the innate potentials of these cells.

9. The implications of these changes are broad. Recurrent disease, following complete response, may indicate population by tumor cells of another type. Such a change may require rethinking of treatment modalities. It is possible that such changes are responsible for the insensitivity of tumors to chemotherapy, following relapse.

10. There is no clear reason to subtype classic small cell tumors. It is important to recognize that a subset of these tumors have large cell components. These tumors are responsive to therapy and should be treated on small cell protocols. Polygonal cell malignancies, predominantly composed of cells with prominent nucleoli, are not small cell tumors and should be excluded from small cell protocols.

REFERENCES

1. Matthews MJ, Rozencweig M, Staquet MJ et al.: Long term survivors with small cell carcinoma of the lung. Eur J Cancer. 16:527-532, 1980.
2. Minna JD, Brereton HD, Cohen MH et al.: The treatment of small cell carcinoma of the lung. Prospects for cure. In: Lung Cancer, Progress in Therapeutic Research, Muggia, F and Rozencweig, M (eds), Raven Press, New York, 1979, p 593-599.
3. Fox W and Scadding JG: Medical Research Council comparative trial of surgery and radiotherapy for primary treatment of small-celled or oat-celled carcinoma of bronchus. Ten-year follow up. Lancet 2:63-65, 1973.
4. Higgins GA Jr, Shields TW and Keehn RJ: The solitary pulmonary nodule. Ten-year follow-up of Veterans Administration Armed Forces cooperative study. Arch Surg 110:570-575, 1975.
5. Matthews MJ: Effects of therapy on the morphology and behavior of small cell carcinoma of the lung. A clinico pathologic study. In: Lung Cancer, Progress in Therapeutic research, Muggia, F and Rozencweig M (eds). Raven Press, New York, 1979, p 155-165.
6. Gazdar AF, Cohen MH, Ihde DC et al.: Bronchial epithelial changes in association with small cell carcinoma of the lung. In: Lung Cancer, Progress in Therapeutic Research, Muggia F and Rozencweig M (eds). Raven Press, New York, 1979, p 167-174.

7. Brereton HD, Matthews MJ, Costa J *et al.*: Mixed anaplastic small cell carcinoma of the lung. Ann Int Med 88:805-806, 1978.

8. Bates M, Hurt R, Levison V *et al.*: Treatment of oat cell carcinoma of bronchus by preoperative radiotherapy and surgery. Lancet 1:1134-1135, 1974.

9. Abeloff MD, Eggleston JC, Mendelsohn G *et al.*: Changes in morphologic and biochemical characteristics of small cell carcinoma of the lung. Am J Med 66:757-764, 1979.

10. Baylin SB, Weisburger WR, Eggleston JC *et al.*: Variable content of histaminase, L-dopa decarboxylase and calcitonin in small cell carcinoma of the lung. Biologic and clinical implications. N Engl J Med 299:105-110, 1978.

11. Silva OL, Becker KL, Primack A *et al.*: Ectopic production of calcitonin by oat cell carcinoma. N Engl J Med 290:1122-1124, 1974.

12. Hattori S, Matsuda M, Tateishi R *et al.*: Oat cell carcinoma of the lung. Clinical and morphologic studies in relation to its histogenesis. Cancer 30:1014-1024, 1972.

13. Gazdar AF, Carney DN, Russell EK *et al.*: Small cell carcinoma of the lung. Establishment of continuous clonable tumorigenic cells having amine precursor uptake and decarboxylation properties. Cancer Res, 1980.

14. Gazdar AF, Carney DN, Baylin S *et al.*: Small cell carcinoma of the lung. Altered morphological, biological and biochemical characteristics in cultured and hetero transplanted tumors. In press.

15. Barnard WG: The nature of the 'oat-celled sarcoma' of the mediastinum. J Path Bact 29:241-244, 1926.

16. Azzopardi JG: Oat cell carcinoma of the bronchus. J Path Bact 78:513-519, 1959.

17. Kreyberg L: Histological Typing of Lung Tumors. International Histological Classification of Tumors, Geneve, World Health Organization, 1967.

18. Spencer H: Carcinoma of the lung, in Pathology of the lung, Pergamon Press, LtD, Oxford, 1962.

19. Spencer H: Carcinoma of the lung, In Pathology of the Lung, Pergamon Press, LTD, Oxford, 1968.

20. Spencer H: Carcinoma of the lung, in Pathology of the Lung, Pergamon Press, LTD, Oxford, 1977.

21. Matthews MJ: Morphologic classification of bronchogenic carcinoma. Cancer Chemother Rep Part 3 4:299-301, 1973.

22. Yesner R, Gerstl B and Auerbach O: Application of the World Health Organization clasification of lung carcinoma to biopsy material. Ann Thorac Surg 1:33-39, 1965.

23. Yesner R and Sobel L: Histological Typing of Lung Tumors. International Histological Classification of Tumors. Geneva, World Health Organization, 1977 (in press).

24. Mackay B, Osborne BM and Wilson RA: Ultrastructure of lung neoplasms. In: Lung Cancer, Clinical Diagnosis and Treatment, Straus, MJ (ed), Grune & Stratton, New York, 1977, p 71-84.

25. Ahmed A: Some ultrastructural observations of haematoxy philvascular changes in oat cell carcinoma. J Pathol 112: 1-3, 1974.

26. Radice P, Matthews MJ, Ihde DC *et al.*: Characterization of mixed histology large cell/small cell lung cancer and its response to combination chemotherapy. Proc Am Assoc Cancer Res and ASCO 20:409, 1979.

27. Carney DN, Radice P, Matthews MJ *et al.*: Small cell carcinoma of the lung: Effects of subtyping on response to therapy and metastatic behavior. JNCI, 1980.

28. Cohen MH, Creaven PJ, Fossieck BE *et al.*: Intensive chemotherapy of small cell bronchogenic carcinoma. Cancer Treat Rep 61:349-354, 1977.

29. Cohen MH, Ihde DC, Bunn P *et al.*: Alternating combination chemotherapy for small cell bronchogenic carcinoma. Cancer Treat Rep 63:163-170, 1979.

30. Zubrod CG, Schneiderman MA, Frei E *et al.*: Appraisal of methods for the study of chemotherapy in man. Comparative therapeutic trial of nitrogen mustard and triethylene thiophosphoramide. J Chron Dis 11:7-23, 1960.

31. Radice P, Matthews MJ, Ihde DC *et al.*: Mixed histology of small cell carcinoma of the lung: Effects on response to therapy and survival. In press.

32. Hansen HH and Hansen MA: A comparison of 3 and 4 drug combination chemotherapy for advanced small cell anaplastic carcinoma of the lung. Proc Am Assoc Cancer Res and ASCO 17:129, 1976.

33. Matthews MJ, Gazdar AF, Ihde DC *et al.*: Histologic subtypes of small cell carcinoma of the lung and their clinical significance. Proc Am Assoc Cancer Res and ASCO 19:392, 1978.

34. Burdon JGW, Sinclair RA and Henderson MM: Small cell carcinoma of the lung. Prognosis in relation to histologic subtypes. Chest 76:302-304, 1979.

35. Hirsch F, Hansen HH, Dombernowsky P *et al.*: Bone marrow examination in the staging of small cell anaplastic carcinoma of the lung with special reference to subtyping. An evaluation of 203 consecutive cases. Cancer 30:2563-2567, 1977.

36. Hansen HH, Dombernowsky P, Hansen M *et al.*: Chemotherapy of advanced small cell anaplastic carcinoma. Superiority of four-drug combination to a three-drug combination. Ann Intern Med 89:177-181, 1978.

37. Reinila A, Dammert K: An attempt to use the WHO typing in the histological classification of lung carcinomas. cta Pathol Microbiol Scand (A) 82:783-790, 1974.

38. Larsson S: Pretreatment classification and staging of bronchogenic carcinoma. Scand J Thorac Cardiovasc Surg 7:(Suppl) 44-56, 1973.

39. Hinson KFW, Miller AB and Tall R: An assessment of the World Health Organization Classification of the histologic typing of lung tumors applied to biopsy and resected material. Cancer 35:399-405, 1975.

40. Wheeler RH, Nishiyama RR, Fayos JV *et al.*: Difference in response to combined modality therapy of small cell undifferentiated carcinoma of the lung according to histologic classification. Proc Am Assoc Cancer Res and ASCO 17:274, 1976.

41. Hattori S, Matsuda M, Idegami H *et al.*: Small cell carcinoma of the lung: Clinical and cytomorphological studies in relation to its response to chemotherapy. Gann 68:321-331, 1977.

42. Nixon DW, Murphy GF, Sewell CW *et al.*: Relationship between survival and histologic type in small cell anaplastic carcinoma of the lung. Cancer 44:1045-1049, 1979.

43. Bunn PA, Cohen MH, Ihde DC *et al.*: Commentary. Advances in small cell bronchogenic carcinoma. Cancer Treat Rep 62:333-241, 1977.

44. Edmondson JH, Legakos SW, Swlawry OS: Cyclophosphamide and CCNU in the treatment of inoperable small cell carcinoma and adenocarcinoma of the lung. Cancer Treat Rep 60:925-932, 1976.

45. Einhorn LH, Bond WH, Hornback N *et al.*: Long term results in combined modality treatment of small cell carcinoma of the lung. Sem Oncol 5:309-313, 1978.

46. Matthews MJ and Gordon PR: Morphology of Pulmonary and Pleural Malignancies, In Lung Cancer Clinical Diagnosis and Treatment, Straus MJ (ed) Grune and Stratton, Inc, New York, 1977, p 49-69.

47. Feinstein AR, Gelfman NA, Yesner R *et al.*: Observer variability in the histopathologic diagnosis of lung cancer. Am Rev Resp Dis 101:671-676, 1970.

48. Yesner R: Spectrum of lung cancer and ectopic hormones, In: Pathology Annual, Part I, Sommers SC and Rosen PP (eds) Appleton Century Croff, New York, 1978, p 217-240.

49. Brigham BA, Bunn PA, Minna JD *et al.*: Growth rates of small cell bronchogenic carcinoma. Cancer 42:2880-2886, 1978.

50. Pearse AGE: The cytochemistry and ultrastructure of polypeptide hormone-producing cells of the APUD series and the embryologic, physiologic and pathologic implications of the concept. J Histochem Cytochem 17:303-313, 1969.
51. Pictet RL, Rall LB, Phelps P *et al.*: The neural crest and the origin of the insulin-producing and other gastrointestinal hormone-producing cells. Science 191:191-192, 1976.
52. Sidhu GS: The endodermal origin of digestive and respiratory tract APUD cells. Am J Pathol 96:5-20, 1979.

Subject Index

ACTH, 163
Acute radiation syndrome, 253
Adjuvant therapy, 39, 134, 171
AHH (aryl hydrocarbon hydroxylase),
  1-23
  activity, 16
  and lung cancer, 14
  as a rate-limiting step, 22
  genetics of, 9
  inducers, 7
  inducibility, 7, 9, 10, 20
  liver, 20
  lung cancer diagnosis, 21
AHH levels
  in lymphocytes from noncancer
    patients, 20
  in lymphocytes in lung cancer, 20
  in PAMs from lung cancer, 20
  in PAMs from noncancer patients, 20
  high, 22
AHH-mediated pulmonary carcinogenesis, theories of, 10
AHH metabolizing capabilities in
  different tissues, 17
AHH system, induction of different
  P-450s of, 7
Alternating non-cross resistant
  regimens, 184
American Joint Committee on Cancer
  Staging and End Results Reporting,
  157
Anaplastic large cell malignancies,
  283, 289, 303
Anti-anergic agent, 56
Antipyrine, 20
  clearance, 20
Aorta tissue, 13
Aortic wall, 102
APUD cells, 301
Aryl hydrocarbon hydroxylase,
  see AHH
Autopsy, 81, 158, 296

Bacillus Calmette-Guerin (BCG),
  38, 53-55, 59, 76
  intralesional, 58, 60
Benzanthracene (BA), 2
Benzo(a)pyrene (BP), 2
  binding protein, 21
  epoxide derivatives of, 5
  metabolism, 5, 19, 23
  ultimate carcinogen of, 5
Biochemical markers, 283

Biologic response modifiers, 45
Blood cells, 11
Bone marrow aspiration
  biopsy, 159
Bone marrow
  examination
    bilateral, 160
    unilateral, 159
  kinetics, 249
  radiobiology, 249
Bone scanning, 160, 161
Boost port isodose curves, 126
Bronchopleural fistula and empyema,
  65
Buccal tissue, 13

C. parvum, 38
Calcitonin, 163
Carbogen, 227
Carcinogenesis, susceptibility to,
  10
  animal studies, 22
Carcinoma
  adeno- 79, 82
  bronchogenic, 75
  epidermoid, 70, 79
  large cell, 79, 82, 283, 284, 290,
    300, 301
  left lung, 90
  non-small cell bronchogenic, 211
  small cell, 35, 169, 210, 283-285,
    291, 294-296, 298, 299, 302
  squamous cell, 71, 117
Cardiac reserve, 104
Carina, 102
Central nervous system,
  see CNS
Chemotherapy, 138
  intensity, 183
  maintenance, 185
  single agent, 175
Chemotherapy and radiation therapy,
  combined, 137, 173
Cigarette smoking, 1, 15
Classification of lung cancer types,
  80
Clinical trials, controlled, 38, 85
CNS metastasis, 161, 200
CNS syndrome, 197
Colon tissue, 13
Combination chemotherapy,
  134, 137, 138, 140, 173, 177, 180-
  182, 187, 201, 210, 267, 270, 272

Computerized tomography, 163, 166
Conjugation reactions, 23
Containment of disease, 104
Continuous courses of therapy,
  83, 131, 239, 242
Control arm, randomized, 43
Corynebacterium parvum,
  see C. parvum
Cultured human bronchus, 15
Cytochrome P-448, 8
Cytochrome P-450, 7, 8
Cytosol receptor proteins, 7

Dilantin, 232
Diol epoxide I, 10, 19
Dissection, 'en bloc', 92
DNA, 3, 15
Dose reduction factor (DRF), 236
Drugs,
  optimal number of, 270
  optimal timing of, 179
Dry-mouth syndrome, 253
Dysphagia, 196

Ectopic markers in the cerebrospinal
  fluid, 163
Endometrium tissue, 12
Environmental carcinogens, 1, 4
Esophagitis, 149, 196
Extensive disease, 158, 170, 293

Fast neutron irradiation, 266, 267
Fetal tissue, 12
Fibrosis, 96, 241
Fractionation schedule, 234, 239, 245
  super or hyper-, 248
  unconventional, 237
  uneven, 243
Freund's adjuvant, 57
Fusiform components of tumors,
  288, 289, 302

Gallium-67 scan, 165
Genetic damage, 120
Genetic factors, 2

Hemibody irradiation (HBI),
  248, 252, 257, 259
  delivery of, 251
  future uses of, 260
  tumor responses, 250
Hollinshead antigen, 44
Horner's syndrome, 66
Host immunocompetence, 51
Hyperbaric oxygen (HBO) therapy,
  226, 245
Hyperthermia, 263
Hypoxia, 224, 226
Hypoxic cells, 214
  cytotoxicity for, 231
  electron-affinic sensitization
    limited to, 229
Hypoxic enhancements, 234
Hypoxic fraction, 217, 246

Immunity, cell-mediated, 51
Immunocompetence, host, 51
Immunopotentiator, 56
Immunosuppression, 51, 53
Immunosurveillance, 4
Immunotherapy, 52, 55, 137, 186
  adjuvant, 52
  non-specific, 56
  specific, 57
  specific active, 44
Interstitial implants, 262
Iodine-125, 67, 143
Iridium-192 , 67
Irradiation
  fast neutron, 266, 267
  hemibody, 248
    (see Hemibody irradiation)
  interstitial, 143, 144
  intraoperative, 262
  postoperative, 80
  preoperative, 103
  prophylactic, 142
  split course, 132, 240, 242
  technique, continuous, 130
  therapy techniques, 103
  to extrathoracic sites, 198
  tolerance, 211
  total body, 248
Isotopes, 67, 263

Kidney tissue, 13

Leptomeninges, 199
Levamisole, 41, 57, 76
Limited disease, 71, 158, 170
Linear energy transfer (LET),
  220-222, 224, 265, 266
Liver function tests, 164
  scans, 164
  tissue, 11
Loco-regional disease, 117
Lower half-body irradiation (LHBI),
  251
Lumbar puncture, 162
Lung cancer
  altered immunity in, 36
  human susceptibility to, 2
  marginally resectable, 67, 71, 101
  pathologic forms of, 209
  resected, 42
  risk, 20
  tumor associated antigens (TAA),
    37
Lung tissue, 12, 17
  alveolar, 12
  bronchus, 12
  human, 22
  macrophages, 12
  PAMs, 12
  surgically-resected, 15
  whole lung, 12
Lymph node
  contralateral, 90
  extent of, 89
  location, 88

SUBJECT INDEX

number, 88
paratracheal, 90
periesophageal, 90
size, 88
spread to, 105
hilar, 78
positive, 65
Lymphocyte, 9, 10, 14, 15, 17, 20,
21, 302
Lymphocyte-like type, 287, 301
Lymphocyte/oat cell subtype, 286

Main stem bronchus, 81, 101
Mediastinoscopy, 166
Mediastinum, 79
hilum, 86
Megavoltage photon, 251
Metastasis, 75
bone, 159
brain, 141, 142
CNS, 161, 200
distant, 82
liver, 163
lymph node, 77
occult distant, 78
sites of, 116
subclinical, 258
Metastatic compartment, subclinical,
259
Metastatic spread, extrathoracic, 158
Metronidazole, 230
Micrometastasis, 77
Mid-body irradiation (MBI), 251
Misonidazole, 230, 233, 234
Mitotic cycle, 219
Mixed beam therapy, 267
Mixed small cell-large cell carcinoma,
291
Morbidity, due to therapy, 212
Myelitis, 150

National Collaborative Study, 64
Natural history of lung cancer, 63
Neuropathy, 233
Nitromidazole sensitizer, 231
Nominal standard dose (NSD) of
radiation, 238
dose-time-relation, 238
Non-small cell types, 35
Nonresectable lesion, 104

Osteoblastic changes, 160
Ototoxicity, 233
Oxygen, 214, 226, 227
Oxygen enhancement ratio (OER), 215
Oxygen mimetic agents, 228
Oxygen radiosensitization, 216
Oxygenated cell killing, 219
Oxygenated curve, 218
Oxygenated-hypoxic curve, 218

Pancreatic duct tissue, 13
Peak plasma concentrations, 232, 233
Peritoneoscopy, 164
Placenta tissue, 11

Pneumonectomy, 71, 86
Pneumonitis, 241
Polycyclic aromatic hydrocarbons
(PAHs), 2, 5, 22
Polygonal cells, 284, 289
Polygonal cell subtype, diagnosis of,
300, 302
Polygonal large cell tumors, 301
PPD, 59
converters, 55
non-converters, 55
skin test, 41
Progenitor cells, 303
Prognostic variables, 119
Prophylactic cranial irradiation
(PCI), 199
Prostate tissue, 13
Pulmonary alveolar macrophages
(PAM), 16, 17, 20, 21
Pulmonary artery, 69, 71

Radiation biology, 119
laboratory, 213
Radiation fibrosis, 148, 149
Radiation field, 68, 127
oblique opposed arrangement, 68
Radiation myelitis, 149
Radiation pneumonitis,
148, 149, 252, 255, 256
Radiation therapy, 138, 195
alone, 114, 173
approaches, 225
decreasing dose schedules, 246
definitive, 105
dose, 93, 195
fractionation, 93
innovations, 272
local, 210, 211
megavoltage, 121
once-a-week treatment, 244
palliative, 145
portals, 100
split course, 84, 96, 129, 130-133,
238, 240, 241, 242, 257
standardized, 93
super and hyperfractionation
schedules, 237, 248
therapeutic ratio, 238
threshold dose, 255
two or three treatments per week,
245
Radiation therapy and chemotherapy,
combined, 137, 173
Radiation therapy versus placebo, 115
Radiation treatment ports, 122
Radiation
adjuvant, 76
continuous, 133
directly ionizing, 220
high LET, 265
indirectly ionizing, 220
interstitial, 144
low LET, 266
megavoltage, 145

non-ionizing, 150
postoperative, 72, 85
preoperative, 63, 64, 114
prophylactic, 141, 142
Radioactive material,
 see Isotopes
Radiobiologic hypoxia, 216
Radiofrequency energy, 265
Radiographic bone survey, 159
Radio-isotopic bone scan, 159
Radioprotection, 235
Radioresistance, 217
Radiosensitization, thermal, 264
Radiosensitizers, 248
Radium, 113
Radon-222, 67, 143
Radon seeds, 113
Relapse, sites of, 185, 198
Relative biologic effectiveness (RBE),
 129, 222, 223, 225
Relative equivalent therapy (RET), 129
Reoxygenation, 219
Resectability rate, 65
Resected patients, 84
Resection
 atrial, 102
 curative, 78
 sleeve, 103
 surgical, 78
Respiratory capacity, 96
Respiratory function, 92
Rest periods, 241, 242

Saturation method, Pfahler, 246
Schedule
 continuous, 239
 decreasing dose, 246
 fractionation, 10
 fractionation, super or hyper-, 248
 unconventional, 237, 245
 uneven, 243
Selective normal tissue protection,
 236
Sensitizer enhancement ratio (SER),
 230
Skin tissue, 11
Solvated electron, 228
Spinal cord, 100, 199, 243
Sputum sample tissue, 13
Staging, 45, 158, 169
Stem cells, 249
Stomach tissue, 13
Stump, bronchial, 81, 101
Sulfhydryl compounds, 235
Superior sulcus tumors, 66, 103
Superior vena cava obstruction,
 treatment of, 185
Superior vena cava syndrome, 146, 147
Supraclavicular disease, 85
Surgical judgment, 91
Surgical procedures, 75

Surgically-resected lung tissue, 15
Survival curves, 217
Survival, 91, 228, 242
 determinants of, 89
 improved, 115
 median, 169
 2-years disease-free, 171

Therapeutic additivity and synergism,
 268
Therapeutic gain factor (TGF), 224
Thermal dose, 264
Thermal radiosensitization, 264
Thoracic wall, 102
Thrombocytopenia, 159
Thymosin, 40
Thymosin fraction V, 202
Time-dose schemes, 150
Tissue damage, 213
Tissue uptake, 236
TNM system, 157
Toxicity, 186, 196, 231
 cardiac, 197
 hematologic, 254
 hematopoietic, 197
 independent, 268
 pulmonary, 197, 254
 pulmonary fibrosis and/or
  pneumonitis, 197
 skin, 196
Tubular components of tumors, 289
Tumor associated antigens (TAA), 37
Tumor control, 83, 213, 271
Tumor extension to the chest wall, 87
Tumor repopulation, 246, 247
Tumor recurrence, 81, 82
Tumor responses
 HBI, 250
 objective, 250
 pathologic, 250
 subjective, 250
Tumor sterilization, 84, 114, 261
Type I inducer, 7
Type II inducers, 8
Type II pneumocyte cells, 255

Ultrasonography, 164
Untreated patients, 114
Upper half-body irradiation (UHBI),
 251

Vaginal scrapings, 13
Veterans Administration Lung Study
 Group (VALG), 284

WHO classification, 284
Working Party for Therapy of Lung
 Cancer, 284
WR-2721, 235

Xenobiotics, 5